A Clinical Guide to Epileptic Syndromes and their Treatment

BASED ON THE NEW ILAE DIAGNOSTIC SCHEME

C P Panayiotopoulos MD PhD FRCP

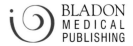

Always refer to the manufacturer's Prescribing
Information before prescribing drugs cited in this
book.

British Library Cataloguing in Publication Data.
A catalogue record for this title is available from the
British Library

ISBN 1-904218-23-72

C P Panayiotopoulos
A Clinical Guide to Epileptic Syndromes and their
Treatment

Design and production:
Design Online Ltd, Oxford

Printed by
Talleres Gráficos Hostench s.a.
Venezuela, 87-93
Barcelona, Spain

Distributed by
Plymbridge Distributors Ltd, Estover Road, Plymouth
PL6 7PY, UK

To my wife Thalia

because

she is a beautiful woman

my muse

the flower, the smile and the angel in my life

ACKNOWLEDGEMENTS

The author wishes to express his gratitude to the following distinguished experts who gave him valuable advice after reading parts or the whole book:
Berkovic, S.F.
Dravet, C.
Duncan, J.S.
Engel, J.Jr.
Fejerman, N.
Ferrie, C.D.
Grünewald, R.A.
Koutroumanidis, M.
Niedermeyer, E.
Oguni, H.
Ohtahara, S.
Plouin, P.
Sander, J.W.A.S.
Scott, R.C.
Watanabe, K.
Zifkin, B.D.

The assistance of S. Rowlinson and S. Sanders, expert EEG technologists, is greatly appreciated.

John Harrison, perfectionist publisher, and Steve Millar, exceptional book designer, worked very hard to publish this book within 6 weeks of receiving the manuscript.

CONTENTS

PREFACE

A major advance in recent epileptology is the recognition of epileptic syndromes that allows an accurate diagnosis and management of seizure disorders. 'Epilepsy' is a common brain disease affecting 1–2% of the population[1] and 4% of children[2] in those developed countries where they have been studied.[3] Lifetime prevalence is 2–5% of the general population[4] and point prevalence is 4–8 per 1000.[5] 'Epilepsy' – a stigmatising word[6] – is not a single disorder but rather a general label for a multitude of different disorders, or syndromes, characterised by underlying aetiology, age at onset, seizure type(s), EEG patterns and prognosis. Accurate diagnosis of the syndrome is necessary for both short- and long-term management. For example, idiopathic generalised and focal epilepsies demand different treatment strategies; certain drugs beneficial to one may be contraindicated in the other.[7]

The standardised classification and terminology for epileptic seizures[8] and syndromes[9] by the International League Against Epilepsy (ILAE) provides a fundamental framework for organising and differentiating them. Such categorisation is essential in clinical practice and research on epilepsies. The current Classification of Epileptic Seizures used is from 1981[8] and the last revision of the Classification of Epilepsies and Epileptic Syndromes was in 1989.[9]

Significant progress made in epileptology in the last decade mandates a revision of the currently used seizure[8] and syndrome classifications.[9] Towards this goal, the ILAE Task Force has recently published 'A proposed diagnostic scheme for people with epileptic seizures and with epilepsy'[10] and a 'Glossary of descriptive terminology for ictal semiology'.[11] Within this diagnostic scheme, a variety of approaches to classification are possible. The proposal includes several definitive changes in concepts and terminology but classifications are considered as examples of what could be devised in the future. A list of seizures and syndromes for application to individual patients was presented by way of example only. The ILAE Task Force views the development of specific classifications as a continuing work in progress. Flexible and dynamic diagnostic classifications will be revised periodically on the basis of emerging new information and resolution of problems that will inevitably be identified through usage.[10]

There are significant changes in this new ILAE Task Force diagnostic scheme[10] that will influence our communication on epilepsies and make currently used terms and diagnostic proposals obsolete. In terminology, for example, focal replaces partial seizures. New syndromes such as familial focal epilepsies are recognised while others are discarded. This knowledge should quickly become disseminated to physicians caring for patients with seizure disorders.

This is the first book to be based on the new diagnostic scheme of the ILAE Task Force.[10] I particularly had in mind practising paediatricians, general physicians, neurologists and epileptologists around the world. I have tried to provide them with a brief and concise clinical guide on epileptic seizures and epileptic syndromes in accordance with the new ILAE diagnostic scheme. Also, in view of the fact that the ILAE Task Force[10] invites physicians to contribute in the shaping of future classification revisions, I have made certain limited propositions that may be considered prior to the final new ILAE classification.

The most appropriate modern treatments are objectively presented for everyday clinical practice.

C P Panayiotopoulos MD PhD FRCP   London 12th August 2002

Former member of the ILAE Task Force on Classification
Department of Clinical Neurophysiology and Epilepsies
St. Thomas' Hospital, London SE1 7EH

OPTIMAL UTILISATION OF EEG AND BRAIN IMAGING

THE DIAGNOSIS OF EPILEPSIES

Patients with epileptic seizures and their families are entitled to a diagnosis, prognosis and management that are specific and precise. The inclusive, monolectic diagnostic label 'epilepsy' is unsatisfactory to patient and physician alike and may result in avoidable morbidity and mortality. 'Epilepsy' is not a single disease entity. Epilepsies are many diseases. The short- and long-term management of epilepsies is syndrome-related and often differs markedly between various disorders manifesting with seizures, emphasising the need for accurate diagnosis. There are two important diagnostic steps towards this aim:

First step: are these epileptic seizures?

Second step: what is their cause and what is the epileptic syndrome?

FIRST STEP: THE DIAGNOSIS OF EPILEPTIC SEIZURES

A.   FITS, FAINTS AND FUNNY TURNS

The first step towards the diagnosis of epilepsies is to establish that a paroxysmal clinical event is an epileptic seizure. The differentiation between seizures and other causes of transient neurological disturbance and collapse is epitomised by the familiar theme 'fits, faints and funny turns'. Distinguishing

---

Definitions

Epileptic seizure: Manifestation(s) of epileptic (excessive and/or hypersynchronous) usually self-limited activity of neurons in the brain.[11]

Epileptic seizure type: An ictal event believed to represent a unique pathophysiological mechanism and anatomic substrate. This is a diagnostic entity with aetiologic, therapeutic and prognostic implications (new concept).[10]

EPILEPSY:[11]
(a) Epileptic disorder: A chronic neurological condition characterised by recurrent epileptic seizures.[11]
(b) Epilepsies: Those conditions involving chronic recurrent epileptic seizures that can be considered epileptic disorders.[11]
Epilepsy: (operational definition) when more than two seizures occur (the type of seizure is not defined). '*Epilepsy* is a liability to clinically manifested seizures of any type' would be my proposal.

Abbreviations:
CT scan = X-ray computed tomography
EEG = electroencephalography
FDG = 18F-fluorodeoxyglucose
FLAIR = fluid-attenuated inversion recovery
FMRI = functional magnetic resonance imaging
GTCS = generalised tonic–clonic seizure
H2150 = 150-water
HV = hyperventilation

ILAE = International League Against Epilepsy
IPS = intermittent photic stimulation
MRI = magnetic resonance imaging
MRS = magnetic resonance spectroscopy
MTR = magnetisation transfer ratio
PET = positron emission tomography
SPECT = single photon emission computed
        tomography

epileptic (*fits*) from non-epileptic disorders, particularly vasovagal (*faints*) or psychogenic attacks (*funny turns*) should be a core skill of all trained physicians.

However, this is not always easy: syncopal attacks are frequently associated with myoclonic jerking, rolling of the eyes and brief automatisms,[12,13] psychogenic attacks often imitate epileptic seizures and particularly those of frontal lobe origin. Conversely, epileptic seizures may manifest with syncopal-like symptoms (page 96), bizarre symptoms mimicking psychogenic attacks (page 181) or migraine-like symptoms (page 200).

The differential diagnosis is much more demanding in babies, toddlers and young children in whom there are many different causes such as hyperekplexia, reflex anoxic seizures, cyanotic breath-holding attacks, gastro-oesophageal reflux, non-epileptic myoclonus, parasomnias, paroxysmal vertigo, episodic ataxias, tics and self-gratification.[14]

Misdiagnosis has serious repercussions. Patients with non-epileptic disorders incorrectly diagnosed as having epileptic seizures are likely to be mistreated with antiepileptic drugs and also denied specific and possibly life-saving treatment. Similarly, patients with epileptic seizures erroneously diagnosed as migraine or other non-epileptic paroxysmal events are deprived of specific treatments that also may be life-saving.

The differentiation of epileptic seizures from non-epileptic events is detailed in any textbook of medicine. Therefore, only some aspects of it are discussed in this book when appropriate.

B.   THE EPILEPTIC SEIZURES

There are numerous types of epileptic seizures that are primarily divided into focal and generalised seizures.[8,10,15]

The new diagnostic scheme of the ILAE Task Force is divided into five parts, or Axes, organised to facilitate a logical clinical approach to the development of hypotheses necessary to facilitate the diagnostic studies and therapeutic strategies to be undertaken in individual patients (Table 1.1). Table 1.2 is the list of seizures provided by the ILAE Task Force. For didactic purposes, I describe them in the relevant epileptic syndromes.

The diagnosis of epileptic seizures is based primarily on clinical information, which should be intelligently and patiently gathered from the patient and witnesses.

Epileptic seizures in their presentation may be minor or dramatic, brief or long, frequent, sparse or isolated. Minor seizures such as brief myoclonic jerks, mild absences, simple or even complex focal seizures may go unnoticed for many years or be ignored as normal variations in a person's life. Even if frequent, these events are unlikely to promote a medical consultation.

Definitions

Focal (synonym = partial): A seizure whose initial semiology indicates, or is consistent with, initial activation of only part of one cerebral hemisphere.[11]

Generalised (synonym = bilateral): A seizure whose initial semiology indicates, or is consistent with, more than minimal involvement of both cerebral hemispheres.[11]

Conversely, a major seizure such as a generalised tonic–clonic convulsion invariably raises concerns and draws medical attention.

Thus, studies on the prognosis and treatment of the 'first seizure' mainly refer to a GTCS, although this may not be the first seizure in the patient's life. Three quarters (74%) of patients with 'newly identified unprovoked seizures' (mainly GTCS) had experienced multiple seizure episodes before their first medical contact.[16]

Table 1.1   Proposed diagnostic scheme for people with epileptic seizures and with epilepsy

---

Epileptic seizures and epilepsy syndromes are to be described and categorized according to a system that uses standardized terminology, and that is sufficiently flexible to take into account the following practical and dynamic aspects of epilepsy diagnosis:
1. Some patients cannot be given a recognized syndromic diagnosis.
2. Seizure types and syndromes change as new information is obtained.
3. Complete and detailed descriptions of ictal phenomenology are not always necessary.
4. Multiple classification schemes can, and should, be designed for specific purposes (e.g., communication and teaching; therapeutic trials; epidemiologic investigations; selection of surgical candidates; basic research; genetic characterizations).

This diagnostic scheme is divided into five parts, or Axes, organized to facilitate a logical clinical approach to the development of hypotheses necessary to determine the diagnostic studies and therapeutic strategies to be undertaken in individual patients:
Axis 1: Ictal phenomenology, from the Glossary of Descriptive Ictal Terminology, can be used to describe ictal events with any degree of detail needed.
Axis 2: Seizure type, from the List of Epileptic Seizures. Localization within the brain and precipitating stimuli for reflex seizures should be specified when appropriate.
Axis 3: Syndrome, from the List of Epilepsy Syndromes, with the understanding that a syndromic diagnosis may not always be possible.
Axis 4: Etiology, from a Classification of Diseases Frequently Associated with Epileptic Seizures or Epilepsy Syndromes when possible, genetic defects, or specific pathologic substrates for symptomatic focal epilepsies.
Axis 5: Impairment, this optional, but often useful, additional diagnostic parameter can be derived from an impairment classification adapted from the WHO ICIDH-2.

From Engel (2001)[10] with permission of the author and the *Journal of Epilepsia*.

Terminological changes in the new diagnostic scheme:[10]

The old term 'focal' is re-introduced to replace 'partial' and 'localisation-related' epileptic seizures, which is understandable.

However, this new scheme abandons the division of focal seizures into 'simple' (without impairment of consciousness) and 'complex' (with impairment of consciousness).[10] The reason given is that this 'inappropriately created the impression that impairment of consciousness had certain mechanistic implications related to limbic system involvement' and that 'complex partial seizures' has been used erroneously as a synonym of 'temporal lobe epilepsy'.[10] Although these statements are correct, there are significant practical reasons (medico-legal cases, driving, job-related performance) for distinguishing seizures with or without impairment of consciousness. Therefore, I have retained the terms 'simple' and 'complex' focal seizures in this book, while emphasising that ictal impairment of consciousness is a symptom of either neocortical or limbic seizures.

Minor seizures are more important than the major ones for an appropriate diagnosis, diagnostic tests and management strategies. They should be thoroughly sought during the clinical evaluation (Figure 1.1). Patients are not supposed to know that these are also epileptic events/seizures. It is the physician's responsibility to find out and evaluate them. Minor seizures include

Table 1.2 Epileptic seizure types and precipitating stimuli for reflex seizures

Self-limited seizure types
  Generalized seizures
    Tonic–clonic seizures (includes variations
        beginning with a clonic or
        myoclonic phase)
    Clonic seizures
      Without tonic features
      With tonic features
    Typical absence seizures
    Atypical absence seizures
    Myoclonic absence seizures
    Tonic seizures
    Spasms
    Myoclonic seizures
    Eyelid myoclonia
      Without absences
      With absences
    Myoclonic atonic seizures
    Negative myoclonus
    Atonic seizures
    Reflex seizures in generalized epilepsy
        syndromes
  Focal seizures
    Focal sensory seizures
      With elementary sensory symptoms
          (e.g., occipital and parietal lobe
          seizures)
      With experiential sensory symptoms
          (e.g., temporoparietooccipital
          junction seizures)
    Focal motor seizures
      With elementary clonic motor signs
      With asymmetric tonic motor seizures
          (e.g., supplementary motor
          seizures)
      With typical (temporal lobe) automatisms
          (e.g., mesial temporal lobe seizures)
      With hyperkinetic automatisms
      With focal negative myoclonus
      With inhibitory motor seizures
    Gelastic seizures
    Hemiclonic seizures
    Secondarily generalized seizures

  Reflex seizures in focal epilepsy syndromes
Continuous seizure types
  Generalized status epilepticus
    Generalized tonic–clonic status epilepticus
    Clonic status epilepticus
    Absence status epilepticus
    Tonic status epilepticus
    Myoclonic status epilepticus
  Focal status epilepticus
    Epilepsia partialis continua of
        Kozhevnikov
    Aura continua
    Limbic status epilepticus (psychomotor
        status)
    Hemiconvulsive status with hemiparesis
Precipitating stimuli for reflex seizures
  Visual stimuli
    Flickering light: colour to be specified
        when possible
    Patterns
    Other visual stimuli
  Thinking
  Music
  Eating
  Praxis
  Somatosensory
  Proprioceptive
  Reading
  Hot water
  Startle

From Engel (2001)[10] with permission of the author and the *Journal of Epilepsia.*

Girl aged 16 with JME and a first GTCS 2 months prior to this EEG

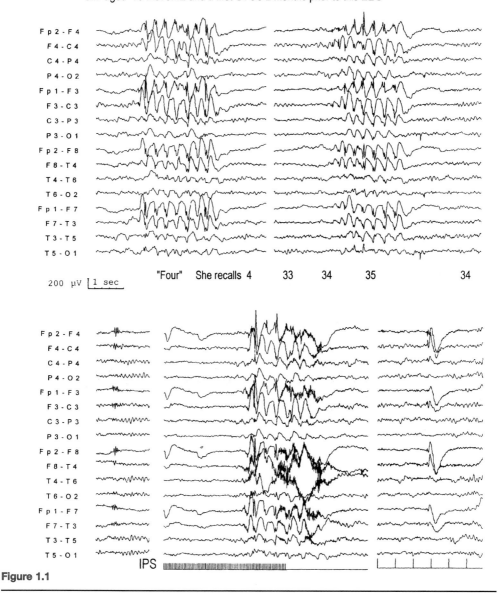

Figure 1.1

Video-EEG of a 16-year-old girl referred for an EEG because of 'a first GTCS' at age 16 years. This happened in the morning on her way to school for exams. She suddenly became vague and nearly simultaneously she fell on the ground with generalised convulsions. On questioning by the EEG technologist, it was revealed that 1 year before the GTCS she had mild jerks of the fingers in the morning interpreted as clumsiness.

The EEG had generalised discharges of 3–4 Hz spike/multiple spike and slow wave. The girl recalled the number shouted to her during the discharge.

However, breath counting during hyperventilation was disturbed during a similar discharge (annotated numbers). In addition there were photoparoxysmal discharges. Brief frontal bursts of polyspikes or spike and slow wave could be erroneously interpreted as 'frontal lobe epilepsy with secondary bilateral synchrony'. On clinical and EEG grounds the diagnosis of juvenile myoclonic epilepsy was established and appropriate treatment was initiated because she had many more seizures (myoclonic jerks and absences) in addition to the single GTCS.

myoclonic jerks (page 117), absences (page 114), simple or complex focal seizures (Chapter 8).

A single GTCS does not require medication, but if the patient also has other, even minor, seizures treatment is usually mandatory. Similarly, it is a medical error to advise withdrawal of medication for a patient with minor seizures even if free of convulsive seizures for many years.

Circadian distribution (on awakening, nocturnal, diurnal) and precipitating factors (flickering lights, sleep deprivation, alcohol indulgence, stress, reading) often provide invaluable clues for the correct diagnosis and may also prompt the appropriate EEG procedure (page 17).

Home video recording (camcorders are widely available) should be used, as seizures are often frequent and sometimes predictable.

Having established that a paroxysmal event is epileptic, the diagnosis by the non-specialist is often limited to excluding structural abnormalities of the brain or predisposing medical disease. However, simply diagnosing 'epilepsy' is insufficient. Defining the type of epilepsy should now be considered mandatory as it offers the best guide to both management and prognosis.[17]

SECOND STEP: THE DIAGNOSIS OF EPILEPTIC SYNDROMES

Syndromic diagnosis of epilepsies provides a firm foundation for short- and long-term therapeutic decisions, and enables natural history, inheritance, treatment efficacy and prognosis of epilepsies to be studied scientifically. The benefits of syndromic diagnosis over seizure/symptom diagnosis or an inclusive diagnosis such as 'epilepsy' far outweigh any morbidity from miscategorisation that may arise in difficult cases.

Some parts of the current ILEA classification[9] remain contentious, some syndromes are ill-defined or broadly defined and require further clarification. There are patients whose clinical and EEG features do not appear to fit neatly into any recognised category or erroneously appear to evolve from one syndrome to another. Some may represent new or 'overlap' syndromes, others may be unusual or atypical forms of known syndromes or cases where clinical history is misleading. However, many syndromes are common, easily diagnosed and well characterised.

The most important milestone in modern epileptology has been the recognition of epileptic syndromes and diseases, most of which are well defined and easy to diagnose. The concept of epilepsies as specific syndromes is old (see for example pyknolepsy = childhood absence epilepsy)[18] and the first attempt to formalise them in an international classification was published in 1970.[19] The current classification originated from a meeting in the Centre Saint-Paul, Marseilles, France in July 1983 and has been the basis of the 'Blue Guide': epileptic syndromes in infancy, childhood and adolescence which now runs an updated 3rd edition,[20] which is highly authoritative and recommended for reading.

The classification and definitions from this meeting were adopted in 1985 by the Commission on Classification and Terminology of the ILAE, 1985[21] and remained essentially the same in the revised proposal of 1989.[9] Recent advances in the clinical-EEG manifestations of previously recognised and newly described syndromes, video-EEG information, functional and structural imaging, investigative procedures and genetics mandated a new thorough and realistic revision of this classification and the definitions of epileptic syndromes.[10] Table 1.3 shows the epileptic syndromes and related

Table 1.3 Epilepsy syndromes and related conditions

Benign familial neonatal seizures
Early myoclonic encephalopathy
Ohtahara syndrome
[a]Migrating partial seizures of infancy
West syndrome
Benign myoclonic epilepsy in infancy
Benign familial infantile seizures
Benign infantile seizures (nonfamilial)
Dravet syndrome
Hemiconvulsion–hemiplegia syndrome
[a]Myoclonic status in nonprogressive encephalopathies
Benign childhood epilepsy with centrotemporal spikes
Early-onset benign childhood occipital epilepsy (Panayiotopoulos type)
Late-onset childhood occipital epilepsy (Gastaut type)
Epilepsy with myoclonic absences
Epilepsy with myoclonic-astatic seizures
Lennox-Gastaut syndrome
Landau-Kleffner syndrome (LKS)
Epilepsy with continuous spike-and-waves during slow-wave sleep (other than LKS)
Childhood absence epilepsy
Progressive myoclonus epilepsies
Idiopathic generalized epilepsies with variable phenotypes
  Juvenile absence epilepsy
  Juvenile myoclonic epilepsy
  Epilepsy with generalized tonic–clonic seizures only
Reflex epilepsies
  Idiopathic photosensitive occipital lobe epilepsy
  Other visual sensitive epilepsies
  Primary reading epilepsy
  Startle epilepsy

Autosomal dominant nocturnal frontal lobe epilepsy
Familial temporal lobe epilepsies
[a]Generalized epilepsies with febrile seizures plus
[a]Familial focal epilepsy with variable foci
Symptomatic (or probably symptomatic) focal epilepsies
  Limbic epilepsies
    Mesial temporal lobe epilepsy with hippocampal sclerosis
    Mesial temporal lobe epilepsy defined by specific etiologies
    Other types defined by location and etiology
  Neocortical epilepsies
    Rasmussen syndrome
    Other types defined by location and etiology
Conditions with epileptic seizures that do not require a diagnosis of epilepsy
Benign neonatal seizures
Febrile seizures
Reflex seizures
Alcohol-withdrawal seizures
Drug or other chemically induced seizures
Immediate and early posttraumatic seizures
Single seizures or isolated clusters of seizures
Rarely repeated seizures (oligoepilepsy)

[a] Syndromes in development

From Engel (2001)[10] with permission of the author and the *Journal of Epilepsia*

conditions as listed in the new diagnostic scheme[10] and Table 1.4 is an example of their group classification.

Table 1.4   An example of a classification of epilepsy syndromes

Groups of syndromes	*Specific syndromes*
Idiopathic focal epilepsies of infancy and childhood	Benign infantile seizures (nonfamilial)
	Benign childhood epilepsy with centrotemporal spikes
	Early-onset benign childhood occipital epilepsy (Panayiotopoulos type)
	Late-onset childhood occipital epilepsy (Gastaut type)
Familial (autosomal dominant) focal epilepsies	Benign familial neonatal seizures
	Benign familial infantile seizures
	Autosomal dominant nocturnal frontal lobe epilepsy
	Familial temporal lobe epilepsy
	Familial focal epilepsy with variable foci[a]
Symptomatic and probably symptomatic focal epilepsies	Limbic epilepsies
	Mesial temporal lobe epilepsy with hippocampal sclerosis
	Mesial temporal lobe epilepsy defined by specific etiologies
	Other types defined by location and etiology
	Neocortical epilepsies
	Rasmussen syndrome
	Hemiconvulsion-hemiplegia syndrome
	Other types defined by location and etiology
	Migrating partial seizures of early infancy[a]
Idiopathic generalized epilepsies	Benign myoclonic epilepsy in infancy
	Epilepsy with myoclonic astatic seizures
	Childhood absence epilepsy
	Epilepsy with myoclonic absences
	Idiopathic generalized epilepsies with variable phenotypes
	Juvenile absence epilepsy
	Juvenile myoclonic epilepsy
	Epilepsy with generalized tonic-clonic seizures only
	Generalized epilepsies with febrile seizures plus[a]
Reflex epilepsies	Idiopathic photosensitive occipital lobe epilepsy
	Other visual sensitive epilepsies
	Primary reading epilepsy
	Startle epilepsy
Epileptic encephalopathies (in which the epileptiform abnormalities may contribute to progressive dysfunction)	Early myoclonic encephalopathy
	Ohtahara syndrome
	West syndrome
	Dravet syndrome (previously known as severe myoclonic epilepsy in infancy)
	Myoclonic status in nonprogressive encephalopathies[a]
	Lennox-Gastaut syndrome
	Landau-Kleffner syndrome
	Epilepsy with continuous spike-waves during slow-wave sleep
Progressive myoclonus epilepsies	See specific diseases
Seizures not necessarily requiring a diagnosis of epilepsy	Benign neonatal seizures
	Febrile seizures
	Reflex seizures
	Alcohol-withdrawal seizures
	Drug or other chemically induced seizures
	Immediate and early post traumatic seizures
	Single seizures or isolated clusters of seizures
	Rarely repeated seizures (oligoepilepsy)

[a] Syndromes in development.

From Engel (2001)[10] with permission of the author and the *Journal of Epilepsia.*

CLASSIFICATION AND SIGNIFICANCE OF EPILEPTIC SYNDROMES

The definition of a medical syndrome is 'a distinct group of symptoms and signs which, associated together, form a characteristic clinical picture or entity', while 'a disease has common aetiology and prognosis despite individual modifications'. Similarly, in the epilepsies, the recognition of non-fortuitous clustering of symptoms and signs requires the study of detailed clinical and laboratory data.

Important clinical features include the type of seizures, their localisation, frequency, sequence of events, circadian distribution, precipitating factors, response to treatment, age at onset, mode of inheritance, and physical or mental symptoms and signs.

Definitions

Epilepsy syndrome: A complex of signs and symptoms that define a unique epilepsy condition. This must involve more than just the seizure type; thus frontal lobe seizures *per se*, for instance, do not constitute a syndrome (changed concept).[10]

Epilepsy disease: A pathological condition with a single specific, well-defined aetiology. Thus progressive myoclonus epilepsy is a syndrome, but Unverricht-Lundborg is a disease (new concept).[10]

Idiopathic epilepsy syndrome: A syndrome that is only epilepsy, with no underlying structural brain lesion or other neurological signs or symptoms. These are presumed to be genetic and are usually age-dependent (unchanged term).[10]

Idiopathic comes from the Greek words idios (meaning self, own, personal) and pathic (suffer, see also pathology, pathological).[22] Idiopathic is not synonymous with benign. There are idiopathic epilepsies with poor prognosis or lifelong duration and conversely there are symptomatic epilepsies with a few seizures that may not even need treatment.

Symptomatic epilepsy syndrome: A syndrome in which the epileptic seizures are the result of one or more identifiable structural lesions of the brain (unchanged term).

Probably symptomatic epilepsy syndrome: Synonymous with, but preferred to, the term cryptogenic, used to define syndromes that are believed to be symptomatic, but no aetiology has been identified (new term).

The number of cryptogenic epilepsies is decreasing in favour of the symptomatic ones with the use of high-resolution MRI, which demonstrates structural cortical lesions previously undetected by CT brain scan or first generations of MRI scanners.

Benign epilepsy syndrome: A syndrome characterised by epileptic seizures that are easily treated, or require no treatment, and remit without sequelae (clarified concept).[10]

Terminological changes in the new diagnostic scheme:[10]

The previous classification of the ILAE was based on two major features:[9]

first, whether the predominant seizure type is focal or generalised and

second, whether the aetiology is idiopathic (with genetic predisposition), symptomatic (structural) or possibly symptomatic (cryptogenic).

These divisions shaped the first two major groups of epileptic syndromes; a third group covered syndromes with seizures of uncertain type (often the case with nocturnal seizures) and a fourth covered seizures associated with a specific situation (fever, drugs, metabolic imbalance).

The new diagnostic scheme maintains focal and generalised epilepsies, does not specify on syndromes of uncertain origin and replaces 'seizures with a specific situation' with 'conditions with seizures that do not require a diagnosis of epilepsy'.[10]

Also, the scheme rightly considers and lists the 'Diseases frequently associated with epileptic seizures or syndromes' (Table 1.5).

Table 1.5 An example of a classification of diseases frequently associated with epileptic seizures or syndromes

Groups of diseases
    Specific diseases

Progressive myoclonic epilepsies
    Ceroid lipofuscinosis
    Sialidosis
    Lafora disease
    Unverricht-Lundborg disease
    Neuroaxonal dystrophy
    MERRF
    Dentatorubropallidoluysian atrophy
    Other

Neurocutaneous disorders
    Tuberous sclerosis complex
    Neurofibromatosis
    Hypomelanosis of Ito
    Epidermal nevus syndrome
    Sturge-Weber syndrome

Malformations due to abnormal cortical developments
    Isolated lissencephaly sequence
    Miller-Dieker syndrome
    X-linked lissencephaly
    Subcortical band heterotopia
    Periventricular nodular heterotopia
    Focal heterotopia
    Hemimegalencephaly
    Bilateral perisylvian syndrome
    Unilateral polymicrogyria
    Schizencephalies
    Focal or multifocal cortical dysplasia
    Microdysgenesis

Other cerebral malformations
    Aicardi syndrome
    PEHO syndrome
    Acrocallosal syndrome
    Other

Tumors
    DNET
    Gangliocytoma
    Ganglioglioma
    Cavernous angiomas
    Astrocytomas
    Hypothalamic hamartoma (with gelastic seizures)
    Other

Chromosomal abnormalities
    Partial monosomy 4P or Wolf-Hirschhorn syndrome
    Trisomy 12p
    Inversion duplication 15 syndrome
    Ring 20 chromosome
    Other

Monogenic mendelian diseases with complex pathogenetic mechanisms
    Fragile X syndrome
    Angelman syndrome
    Rett syndrome
    Other

Groups of diseases
    Specific diseases

Inherited metabolic disorders
    Nonketotic hyperglycinemia
    D-Glyceric acidemia
    Propionic acidemia
    Sulphite-oxidase deficiency
    Fructose 1-6 diphosphatase deficiency
    Other organic acidurias
    Pyridoxine dependency
    Aminoacidopathies (maple syrup urine disease, phenylketonuria, other)
    Urea cycle disorders
    Disorders of carbohydrate metabolism
    Disorders of biotin metabolism
    Disorders of folic acid and B12 metabolism
    Glucose transport protein deficiency
    Menkes' disease
    Glycogen-storage disorders
    Krabbe disease
    Fumarase deficiency
    Peroxisomal disorders
    Sanfilippo syndrome
    Mitochondrial diseases (pyruvate dehydrogenase deficiency, respiratory chain defects, MELAS)

Prenatal or perinatal ischemic or anoxic lesions or cerebral infections causing nonprogressive encephalopathies
    Porencephaly
    Periventricular leukomalacia
    Microcephaly
    Cerebral calcifications and other lesions due to toxoplasmosis, CVI, HIV, etc.

Postnatal infections
    Cysticercosis
    Herpes encephalitis
    Bacterial meningitis
    Other

Other postnatal factors
    Head injury
    Alcohol and drug abuse
    Stroke
    Other

Miscellaneous
    Celiac disease (epilepsy with occipital calcifications and celiac disease)
    Northern epilepsy syndrome
    Coffin-Lowry syndrome
    Alzheimer's disease
    Huntington disease
    Alpers' disease

MERRF, myoclonus epilepsy with ragged red fibers; DNET, dysembryoplastic neuroepithelial tumor; MELAS, mitochondrial encephalomyopathy, lactic acidosis, and stroke-like symptoms; CVI, cerebrovascular incident; HIV, human immunodeficiency virus.

From Engel (2001) with permission of the author and *Journal of Epilepsia*.

Although some symptoms predominate and may indicate the underlying disease, no single symptom or sign can be considered entirely pathognomonic. The process of differential diagnosis requires close scrutiny of the clinical data before a list of possible diagnoses can be drawn up and the final diagnosis reached. It should be realised that some epilepsies are easy to diagnose and some more difficult, but this is not unusual in medicine.

Of the laboratory tests EEG (mandatory for all patients) and brain imaging (structural and sometimes functional) are the most important. Biochemical and haematological investigations, other blood and urine tests aiming to identify specific disorders, and sometimes tissue biopsy may be needed. The significance of the EEG and its optimal use in the diagnosis of the epilepsies is detailed on page 13. Molecular genetics are already making decisive discoveries in the identification of epilepsies.

IMPORTANCE OF ACCURATE DIAGNOSIS

The significance of the syndromic diagnosis of epilepsies has been detailed.[23,24] The results to be expected from syndromic diagnosis of epilepsies can be compared with the advances which have accrued from the widespread acceptance of syndromic diagnosis of connective tissue and neuromuscular diseases. If diagnosed on a few symptoms alone, distinction would often be impossible between rheumatoid disease, ankylosing spondylitis and psoriatic arthropathy, diseases with different (although unknown) aetiology, management, inheritance and prognosis. Similarly, most neuromuscular disorders are mainly characterised by muscle weakness and atrophy. Despite the occasional occurrence of 'overlap syndromes', syndromic classification allows the scientific analysis of the underlying disease processes and their specific clinicopathological features and genetics, and provides a framework for clinical trials aimed at optimising treatment.

The danger of a unified diagnosis of 'epilepsy' or a symptom diagnosis of 'seizures' is exemplified by three common epileptic syndromes: benign childhood focal seizures, juvenile myoclonic epilepsy and temporal lobe epilepsies comprise more than 40% of all epilepsies. They are entirely different in presentation, causes, investigative procedures, short- and long-term treatment strategies and prognosis.

Benign childhood focal seizures (Chapter 5), like febrile convulsions, are age-related, show genetic predisposition, may be manifested by a single seizure, remit within a few years of onset, and may or may not require a short course of antiepileptic medication. The risk of recurrent seizures in adult life (1–2%) is less than in febrile convulsions (4%). Recognition of the characteristic clinical and EEG features of benign childhood focal epilepsies will enable the parents to be reassured of the invariably benign prognosis with spontaneous resolution of the disorder by the middle teens.

Juvenile myoclonic epilepsy (page 139), an idiopathic epileptic syndrome with myoclonic jerks on awakening, GTCS and, more rarely, absences, has a prevalence of 8–10% among adult patients with seizures. The management of juvenile myoclonic epilepsy differs from standard medical practice for the treatment of seizures in several important respects. Recommendations not to treat after the first seizure are usually inappropriate, not only because affected patients have usually experienced other epileptic events (e.g. myoclonic jerks, absences) for many months or years before the first GTCS, but also because juvenile myoclonic epilepsy is a lifelong disease with a high risk of major and minor seizures, particularly after sleep deprivation, fatigue and alcohol indulgence. Emphasising avoidance of precipitating factors in juvenile myoclonic epilepsy is part of the management strategy. Withdrawal of medication after 2–3 seizure-free years and substitution of carbamazepine instead of sodium valproate are also inappropriate, because relapses are inevitable.

Temporal lobe epilepsies (page 170), comprising more than 30% of epilepsies in adults, are mostly due to progressive or non-progressive structural lesions of the temporal lobe and hippocampal sclerosis, shown with high–resolution MRI. Seizures can begin at any time between infancy and old age but usually start in the mid-teens. The diagnosis is often easy on clinico-EEG grounds. Complex focal seizures are the commonest type of fits and approximately half of these patients also have secondarily GTCS. Remission may occur in 30% of the patients but 20% may become medically intractable.

Even the most sceptical physicians, among those who doubt the clinical or practical significance of the syndromic diagnosis of epilepsies, have to accept that benign childhood focal epilepsies, juvenile myoclonic epilepsy and symptomatic temporal lobe epilepsy have nothing in common other than the fact that they may all be manifested by GTCS, which are primary in juvenile myoclonic epilepsy and secondary in benign childhood focal epilepsies and symptomatic temporal lobe epilepsy. Furthermore, the short- and long-term treatment strategies are entirely different for each disorder: benign childhood focal epilepsies may or may not require drug treatment, mainly with carbamazepine, for a few years; sodium valproate is the drug of choice in juvenile myoclonic epilepsy and treatment is lifelong; and cryptogenic/symptomatic temporal lobe epilepsy may be resistant to the drugs of choice such as carbamazepine and may require neurosurgical resection of the affected area of the temporal lobe.

It should not be difficult to distinguish an intelligent child with benign focal seizures or childhood absence epilepsy from a child with Kozhevnikov-Rasmussen, Down or Sturge-Weber syndrome, or a child with severe post-traumatic cerebral damage, brain anoxia, trisomy and deletion of chromosome 4p or Baltic myoclonic epilepsy. Diagnosing all these children as simply having epilepsy just because they have seizures offers no more benefit than a diagnosis of a febrile illness irrespective of cause, which may be a mild viral illness, bacterial meningitis or malignancy.

Significant progress is expected if emphasis is directed towards 'how to diagnose epilepsies' rather than the current theme of 'how to treat epilepsy'.

THE SIGNIFICANCE OF THE EEG IN THE DIAGNOSIS AND MANAGEMENT OF EPILEPSIES [25–27]

The electroencephalogram (EEG), entirely harmless and relatively inexpensive, is the most important investigation in the diagnosis and management of epilepsies providing that it is properly performed by experienced technicians, carefully studied and interpreted in the context of a well-described clinical setting by experienced physicians.
The EEG is an integral part of the diagnostic process in epilepsies and this should not be under-rated.

More than half of children and adults presently referred for a routine EEG are suspected or suffer from epilepsies. The EEG is indispensable in the correct syndromic diagnosis of these patients.

THE VALUE OF ROUTINE INTERICTAL OR ICTAL EXTRACRANIAL EEG IN EPILEPSIES SHOULD NEITHER BE UNDERESTIMATED NOR OVER-RATED

The EEG in epilepsies is over-rated by some and undervalued by others. The truth is in between.

The EEG should not be underestimated because:

- The EEG is the only available investigation to record and evaluate the paroxysmal discharges of cerebral neurones causing seizures. The appropriate evaluation of patients with epileptic disorders is often impossible without EEG. In the majority of the cases the clinical diagnosis is concordant with the EEG findings. However, it is often with the help of EEG that the correct diagnosis is established, particularly if the clinical information is inadequate or misleading (Figure 1.2). On other occasions, the clinical data are more sound than the EEG analysis, particularly if this is non-specific or in chronic cases of treated epilepsies.
- The seizure and epileptic syndrome classifications are based on combined clinico-EEG manifestations. Epileptic syndromes, the most important advance of recent epileptology, were mainly identified because of their EEG manifestations.
- Focal and generalised epilepsies are often difficult to differentiate without EEG even by the most experienced epileptologists (Figure 1.2).
- It is the EEG that will often demonstrate beyond any doubt that the 'daydreaming' of a child is due to absence seizures (Figure 1.3), that long-lasting episodes of behavioural changes are due to non-convulsive status epilepticus, that the 'eyelid tics' are due to eyelid myoclonia with

photosensitivity, that the clumsiness on awakening is due to myoclonic jerks, that periodic bed-wetting is due to nocturnal seizures.
- The EEG in neonatal seizures is the most powerful investigative tool (page 38).

The EEG should not be overvalued because:
- The EEG may be oversensitive in conditions such as the benign childhood seizure susceptibility syndrome and sightless in others such as frontal or often temporal lobe epilepsies. Rarely, even ictal events may be undetected in surface EEG (some frontal seizures are typical examples of this). Patients mainly with focal epilepsies may have a series of normal EEG and the EEG localisation is not always concordant with ictal intracranial recordings. More than 40% of patients with epileptic disorders may have one normal interictal EEG, although this percentage falls dramatically to 8% with a series of EEG and appropriate activating procedures, particularly sleep.[28]
- The frequency of seizures is not proportional to the EEG paroxysmal 'epileptogenic' discharges. Severely 'epileptogenic' EEG may be recorded from patients with infrequent or controlled clinical seizures and vice versa. The EEG abnormalities do not reflect the severity of the epileptic disorder.[25]
- More than 10% of normal people may have non-specific EEG abnormalities and around 1% may have 'epileptiform paroxysmal activity' without seizures.[26] The prevalence of these abnormalities is higher in children, with 2–4% having functional spikes.[25]
- Paroxysmal epileptiform activity is high in patients with non-epileptic, neurological or medical disorders or with neurological deficits. For example, children with congenital visual deficits frequently have occipital spikes and patients with migraine have a high incidence of sharp paroxysmal activity.[25]

FACTORS OF ERROR IN EEG

Even the most reliable investigative tools in medicine cannot escape severe errors either because of poor technical quality (equipment, personnel, or both), interpretation by poorly qualified physicians, or both. A competent report should not only accurately spot the EEG abnormality but also provide its significance and meaning in accordance with a well-described clinical setting.[25]

Failing to achieve this leads to severe errors and erroneous criticism such as 'Routine interictal EEG is one of the most abused investigations in clinical medicine and is unquestionably responsible for great human suffering'.[29] Anything in medicine, clinical or laboratory, may be harmful if misinterpreted – raising standards, not abandoning the service, is the appropriate answer (Figure 1.2).[30]

Providing that the EEG is technically correct, in my opinion the following are the most important factors of error listed in order of significance:

1. The single most significant source of error is that the EEG is often interpreted out of the clinical context. There are two reasons for this. First, the referring physician provides inadequate information regarding the events – e.g. 'Patient with loss of consciousness or grand mal seizures', 'Black-outs. Epilepsy?', 'Unexplained aggressiveness. Temporal lobe

The use and abuse of the EEG

Girl aged 13 with 2 seizures described as simple focal motor "eyes and head turned to the left" for 2 minutes with no impairment of consciousness

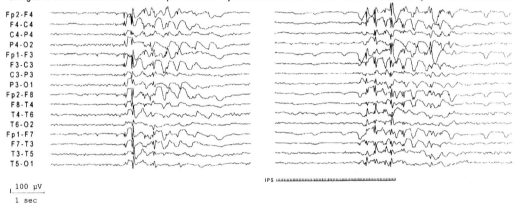

Girl aged 13 with frequent brief absences of eyelid flickering

This EEG was reported as normal because the discharges were considered as artefacts due to "eye movements"

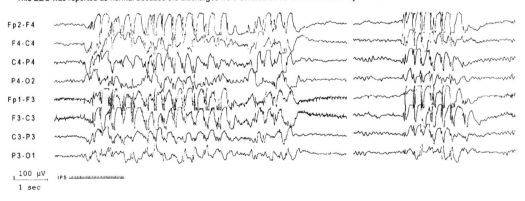

Figure 1.2 Two girls with similar EEG abnormalities of generalised spike/multiple spike and slow wave discharges either spontaneously or IPS-elicited.

Top: Usefulness of the EEG.
This girl gave a clear-cut history of two seizures that on clinical grounds had all the elements of focal motor seizures. Her eyes first and then the head turned to the left and she 'could not bring them back to normal' for 2 minutes. EEG clearly documented that she had generalised, not focal, epilepsy.

Bottom: EEG abuse.
A 26-year-old woman with IGE had onset of seizures at age 13. These consisted of brief absences with eyelid jerking. Her first EEG documented the epileptic nature of the attacks but the reporting physician and the EEG technologist considered the discharges as artefacts produced by the concurrent eyelid jerking.

epilepsy?' – and often fails to mention other medical conditions or drugs which may significantly affect the EEG and its interpretation. Second, the reporting clinical neurophysiologist prefers a convenient but rather unhelpful and uncommitted abbreviation of the factual report, e.g. 'normal EEG', 'an abnormal EEG with active spike in the occipital regions', 'focal episodic left temporal slowing without genuine epileptiform activity'. In St Thomas' Hospital, I am in the advantageous position of being the referring and the reporting physician and this practice may expand to other clinics for epilepsies. Further, our EEG technologists are well trained as regards the need to obtain the missing clinical information (see page 21).

2. Non-specific EEG abnormalities are overemphasised without suggesting means of clarifying their significance with a sleep-deprived EEG, for example, or after obtaining more clinical data. Episodic focal slow waves are non-specific and may occur in a normal person, a patient with migraine, with mild cerebrovascular disease or even cerebral tumours. They may be of lateralising significance even if they are infrequent and of small amplitude in a patient with well-established clinical history of temporal lobe seizures.

3. EEG during hyperventilation, drowsiness and sleep may produce significant changes, which are often difficult to interpret even by experienced neurophysiologists. EEG in babies and children is even more complex and demanding. Non-epileptic episodic transients such as benign epileptiform transients of sleep, 6 and 14 per second positive spikes, rhythmic mid-temporal discharges may often be misinterpreted as evidence of 'epilepsy'.[26]

4. Previous EEG records and results are lost, destroyed or not sought. This is significant in the re-evaluation of patients with long-standing epilepsy. EEGs recorded at the initial stages of the disease and particularly before treatment are usually diagnostic. These patients are mainly referred for treatment modifications because, for example, they are free of seizures and still on medication, they had a recent convulsion after a long seizure-free period, seizures are not controlled with long-standing medication, adverse reactions to their medication or appropriateness to change to new anti-epileptic drugs, or anticipated pregnancy in women. The answer in all these cases is difficult. It requires a thorough clinical evaluation, review of previous medical and EEG records and the establishment of the appropriate epileptic syndrome. It does not depend on the findings of a new EEG, which may be misleading – for example, it may be normal in a patient with idiopathic generalised epilepsy who is on sodium valproate or may show focal slow wave paroxysms in a patient with well-documented generalised spike and polyspike discharges in early EEG. However, on other occasions this recent EEG may prompt the correct advice on documenting mild epileptic seizures such as myoclonic jerks or absences in a patient 'free of seizures' or of 'continuing focal seizures' inadequately treated with carbamazepine.

5. Alteration of the EEG by drugs (such as neuroleptics or antiepileptics) or co-existing medical conditions (cerebrovascular disease, electrolyte disturbances, previous head injury).

The fact that a patient with a brain tumour may not have clinical signs does not invalidate the clinical examination and the same is true for the EEG. The main cause of concern and suffering is that physicians, including epilepsy authorities, have misunderstood EEG, its value and its limitations. The ILAE Commissions may consider issuing updated recommendations on the use of EEG in clinical practice as they rightly did for neuro-imaging.[31–33]

ACTIVATING PROCEDURES

These intend to improve the EEG diagnostic yield by inducing or enhancing epileptogenic paroxysms. Hyperventilation (HV) and intermittent photic stimulation (IPS) are the only activating procedures applied in routine waking EEG. Drowsiness, sleep and awakening are very important activating procedures.

Hyperventilation often induces physiological changes such as diffuse and paroxysmal slow activity, particularly in healthy young persons who overbreathe well. They do not last for more than 60 seconds after cessation of HV and they should not be confused with abnormal epileptogenic disturbances, which are also activated by HV. The 3–4 Hz generalised spike and slow wave, which is the electrical accompaniment of typical absences, is nearly invariably (>90% of untreated patients) induced or enhanced by HV.

Cognition during generalised discharges can be practically evaluated in routine EEG by asking the patient to count his breaths during HV (Figure 1.1). Breath counting during HV is just a simple modification of the routine EEG technique (hyperventilation). It allows accurate identification of even mild transient cognitive impairment during generalised spike/multiple spike wave discharges.[34] It is powerful because breath counting during hyperventilation simultaneously tests attention, concentration, memory, sequence and language function. It could not be simpler.

Intermittent photic stimulation is significant for the detection of photosensitive patients. Photoparoxysmal discharges, which are often initiated from the occipital regions, indicate a genetically determined photosensitivity and may occur in more than 1% of healthy subjects.

Other forms of appropriate activation should be used – and they are as much fascinating as rewarding in patients with reflex seizures – such as reading, pattern, musicogenic, proprioceptive or noogenic epilepsy. Their detection is of significance regarding diagnosis and management. Avoidance of precipitating factors may be all that is needed in certain patients with reflex seizures.

It is important to study drowsiness, sleep and awakening in patients with epileptic disorders, particularly those who produce a normal routine awake EEG and their seizures are consistently associated with these physiological stages. However, drowsiness and sleep are associated with dramatic physiological EEG changes, which may imitate epileptogenic paroxysms; their interpretation should be left to highly experienced clinical neurophysiologists, otherwise significant errors are inevitable. Sleep recording should always include the awakening stage, as it is well known that in certain epileptic syndromes such as idiopathic generalised epilepsies, seizures and EEG paroxysms may only occur at this stage.

Partial instead of all-night sleep deprivation should be preferred.

The recording should continue after awakening – which is not a common practice in most EEG laboratories.

All-night sleep deprivation is a well-known activating procedure in epilepsies. However, it causes significant inconvenience to the patient and family, may jeopardise the diagnosis because it is associated with a higher incidence of EEG abnormalities in normal people and may unnecessarily induce seizures in susceptible individuals. We have adopted a rather practical, more natural, less disturbing and equally rewarding approach. We ask the patient to go to sleep 1–2 hours later and wake 1–2 hours earlier than his routine practice. The EEG is recorded the next day after lunch, the patient is allowed to sleep for an hour and the recording continues for another 30 minutes after awakening; where HV and IPS are also performed. The awakening state is as important as the sleep state (Figure 1.4).

A REQUEST FOR AN EEG SHOULD DESCRIBE THE CLINICAL PROBLEM WELL

Although not a substitute for the clinical examination, the EEG is an integral part of the diagnostic process in epilepsies.[25]

Epilepsies are usually easy to diagnose. However, as with any other medical condition, they are sometimes difficult and challenging. I use the EEG as an integral part of the diagnostic process. In this sense, there is more than enough justification to have an EEG after the first suspected seizure. The EEG may be the only means of an incontrovertible syndromic diagnosis. The fact that the patient may not need treatment[35] is not a convincing argument against such a practice; the prime aim in medicine is the diagnosis, which determines treatment strategies.

EEG aspects: The role of the EEG is to help the physician to establish an accurate diagnosis. In most conditions (infantile spasms, myoclonic epilepsies, symptomatic generalised epilepsies, idiopathic generalised epilepsies, temporal lobe epilepsy, Landau-Kleffner syndrome, benign childhood focal seizures, photosensitive and other reflex epilepsies) the EEG may specifically confirm or may specifically direct towards such a diagnosis if this is clinically uncertain (Figure 1.3). In other situations it may not be helpful with normal rhythms or some non-specific diffuse or paroxysmal slow activity. These cases may need an EEG during sleep, awakening or both, and again it may not reveal specific changes in approximately 10% of the patients. However, even a normal EEG in an untreated patient may be useful as it may exclude some of the above conditions where EEG abnormalities are expected to be high – such as in idiopathic generalised epilepsies (IGE) with typical absence seizures.

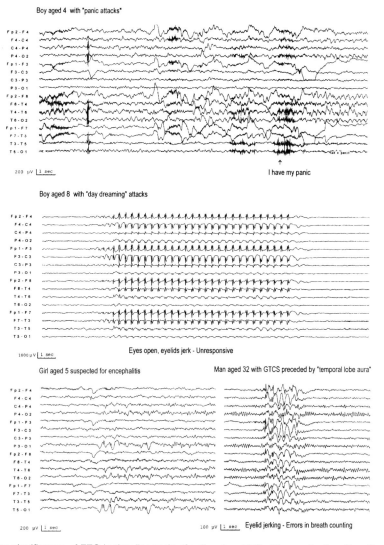

Figure 1.3 The significance of EEG in the diagnosis of epilepsies; EEG of four patients with epileptic diseases.

Top: Ictal EEG of a 4-year-old boy who had frequent brief episodes of 'panic' without impairment of consciousness or convulsive features. The resting EEG was normal but a 'panic' attack was video-EEG recorded with ictal EEG changes of 2 minutes, mainly involving the right temporal regions. The child accurately answered all questions and communicated well with the technician during the ictus. This EEG unequivocally established the diagnosis and dictated the appropriate management. MRI showed right hippocampal sclerosis.

Middle: Video-EEG of a child aged 8 years with frequent episodes of 'blanks and daydreaming' for 2 years. Frequent typical absence seizures were recorded and appropriate treatment was initiated with complete control of the seizures.

Bottom left: Interictal EEG of a 5-year-old child 2 days after a prolonged autonomic status epilepticus suspected and treated for encephalitis (case 47 in ref [36]). EEG showed scattered right central and bi-occipital spikes. The diagnosis of Panayiotopoulos syndrome was established and the child was discharged home.

Lower right: Video-EEG of a 32-year-old man with three or four GTCS every year from age 16 (case 1 in ref [37]). All GTCS were preceded by absence status diagnosed as 'prodrome' or 'temporal lobe aura'. Treatment included inappropriate use of phenytoin and even vigabatrin. Brief generalised discharges of 3–4 Hz spikes/multiple spikes and slow waves were recorded during hyperventilation. These were associated with brief rhythmic myoclonic jerks of the eyelids (which would be impossible to detect without video) and minor errors in breath counting. The correct diagnosis of IGE with phantom absences was established and treatment was changed to sodium valproate. No further seizures occurred in the next 5 years of follow-up.

19

The EEG should be tailored to the specific circumstances of the individual patient. The technician should be alerted to apply the appropriate stimulus such as in reading epilepsy, proprioceptive or fixation–off sensitivity.

Patients with idiopathic generalised epilepsies having generalised convulsions after awakening may have a normal or non–specific routine EEG.

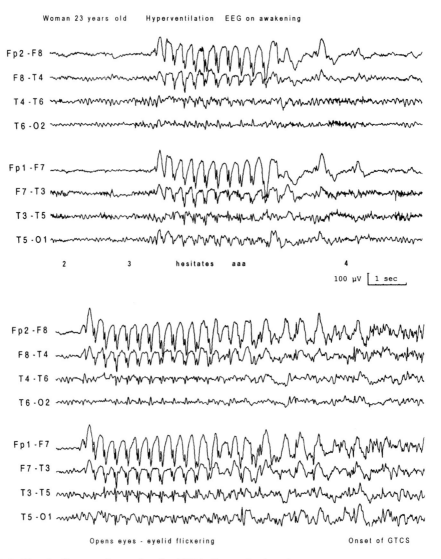

Figure 1.4 The significance of recording the EEG in the awakening stage.

From video-EEG of a 23-year-old woman with IGE and absence seizures. She was thought to be free of seizures. A long EEG the previous day, including two sessions of well-performed overbreathing was normal. She slept for 5 hours in the same night (not an unusual situation for a young person at her age) and the EEG was recorded in the middle of the next day. This showed, upon awakening, numerous absence seizures which ended with a GTCS.

From Panayiotopoulos (2000)[38] with the permission of the Editor of *Epilepsia*.

An EEG after partial sleep deprivation with video-EEG recording during sleep and awakening frequently reveals clinical and EEG ictal events which are important for diagnosis and treatment (Figure 1.4). The same applies to patients with nocturnal seizures who may have a normal EEG while awake.

EEG in chronic or treated patients may be uninformative and misleading. Obtaining previous medical and EEG reports is essential.

TECHNICIANS

The principal role of the EEG technologists is to provide a competent EEG recording and factual report. However, their role should be more than this, considering that:

- Currently ~70% of EEG referrals are for epileptic disorders
- Referrals commonly come from general paediatricians/general physicians who may not be familiar with the syndromic diagnosis of epilepsies
- Information in the request form is usually inadequate
- An EEG technologist spends 15–20 minutes preparing the patient for the recording, which may be valuably used to obtain information regarding minor seizures, precipitating factors, circadian distribution and other aspects of the particular individual
- The interpretation of the EEG depends on clinical history, which often is poor or missing
- Nurses and other non-medical health professionals are involved in the management of epilepsies.

A well-qualified EEG technician is expected to have and should be trained to have thorough knowledge of seizures and epileptic syndromes.

In my department, technicians often provide me with the correct syndromic diagnosis of our patients based on such a dual clinico-EEG approach. Even the interpretation of a normal EEG may be significantly different according to clinical information.

VIDEO-EEG SHOULD BE MADE ROUTINE PRACTICE

Video-EEG machines are relatively inexpensive today and their use should be mandatory in the evaluation of patients suspected or having seizures. An EEG discharge is of great diagnostic and therapeutic significance if it is associated with a minor jerk or impairment of consciousness, which often escape recognition in routine EEG without video recordings (Figures 1.1, 1.2 and 1.3).

Video-EEGs are particularly important in the identification and categorisation of absences, which are easily elicited by hyperventilation, myoclonic jerks which may be inconspicuous, pseudoseizures and particularly those of the hyperventilation syndrome, focal seizures or other convulsive seizures which may occur incidentally during the EEG or may be predictably recorded based on their circadian distribution and the precipitating factors.

Video-EEG is probably mandatory during hyperventilation, photic stimulation, sleep and awakening.

Seizures or other paroxysmal events may occur at any stage during the EEG (Figures 1.1, 1.2 and 1.3). Therefore, it is advisable to start and continue video recording during the whole procedure of EEG preparation. Vasovagal attacks often occur during the EEG electrode placement and fraudulent or other pseudoseizures may occur during the disconnection period, particularly when the patient is reassured that the EEG is normal. Other types of non-epileptic paroxysmal disorders such as paroxysmal kinesiogenic choreoathetosis may also be captured with video-EEG and prompt the correct diagnosis.

AN EEG REPORT SHOULD BE HELPFUL AND COMMITTED; IT SHOULD NOT BE AN ABBREVIATED FACTUAL REPORT

One of the most important factors of error in EEG is that the reporting clinical neurophysiologist prefers a convenient but rather unhelpful and uncommitted approach, which is often an abbreviation of the factual technical report – e.g. 'normal EEG', 'an abnormal EEG with active spike in the occipital regions', 'focal episodic left temporal slowing without genuine epileptiform activity', 'an abnormal EEG with normal background and generalised discharges of spike wave with a frontal onset'. This is inadequate, often uninformative and sometimes misleading. The receiving physician is often unfamiliar with these EEG terms and their significance. My approach is to provide as much information as possible, supplementing the traditional conclusion with an opinion and often a comment, which improves the EEG contribution. Let me take a few examples.

Routine EEG may be normal but the clinical information is such that it requires a new appropriately tailored EEG. These are just a few examples.

1. **Normal routine EEG of a teenager with a single GTCS on awakening.**

    'The EEG is normal but because the patient's seizure occurred on awakening after significant precipitating factors, we have arranged an EEG after partial sleep deprivation.' This was normal in all other stages but on awakening there were brief (1–2 seconds) asymptomatic generalised discharges during hyperventilation, thus documenting a low threshold to IGE. The patient was advised regarding precipitating factors; no drug treatment was given.

2. **Normal routine EEG of an 8-year-old child with a GTCS during sleep.**

    'The EEG is normal but because this is a child with a nocturnal convulsive seizure, a sleep EEG is indicated.' This showed Rolandic spikes during sleep thus securing an excellent prognosis.

3. **Normal routine EEG of a woman with prolonged episodes of mild confusion pre-menstrually.**

   'The EEG is normal but because the episodes of confusion may be non-convulsive status epilepticus, an EEG will be performed in a pre-menstrual period.' This showed frequent generalised discharges of 3–4 Hz spike and slow waves associated with mild impairment of consciousness and eyelid blinking.

Abnormal EEG

There are numerous examples in diverse cases of epileptic or non-epileptic disorders where the reporting physician may make a significant contribution. I will illustrate only a few of them.

1. **EEG with occipital spikes of a 6-year-old child referred because of 'a prolonged episode of loss of consciousness with convulsions':**

   Conclusion. The EEG is of good organisation with well-formed alpha rhythm, which is often interrupted by clusters of high amplitude bi-occipital sharp and slow waves.

   Opinion. The EEG abnormality of this type of occipital spikes is often associated with benign seizures in this age group. From the clinical description, this child may suffer from 'Panayiotopoulos syndrome' whereby seizures are often solitary or infrequent as detailed in the attached paper (I enclose a brief report if the referring physician is not aware of the condition). However, occipital paroxysms may also occur in 1% of normal children or more in children with congenital visual abnormalities (strabismus, amblyopia) and other conditions with or without seizures.

   Comment: This EEG should be interpreted in accordance with the clinical manifestations of this child.★ In particular, was the event nocturnal or diurnal? what were the symptoms that preceded the convulsions and what was their duration? did he have autonomic disturbances, eye deviation or vomiting? is this a normal child with normal vision and development? Please let me know, as treatment may not be needed.

   ★*Note: This information could be obtained by the technologist (page 21)*

2. **EEG with brief generalised discharges in a 30-year-old man referred because of a first GTCS.**

   Conclusion. The EEG is of good organisation with well-formed alpha rhythm. It is abnormal because of brief generalised discharges of 3–4 Hz small spike and wave, which are facilitated by hyperventilation. These are not associated with any ictal clinical manifestations tested with video-EEG and breath counting.

   Opinion. The EEG abnormality indicates a low threshold to IGE. This is consistent with the clinical information that the recent GTCS occurred in the morning after sleep deprivation and alcohol consumption. The patient is not aware of absences or myoclonic jerks.

There is a remote possibility that these abnormalities are due to frontal lesions or subependymal heterotopia (a distinct neuronal migration disorder associated with epilepsy). This may indicate the need for high-resolution MRI, although I expect it to be normal.

Comment: This patient may not need any drug treatment but should be advised regarding precipitating factors.

MRI was normal and the patient did not have any other seizures in the next 10 years of follow-up.

3. **A 35-year-old woman was referred because of prolonged confusional episodes premenstrually.**

    Conclusion. The EEG is of good organisation with well-formed alpha rhythm. It is suspiciously but not definitely abnormal because of a brief and inconspicuous burst of larval spikes and theta waves.

    Opinion. The EEG abnormality is mild and not conclusive. We have organised an EEG during her vulnerable menstrual periods because the confusional episodes may be non-convulsive status epilepticus.

    This was performed and showed definite and frequent generalised discharges of 3–4 Hz spike/multiple spike and slow wave associated with impairment of consciousness and eyelid flickering.

    No further confusional episodes occurred after treatment with sodium valproate.

4. **A 17-year-old man was referred because of a 'single episode of loss of consciousness and convulsions. Epilepsy?'**

    Conclusion. The EEG is of good organisation with well-formed alpha rhythm. It is abnormal because of brief runs of monomorphic theta waves around the left anterior temporal regions.

    Opinion. The EEG abnormality is mild but definite though does not show conventional epileptogenic features. However, because it is strictly unilateral a high-resolution MRI is indicated. This is also mandated because according to the information gathered by our EEG technologist, the recent convulsive episode was preceded by an ascending epigastric sensation and fear, which also occurred in isolation over the last 2 years. These raise the possibility of hippocampal epilepsy.

    MRI confirmed left hippocampal sclerosis and a sleep EEG showed a clear-cut sharp and slow wave focus in the left anterior temporal electrode.

There are numerous similar examples that this type of communication between electroencephalographers and clinicians is essential for a better diagnosis and management of patients with epilepsies. The problems become even more complicated and demanding of EEGs for patients with migraine, psychiatric diseases, cerebrovascular insufficiency and so forth. It is often important to state that the EEG 'although abnormal may be misleading in view of the migraine, psychiatric or previous head injuries of the patient. It cannot be taken as evidence or not of epilepsy'.

THE SIGNIFICANCE OF THE EEG AFTER THE FIRST AFEBRILE SEIZURE

Routine EEG is a standard recommendation for the diagnostic evaluation of a child after a first non-febrile seizure.[39] This comes from the Quality Standards Subcommittee of the American Academy of Neurology based on analysis of evidence.[39] However, in the UK, EEG is not recommended after the first afebrile seizure, a practice that may have significant adverse implications in the correct diagnosis and management (see ref [30] and associated commentary[35]).

THE FIRST SEIZURE

Most of the epilepsies manifest with primarily or secondarily generalised tonic-clonic seizures (GTCS), which may herald the onset or occur long after the beginning of the disease. Studies on the prognosis and treatment of the 'first seizure' mainly refer to a GTCS although this may not be the first seizure in the patient's life.[40] Myoclonic jerks, absences and focal seizures are less dramatic but more important than a GTCS for diagnosis. In one study, 74% of patients with newly identified unprovoked seizures had experienced multiple seizure episodes before their first medical contact.[16]

The recurrence rate after a first convulsive seizure varies from 27% to 81%, reflecting significant differences in selection, treatment and methodological criteria.[25,30] An abnormal EEG and particularly generalised spike wave discharges has been reported as a consistent predictor of recurrence in all[16,41–44] but one study,[45] which was in adults (see for review refs[25,30]). In a meta-analysis of 16 publications on the risk of recurrence after a first fit, seizure aetiology and EEG were the stronger predictors of recurrence.[41] This was confirmed in a more recent study of 407 children with a first unprovoked afebrile seizure.[44] In idiopathic and cryptogenic seizures the EEG was the most important predictor of outcome, with 52% risk of recurrence at 2 years in those with abnormal versus 28% in those with a normal EEG.[44] The EEG showed specific abnormalities of focal spikes or generalised discharges in 32.5% of 268 children after their first idiopathic seizure.[43]

In other studies of patients with a syndromic classification, it was possible to predict an excellent prognosis in children with benign childhood focal epilepsies with more than 98% remission within 1 year from onset or in their late teens. In other syndromes such as juvenile myoclonic epilepsy there is a lifelong liability to seizures.

WHY AN EEG AFTER THE FIRST AFEBRILE SEIZURE?

The fact that an epileptiform EEG is associated with a 2–3 times higher risk for recurrence than a normal EEG is well established.[16,25,30,41–44] However, the most significant reasons for having an EEG after a single afebrile convulsion are four-fold.

1. It is possible to recognise children with the features of specific epileptic syndromes. Ten to forty percent of children with benign childhood focal

seizures may not have more than a single fit, thus depriving them from receiving a precise diagnosis and prognosis under the current practice. On other occasions, a symptomatic generalised epilepsy may be established that requires early attention.

2. Minor seizures such as absences and myoclonic jerks may be recorded that also have significant implications for diagnosis and treatment.

3. The EEG is imperative in establishing seizure precipitating factors such as video games or television, thus leading to early and appropriate advice.

4. An EEG in an untreated stage of an epileptic syndrome is imperative. This is most likely to happen if the EEG is requested after the first seizure. Many paediatricians would be reluctant to withhold treatment after a second and possibly more seizures, which are expected to occur in a quarter of children within 3 months of their first fit. Requesting an EEG at that stage may be late. Masking or altering the EEG with antiepileptic drugs may be detrimental even for a seizure diagnosis of an epilepsy condition that may need long-term and expensive medication, which is often seizure-specific.

A convulsive seizure is a dramatic event in a child's life and family.[46] As in all other fields of medicine, they are entitled to a diagnosis, prognosis and management, that is specific and precise.[25,40] Even for the benefit of the few patients where this is possible after the first seizure an EEG should be requested.[39]

BRAIN IMAGING IN THE DIAGNOSIS AND MANAGEMENT OF EPILEPSIES

Contemporary magnetic resonance imaging (MRI) scanners are of sufficiently high resolution to allow in vivo visualisation of structural causes of epilepsies such as hippocampal sclerosis and malformations of cortical development.
MRI is much superior to X-ray computed tomography (CT) in terms of sensitivity and specificity for identifying lesional epilepsies.
In clinical practice, mainly neurosurgical cases, functional brain imaging is currently supplementary to MRI.

Modern structural and functional brain imaging methodologies have made a colossal impact in the diagnosis and management of epilepsies.[31–33,47–59] A high degree of anatomical and metabolic information is now provided with different brain imaging techniques.

The ILAE has recently produced recommendations for the neuroimaging of persons with epilepsy in general,[31] with intractable seizures in their presurgical evaluation[32] and more recently for functional neuroimaging.[33] The following is a brief reminder of these recommendations.[31–33]

RECOMMENDATIONS FOR NEUROIMAGING OF PATIENTS WITH EPILEPSY

AIMS AND RATIONALE OF NEUROIMAGING

1. To identify underlying pathologies such as tumours, granulomas, vascular malformations, traumatic lesions, or strokes that merit specific treatment.
2. To aid the formulation of syndromic and aetiological diagnoses and to give patients, their relatives, and physicians an accurate prognosis.

TECHNIQUES

Scans must be interpreted in the context of the entire clinical situation. Images must be reviewed by a specialist in neuroimaging who has training and expertise in the neuroimaging of epilepsy.

Magnetic resonance imaging (MRI) is the superior investigative tool of choice.[31,32] It is superior to radiographic CT in terms of both sensitivity and specificity for identification of small lesions and abnormalities of the cerebral cortex. Even when a CT scan reveals an epileptogenic lesion, MRI often adds new and important data.

The principal role of MRI is in the definition of structural abnormalities that underlie seizure disorders. Hippocampal sclerosis may be identified reliably (Figure 1.5), quantitative studies are useful for research and, in

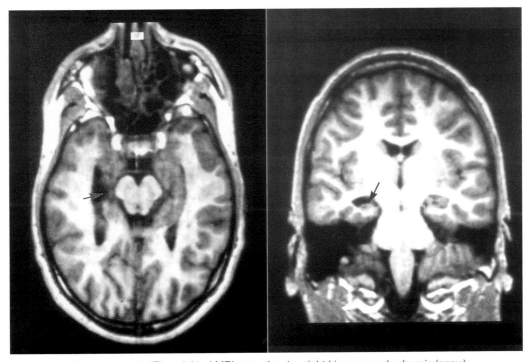

Figure 1.5   Coronal and axial T1-weighted MRI scan showing right hippocampal sclerosis (arrow).

Figure courtesy of Dr Rod C. Scott, Institute of Child Health, London.

equivocal cases, for clinical purposes. A range of malformations of cortical development may be determined (Figures 1.6, 1.7 and 1.8). The proportion of cryptogenic cases of epilepsy has been dramatically decreased with

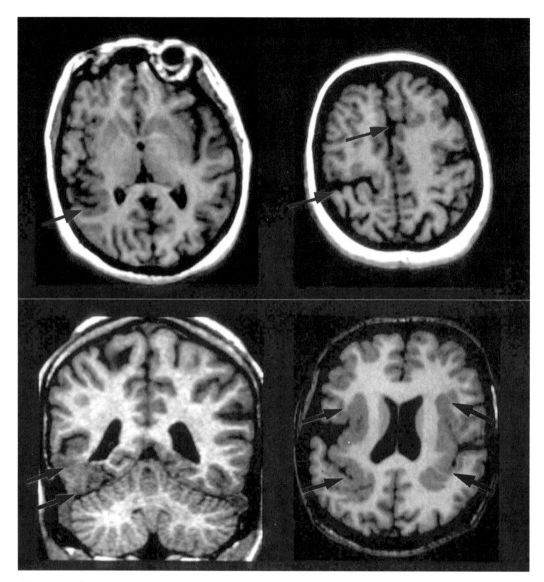

Figure 1.6 Examples of malformations of cortical development documented with MRI.

Top: Axial T1-weighted MRI scan showing bilateral schizencephaly (arrows).

Lower left: Coronal T1-weighted MRI scan showing right focal cortical dysplasia (arrows).
Lower right: Axial T1-weighted MRI scan showing bilateral perisylvian polymicrogyria (arrows).

Figure courtesy of Professor John S. Duncan and the National Society for Epilepsy MRI Unit.

improvements in MRI hardware, signal acquisition techniques and post-processing methodologies (Figure 1.9).

Both T1–weighted and T2–weighted images should be obtained, with slices as thin as possible. 3-D volume acquisition is preferable, but coronal as

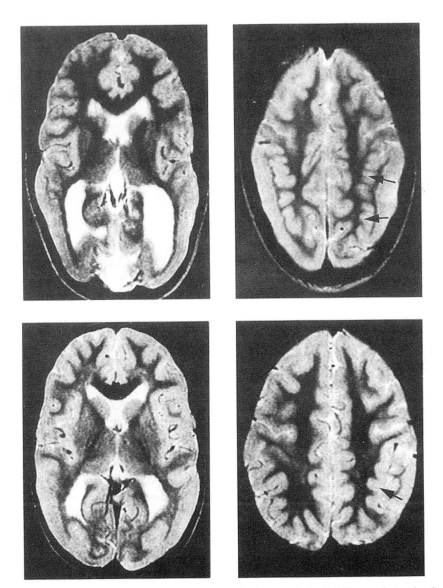

Figure 1.7   Posterior agyria-pachygyria with polymicrogyria documented with MRI scan in two brothers.[60]

Axial T2-weighted MRI scan from older (top) and younger (bottom) brother.

These show marked posterior agyria-pachygyria with areas of polymicrogyria in the parietal cortex.

From Ferrie et al. (1995)[60] with the permission of the authors and the Editor of *Neurology*.

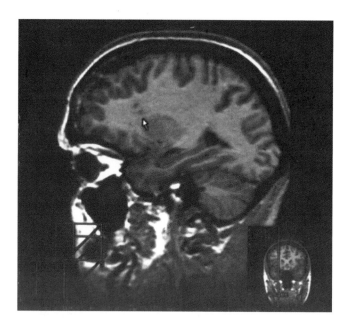

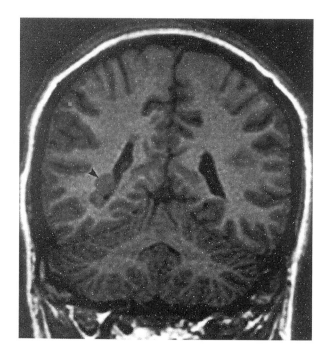

Figure 1.8

Top: Sagittal T1-weighted MRI scan showing frontal focal cortical dysplasia (arrow).

Bottom: Coronal T1-weighted MRI (Ir SPGR) showing nodular subependymal heterotopia in the inferior-lateral wall of the right lateral ventricle (arrow).

Figure courtesy of Professor John S. Duncan and the National Society for Epilepsy MRI Unit.

From Duncan (1997)[47] with the permission of the author and the Editor of *Brain*.

well as axial slices should be obtained in all cases. Gadolinium contrast enhancement is not necessary in routine cases but may be helpful in selected cases if the non-contrast-enhanced MRI scan is not definitive. In the first 2 years of life, myelination is incomplete, resulting in a poor contrast between white and grey matter and thus in difficulties in detecting cortical abnormalities. In contrast, white matter disorders are better recognised because the normal signal of myelin (which varies according to age) and the topography of the brain are well known. In such young patients, MRI scans may not reveal lesions and scans may have to be repeated again after 1–2 years.[31]

Other sequences such as FLAIR (fluid-attenuated inversion recovery) may have a role in selected cases (e.g. if standard imaging is normal, or to clarify the significance of a possible focal abnormality).

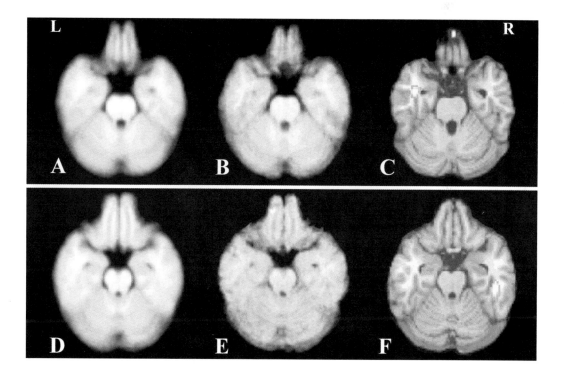

Figure 1.9

Axial images. Magnetisation transfer ratio (MTR) maps for 30 control subjects (A and D) and patients with normal conventional MRI and left temporal lobe epilepsy (B) and right temporal lobe epilepsy (E). Statistical analysis showing areas of significantly reduced MTR in patient groups (C) and (F).

Figure courtesy of Professor John S. Duncan and the National Society for Epilepsy MRI Unit.

In addition to careful qualitative evaluation of the hippocampus, quantitative assessment can be useful. Hippocampal volumetry requires side-to-side ratios as well as absolute volumes corrected for intracranial volume, which must be compared with appropriate controls from the same laboratory. T2 relaxometry also quantifies hippocampal abnormalities and may show evidence of bilateral disease.[31]

X-ray CT scanning can detect certain structural lesions, but will miss many small mass lesions including tumours and vascular malformations and most instances of hippocampal sclerosis and developmental cortical malformations.[31] A negative CT scan conveys little information. For this reason, CT should not be relied on and usually does not need to be performed when MRI is available. Occasionally, CT may be useful as a complementary imaging technique in the detection of cortical calcifications, particularly in patients with congenital or acquired infections (e.g. cysticercosis).[31]

Also, in the acute situation of seizures developing in the context of a neurological insult such as head injury, intracranial haemorrhage or encephalitis, radiographic CT scan is an appropriate initial investigation if MRI is not readily available or cannot be performed for technical reasons (e.g. a patient who has a cardiac pacemaker or who is dependent on a respirator) or if there is a need to have ready access to the patient during scanning.[31]

Conventional isotope brain scans do not provide sufficient information about brain structure to identify many lesions associated with seizures, and their use is not recommended.[31]

The functional imaging modalities **single photon emission computed tomography (SPECT)** and **positron emission tomography (PET)** are also inadequate for assessment of brain structure.[31]

THE NON-ACUTE SITUATION

Ideal practice

In the non-acute situation, the ideal practice is to obtain structural neuroimaging with MRI in all patients with epilepsy, except in patients with a definite electroclinical diagnosis of idiopathic generalised epilepsy or benign focal epilepsy of childhood.[31]

MRI is particularly indicated in patients with one or more of the following:

- Onset of seizures at any age with evidence of focal onset on history or EEG
- Onset of unclassified or apparently generalised seizures in the first year of life or in adulthood
- Evidence of a focal fixed deficit on neurological or neuropsychological examination
- Difficulty in obtaining control of seizures with first-line antiepileptic drug treatment
- Loss of control of seizures with antiepileptic drugs or a change in the seizure pattern that may imply a progressive underlying lesion.

Minimum standards

Appropriate minimum standards vary between different countries and societies, according to economic and geographical factors and the system for providing health care.[31]

- Radiographic CT scanning is an alternative procedure if MRI is not available or cannot be performed for technical reasons. Radiographic CT scans will usually identify large structural abnormalities but may often miss hippocampal sclerosis, small lesions, and developmental brain abnormalities, particularly in the temporal lobe.

- The following are regarded as essential indications for the performance of MRI scans:

  Partial or secondarily generalized seizures, and apparently generalized seizures, that do not remit with antiepileptic drug treatment.

  Development of progressive neurological or neuropsychological deficits.

FUNCTIONAL NEUROIMAGING IN CLINICAL PRACTICE [33]

The Neuroimaging Subcommission of the ILAE has recently re-assessed the roles of the traditional functional imaging techniques of positron emission tomography (PET) and single photon emission computed tomography (SPECT) in clinical practice and research.[33] The place of these methods, and of the emerging MR-based functional imaging methods of functional magnetic resonance imaging (fMRI) and magnetic resonance spectroscopy (MRS), also needed to be considered in the light of the advances in structural imaging with MRI.

The Neuroimaging Subcommission of the ILAE[33] considered fMRI, MRS, SPECT and PET in turn, according to the following format:

1. Indications in clinical practice and research potential.
2. Relation to structural imaging.
3. Minimum and optimal standards if the investigation is to be carried out, with regard to equipment, clinical protocol and logistics, and reporting and interpretation.
4. Misuse and pitfalls.

The conclusions regarding clinical applications of functional neuroimagings are:[33]

- *Functional MRI:* There is no currently approved or universally accepted clinical indication for functional MRI.[33]

- *Magnetic resonance spectroscopy (MRS):* MRS has been evaluated primarily in temporal lobe epilepsy. Proton MRS provides a useful lateralisation of metabolic dysfunction. Sensitivity is around 90%, but bilateral temporal abnormalities are common, and abnormalities may be reversible. MRS may be useful in patients who have otherwise normal MRI studies. Phosphate

(35P) MRS has moderate sensitivity for lateralisation based on abnormal elevations of inorganic phosphate. Abnormalities of pH have been controversial, and so cannot be considered to be reliable for lateralisation. MRS has been reported to be useful in extratemporal epilepsies, but the present limitation of spatial coverage limits clinical utility.[33]

- *Single photon emission computed tomography* (SPECT) with cerebral blood flow agents is useful to support the localisation of focal epilepsy when it is performed in a carefully monitored ictal (Figure 1.10) or early post-ictal examination compared with an interictal scan. This may be used as part of the presurgical evaluation, and may help to guide the placement of intracranial electrodes if other data including structural imaging are equivocal or non-concordant. In apparently generalised epilepsies, ictal SPECT may be helpful to identify a focal component.[33]

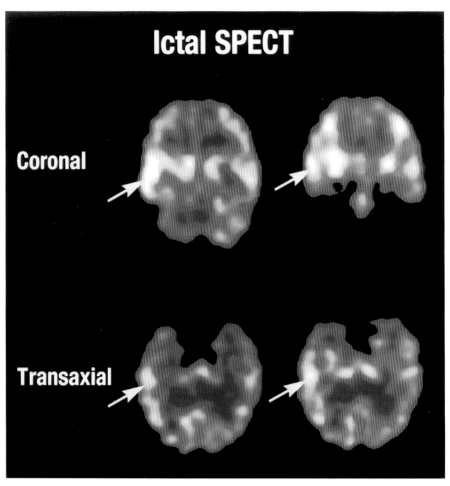

Figure 1.10 Coronal and axial 99Tc HMPAO SPECT images from a child with mesial temporal sclerosis showing an increase in perfusion in the anterior right temporal lobe as indicated by the arrows.

Figure courtesy of Dr Rod C. Scott, Institute of Child Health, London.

- *Positron emission tomography (PET) with 18F-fluorodeoxyglucose (FDG) and 150-water (H2150).* Interictal FDG–PET may have a role in determining the lateralisation of temporal lobe epilepsy, without intracranial EEG recording of seizures, in patients in whom there is not good concordance between MRI, EEG and other data. This role has decreased with the wider availability of high-quality MRI. In patients with normal or equivocal MRI, or discordance between MRI and other data, such that intracranial electrodes are required, FDG–PET may be useful for planning the sites of intracranial electrode placement for recording ictal onsets in temporal and extratemporal epilepsies. FDG–PET may have a useful role in apparently generalised epilepsies, to try to define a focal abnormality, and when resection may be contemplated. For practical purposes, the clinical and research uses of H2150 PET for mapping areas of cerebral activation have been superseded by fMRI.[33]

- *Positron emission tomography with specific ligands.* There are no proven indications for ligand PET in clinical epileptological practice. A role that is being evaluated is in the presurgical evaluation of patients with refractory partial seizures. In patients with mesial temporal lobe epilepsy and negative MRI, 11C-flumazenil PET may have some advantages over FDG, offering more precise localisation of the epileptogenic region, but it does not appear to be superior for lateralisation. In MRI-negative patients with neocortical seizures, the identification of focal abnormalities by 11C-flumazenil PET may be useful to guide the placement of intracranial EEG electrodes.[33]

- *Near infrared spectroscopy* is a recently developed technique for making regional measurements of cerebral blood flow. There is no proven clinical indication at present, but there is research potential for monitoring of spontaneous seizures.[33]

Chapter 1 is updated from Panayiotopoulos (1999)[25] with permission of the publisher John Libbey.

NEONATAL SEIZURES AND NEONATAL SYNDROMES

NEONATAL SEIZURES [61–75]

Neonatal seizures occur from birth to the end of the neonatal period (28 days) with 80% occurring in the first 1–2 days to the first week of life.

Demographic data: Prevalence is ~ 1.5% and overall incidence ~3 per 1000 live births. Incidence in pre-term infants is very high (57–132 per 1000 live births).

Clinical manifestations: Neonatal seizures are usually subtle and manifest with motor, behavioural and autonomic symptoms, alone or in combination.[61–76] The most widely used scheme is by Volpe[76] of five main types of neonatal seizures:

● Subtle seizures (50%)

● Tonic seizures (5%)

● Clonic seizures (25%)

● Myoclonic seizures (20%) and

● Non-paroxysmal repetitive behaviours.

GTCS are exceptional. However, it should be emphasised that nearly one quarter of infants experience several seizure types (Figure 2.1) and that the same seizure may manifest with subtle, clonic, myoclonic autonomic or other symptoms (Figure 2.1).

Subtle seizures are far more common than other types of neonatal seizures. They are described as ***subtle*** because the clinical manifestations are frequently overlooked. They imitate normal behaviours and reactions. These include tonic horizontal deviation of the eyes with or without jerking, eyelid blinking or fluttering, sucking, smacking, or other buccal-lingual oral movements, swimming or pedalling movements and apnoeic spells.

Tonic, clonic or myoclonic are the main motor seizure types. These may be regional, fragmented or generalised, focal or multifocal, alternating or migrating, symmetrical or asymmetrical. Facial, limb and axial muscles and the diaphragm are involved. Motor automatisms include stepping, bicycling, rowing, swimming and paddling movements. Autonomic manifestations of

---

Definition

The neonatal period is arbitrarily defined as the first 28 days of life of a full-term infant (40 weeks gestational age). In prematurely born infants the neonatal period starts at a conceptual age of 40 weeks. Conceptual is the combined gestational (duration of pregnancy) and chronological (actual legal age from the time of birth) age.

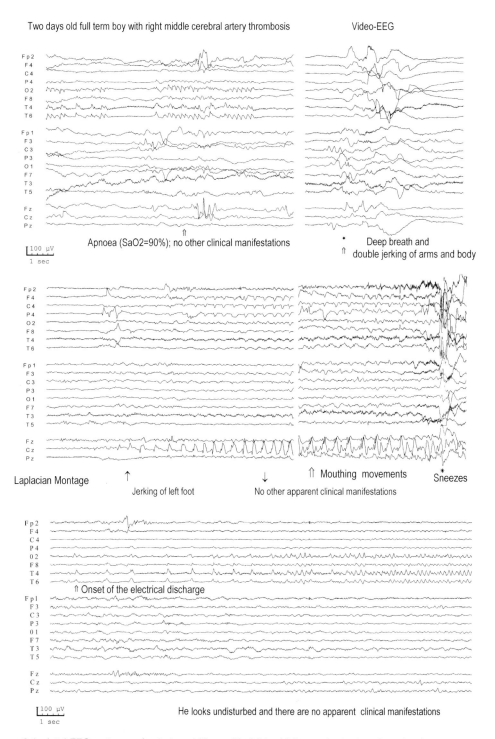

Figure 2.1 Ictal EEG patterns of a 2-day-old boy with right middle cerebral artery thrombosis.

Top and middle: Apnoeic, myoclonic, clonic and subtle seizure of motor automatisms associated with various ictal EEG patterns and locations.

Bottom: 'Electroclinical dissociation': the electrical discharge is not associated with apparent clinical manifestations.

heart rate, respiration, systemic blood pressure, salivation and pupillary changes are associated with motor manifestations in one third of cases.

There is no recognisable post-ictal state.

Neonatal seizures are usually brief (10 seconds to 1–2 minutes) but status epilepticus develops more readily at this age.

Aetiology: This is extensive and diverse (Table 2.1). Severe causes and mainly hypoxic–ischaemic encephalopathy predominate. Intracranial haemorrhage, cerebral infarction, infection and malformations of brain development are prominent. Acute metabolic disturbances such as electrolyte, glucose and calcium abnormalities are now rare.

Diagnostic procedures: Neonatal seizures represent one of the very few emergencies in the newborn. Confirmation of neonatal seizures should initiate appropriate clinical and laboratory evaluation for the aetiological cause (Table 2.1) and treatment. A thorough physical examination of the neonate should be coupled with urgent and comprehensive biochemical tests for correctable metabolic disturbances. More severe inborn errors of metabolism should be considered for diagnosis and possible treatment.

Cranial ultrasonography,[77] brain imaging with CT scan and preferably MRI[78,79] should be utilised for the detection of structural abnormalities such as malformations of brain development, intracranial haemorrhage, hydrocephalus and cerebral infarction.

Electroencephalography: Neonatal EEG is probably one of its best and most useful applications. However, neonatal EEG recordings and interpretations

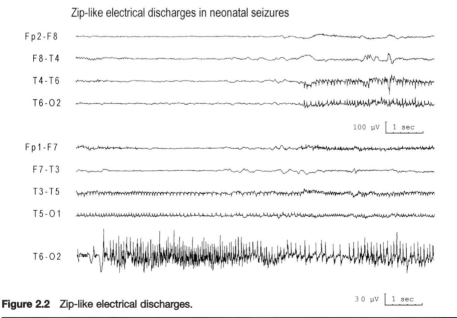

Zip-like electrical discharges in neonatal seizures

Figure 2.2 Zip-like electrical discharges.

Electrical discharges of a neonate with severe brain hypoxia.

Zip-like electrical discharges indicate a poor prognosis.

require the special skills of well-trained technologists and physicians. Polygraphic studies with simultaneous video-EEG recording are essential. Interictal EEG 'epileptogenic' spikes or sharp slow wave foci are not reliable markers in this age group. Certain interictal and background EEG patterns may have diagnostic and prognostic significance (Figures 2.2 and 2.3).[64,71]

Table 2.1 Main causes of neonatal seizures   *Frequency*

Hypoxia-ischaemia   +++++++
  prenatal (toxaemia, fetal distress, abruptio placentae, cord compression)
  perinatal (iatrogenic, maternal haemorrhage, fetal distress)
  postnatal (cardio-respiratory causes such as hyaline membrane disease, congenital heart disease, pulmonary hypertension)

Haemorrhage and intracerebral infarction   ++++
  intraventricular and periventricular (mainly preterm neonates)
  intracerebral (spontaneous, traumatic)
  subarachnoid
  subdural haematoma
  cerebral artery and vein infarction

Trauma   ++++
  intracranial haemorrhage
  cortical vein thrombosis

Infections   ++++
  encephalitis, meningitis, brain abscess
  intrauterine (rubella, toxoplasmosis, syphilis, viral – such as cytomegalovirus, herpes simplex, human immunodeficiency virus, coxsackie virus B)
  postnatal (beta-haemolytic streptococci, *Escherichia coli* infection, herpes simplex, mycoplasma)

Metabolic   ++
  hypoglycaemia (glucose levels <20 mg/d in preterm, <30 mg/d in full-term babies as indicating hypoglycaemia; mainly associated with prenatal or perinatal insults)
  neonates of diabetic and toxaemic mothers
  pancreatic disease
  glucogen storage disease (idiopathic)
  hypocalcaemia (early, at first 2–3 days, mainly in preterm neonates with prenatal or perinatal insults; late, at 5–14 days, is mainly nutritional; maternal hyperparathyroidism; DiGeorge's syndrome)
  hypomagnesaemia (may accompany or occur independently of hypocalcaemia)
  hyponatraemia (mainly associated with prenatal or perinatal insults; inappropriate secretion of antidiuretic hormone)
  hypernatraemia (mainly nutritional or iatrogenic)
  inborn errors of metabolism (amino acid and organic acid disorders, hyperammonaemias; they usually manifest with peculiar odours, protein intolerance, acidosis, alkalosis, lethargy, or stupor)
  pyridoxine dependency

Malformation of cerebral development   ++
  all disorders of neuronal induction, segmentation, migration, myelination and synaptogenesis such as polymicrogyria, neuronal heterotopias, lissencephaly, holoprosencephaly, and hydranencephaly

Neurocutaneous syndromes   ++++
  (tuberous sclerosis, incontinentia pigmenti)

Drug withdrawal and toxic   +++
  (withdrawal from narcotic-analgesics, sedative-hypnotics, and alcohol; heroin- and methadone-addicted mothers; barbiturates)

Inadvertent injections of local anaesthetics during delivery   ++
Idiopathic benign neonatal seizures (familial and non-familial)   ++

Ictal EEG is often mandatory in view of the subtle clinical ictal manifestations (Figure 2.1). EEG ictal activity at various frequencies may be focal or multifocal appearing in a normal or abnormal background. The EEG ictal activity depends on the type of clinical seizures. Clonic, tonic and subtle seizures are usually associated with focal EEG ictal discharges while myoclonic jerks and spasms usually have generalised ictal EEG accompaniments. The same EEG may show focal or multifocal ictal discharges that may occur simultaneously or independently in different brain locations.

Electroclinical dissociation or decoupling is a common phenomenon in neonates: EEG electrical seizure activity occurs without apparent clinical manifestations. This is more common after initiation of antiepileptic drugs that may suppress the clinical manifestations of seizures but not the EEG ictal discharge.

Prognosis: This is cause-dependent. Despite high mortality (~15%) and morbidity (~30%), half of neonates with seizures achieve a normal or near normal state. One third of the survivors develop epilepsy.

Differential diagnosis: Neonatal seizures may impose significant difficulties in their recognition and differentiation from normal or abnormal behaviours of the pre-term and full-term neonate.[64,71] As a rule any suspicious repetitive and stereotypical events should be considered as possible seizures.

Amongst normal behaviours neonates may stretch, exhibit spontaneous sucking movements, and have random and non-specific movements of the limbs. Intense physiological myoclonus may occur during REM sleep. Jitteriness or tremulousness of the extremities or facial muscles is frequent in

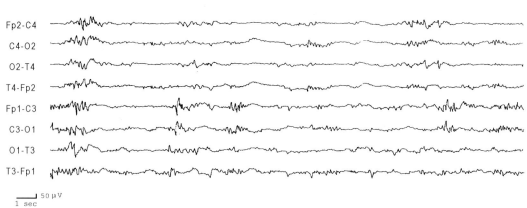

Theta pointu alternant pattern in a baby with benign neonatal (non-familiar) seizures

Figure 2.3   Interictal EEG in a neonate with benign neonatal (non-familial) seizures. Theta pointu alternant pattern is usually associated with good prognosis.

From Plouin (1992)[93] with permission of the author and publisher John Libbey.

normal or abnormal neonates. Tremor has a symmetrical 'to and fro' motion, is faster than clonic seizures, mainly affects all four limbs and will stop when the limb is restrained or by repositioning of the extremity. Conversely, clonic seizures usually have a rate of 3–4 Hz or slower, decelerate in the progress of the attack and are mainly focal.

Among abnormal behaviours of neonates with CNS disorders are episodic and repetitive oro-buccal-lingual movements. These are often reproducible with tactile or other stimuli and interrupted by restraint. Conversely, neonatal seizures persist despite restraint and they are rarely stimulus-sensitive.

Neonatal seizures should be differentiated from benign neonatal sleep myoclonus, hyperekplexia and other non-epileptic conditions (see Appendix 1; pages 47-49).

Significant impairment of vital signs, that may be periodic, is mainly due to non-neurological causes. Changes in respiration, heart rate and blood pressure are exceptional sole manifestations of neonatal seizures.

Management: This demands accurate aetiological diagnosis and treatment of their cause if applicable. Metabolic disturbances are treatable and reversible but most others are not. A trial of pyridoxine is needed if pyridoxine dependency is suspected.

Drug treatment of neonatal seizures is empirical with significant variations among physicians. Phenobarbital first and then phenytoin are the most commonly used, although diazepines are gaining ground. Loading large doses are followed by a maintenance scheme for a variable time. Newer generation antiepileptic drugs such as lamotrigine may be useful.[80] Maintenance treatment may not be needed or may be brief as the active seizure period in neonates is usually short. Less than 15% of infants with neonatal seizures will have recurrent seizures after the newborn period.[81.] A normal EEG[82] and other predictors of good outcome[83] may encourage early discontinuation of treatment.

EPILEPTIC SYNDROMES IN NEONATES

The new diagnostic scheme[10] recognises the following epileptic syndromes in neonates (Tables 1.3 and 1.4):

I. CONDITIONS WITH EPILEPTIC SEIZURES THAT DO NOT REQUIRE A DIAGNOSIS OF EPILEPSY
   Benign familial neonatal seizures
   Benign neonatal seizures (non-familial)

II. EPILEPTIC ENCEPHALOPATHIES (IN WHICH THE EPILEPTIFORM ABNORMALITIES MAY CONTRIBUTE TO PROGRESSIVE DYSFUNCTION)
   Early myoclonic encephalopathy
   Ohtahara syndrome

BENIGN FAMILIAL NEONATAL SEIZURES[84–86]

Benign familial neonatal seizures constitute a rare dominantly inherited syndrome characterised by frequent brief seizures within the first days of life.

Demographic data: Onset is commonly in the first week of life, but in one third this may be in the first 1–2 months. Boys and girls are equally affected. The syndrome appears to be rare but this may be under-recognised or not reported by the families who know the benign character of this syndrome by their own experience. There are reports of 44 families with 355 affected members.[84]

Clinical manifestations: Seizures mainly occur on the second or third day of life in full-term normal neonates after a normal pregnancy and delivery and without precipitating factors. Seizures are brief (1–2 minutes) and may be as frequent as 20–30 per day.

Most seizures start with tonic motor activity and posturing with apnoea followed by vocalisations, ocular symptoms, other autonomic features, motor automatisms, chewing and focal or generalised clonic movements. The clonic components of the later phase are usually asymmetrical and unilateral. Focal and clonic seizures are described but are considered rare.

Aetiology: The disease is caused by mutations in one of two recently identified voltage-gated potassium channel genes, KCNQ2 on chromosome 20q (EBN1) or KCNQ3 (EBN2) on chromosome 8q.[73,87–91]

Diagnostic procedures: All relevant biochemical, haematological, metabolic screening and brain imaging tests are normal.

Electroencephalography: Interictal EEG may be normal or mildly/moderately abnormal with focal and multifocal abnormalities. Ictal EEG starts with a brief flattening followed by asymmetrical spike and waves of 1–2 minutes duration.[85]

Differential diagnosis: A family history of similar convulsions, a prerequisite for the diagnosis of benign familial neonatal seizures, eliminates the possibility of other diseases. However, other causes of neonatal seizures should be excluded.

Prognosis: Seizures remit between 1 and 6 months from onset, and in 68% during the first 6 weeks. Psychomotor development is normal but 10–14% may later develop other types of febrile or afebrile seizures.

Management: There is no consensus regarding treatment as convulsions usually remit spontaneously without medications. The use of antiepileptic medication does not influence the eventual outcome.

BENIGN NEONATAL SEIZURES (NON-FAMILIAL) [84,86,92,93]

Benign neonatal seizures (non-familial) constitute a short-lived and self-limited benign syndrome.

Demographic data: Age at onset is characteristically between the first and seventh day of life. It occurs most frequently (90%) between the fourth and sixth day – for which the synonym 'fifth day fits' was coined.[92] Boys (62%) are slightly more affected than girls. Prevalence is 7% of neonatal seizures.[84,93]

Clinical manifestations: There is a one-off repetitive seizure–clonic status epilepticus event that occurs in otherwise normal full-term neonates. This consists of successive clonic convulsions that are usually unilateral affecting face and limbs, may change side and may also less often be bilateral. Apnoea is a common concomitant in one third of these clonic fits. Each seizure lasts for 1–3 minutes, repeating at frequent intervals and cumulating to discontinuous or continuous clonic status epilepticus. The whole seizure-status event lasts for between 2 hours and 3 days with a median of about 20 hours. It does not recur. Tonic seizures are incompatible with this syndrome.

Aetiology: This is unknown but probably environmental.

Diagnostic procedures: By definition all other than EEG relevant tests for causative factors of neonatal seizures are normal. There are reports of acute zinc deficiency and rotavirus infection.

Electroencephalography: The interictal EEG often shows a 'theta pointu alternant pattern' although this is not specific (Figure 2.3). This pattern consists of runs of a dominant theta wave activity intermixed with sharp waves often of alternating side. It is not reactive to various stimuli. It may occur on awake and sleep. It may persist for 12 days after the cessation of convulsions. It is not specific, as it may be recorded in other conditions such as hypocalcaemia, meningitis, subarachnoid haemorrhage and benign familial neonatal seizures.

The ictal EEG consists of rhythmic spikes or slow waves mainly in the Rolandic regions although they can also localise anywhere else. The EEG ictal paroxysms may be unilateral, generalised, or first localised and then generalised.

Differential diagnosis: The diagnosis can be made only after other causes of neonatal seizures have been excluded. Aetiologies of neonatal seizures with favourable outcome include late hypocalcaemia, subarachnoid haemorrhage and certain meningitides.[84,93] There are significant differences between benign neonatal seizures (non-familial) and benign familial neonatal seizures despite the artificially similar names[10] and the fact that they have a similar age at onset (Table 2.2).

Table 2.2 Benign (non-familial) neonatal seizures versus benign familial neonatal seizures

	Benign (non-familial) neonatal seizures	**Benign familial neonatal seizures**
Main seizures	Mostly clonic	Tonic-clonic
Onset	Fifth day of life	Second or third day of life
Duration of seizures	Status epilepticus (median 20 hours)	Repetitive isolated seizures
Main causes	Unknown, probably environmental	Autosomal dominant
Subsequent seizures	Practically nil (0.5%)	Relatively high (11%)
Ictal EEG	Usually localised spikes	Usually generalised flattening
Interictal EEG	Usually theta pointu alternant	Normal or focal abnormalities
Psychomotor deficits	Minor	Practically non-existent

Prognosis: The prognosis is excellent with normal development and no recurrence of seizures. Some minor psychomotor symptoms may occur.

Management: Convulsions usually remit spontaneously without medication. Prolonged seizures may be shortened or terminated with intravenous administration of diazepines or phenytoin.

EARLY MYOCLONIC ENCEPHALOPATHY [94–97]

Early myoclonic encephalopathy is a dreadful and rare disease of the first days and weeks of life.

Demographic data: Early myoclonic encephalopathy usually starts in the first days of life, sometimes immediately after birth; more than 60% start before 10 days of age and rarely after the second month. Boys and girls are equally affected. The prevalence and incidence of early myoclonic encephalopathy are not known. There are approximately 80 reported cases but this may be an underestimation as many newborn babies with such a severe disease and early death may escape clinico-EEG diagnosis.

Clinical manifestations: The syndrome manifests with a triad of intractable seizures with myoclonic jerks appearing first followed by simple focal seizures and later by tonic infantile spasms. Erratic or fragmentary myoclonus is the defining seizure type that sometimes may appear immediately after birth. Erratic myoclonus affects face or limbs, often restricted in a finger, a toe, eyebrows, eyelids or lips occurring in the same muscle group and often migrating elsewhere usually in an asynchronous and asymmetrical fashion. They are brief, single or repetitive, very frequent and nearly continuous. It is exceptional for a baby with early myoclonic encephalopathy to have mild and infrequent jerks.

Massive, usually bisynchronous axial myoclonic jerks may start from the onset of the disease or occur later, often interspersed with erratic myoclonias.

Simple focal seizures, often clinically inconspicuous, manifest with eye deviation or autonomic symptoms such as flushing of the face or apnoea.

Infantile tonic spasms develop usually within 2–4 months from onset of myoclonias and may be more frequent during alert than sleep stages.

Psychomotor development may be abnormal from onset of seizures or arrests and deteriorates rapidly afterwards. There may be marked truncal hypotonia, limb hypertonia, disconjugate eye movements, dyspnoea, opisthotonic or decerebrate posturing. All patients have bilateral pyramidal signs. Practically, there is no trace of mental activity.

Aetiology: Early myoclonic encephalopathy is a multifactorial disease with some reports suggesting an autosomal hereditary disorder because of affected siblings, inborn errors of metabolism such as non-ketotic hyperglycinaemia and lesional abnormalities of the brain.

Diagnostic procedures: These are the same as those for neonatal seizures, attempting to find an aetiological cause. Brain imaging may be normal or may show asymmetrical enlargement of one hemisphere, dilatation of the corresponding lateral ventricle, cortical and periventricular atrophy and more rarely malformations of cortical development.

Considering the relatively high rate of inborn errors of metabolism and mainly non-ketotic hyperglycinaemia, a thorough metabolic screening is mandatory. This should include serum levels of amino acids – especially glycine and glycerol metabolites, organic acids and amino acids in the cerebrospinal fluid.

Electroencephalography: The interictal EEG of early myoclonic encephalopathy is a repetitive suppression-burst pattern without physiological rhythms (Figure 2.4). Bursts of high amplitude spikes, sharp and slow waves last for 1–5 seconds followed by periods of flat EEG lasting 3–10 seconds.

Erratic myoclonias usually do not have an ictal EEG expression and may follow the bursts.

The suppression-burst pattern transforms to atypical hypsarrhythmia or multifocal spikes and sharp waves 3–4 months from onset of the disease.

Prognosis: Early myoclonic encephalopathy is one of the most dreadful diseases. More than half the patients die weeks or months from onset and the others develop permanent severe mental and neurological deficits.

Management: There is no effective treatment. Adrenocorticotropic hormone therapy and antiepileptic medication (clonazepam, nitrazepam, valproate, phenobarbitone and others) are of no benefit. The effect of vigabatrin and other newer drugs is not known.

Patients with non-ketotic hyperglycinaemia may benefit from a reduction of dietary protein and administration of sodium benzoate 120 mg/kg daily.

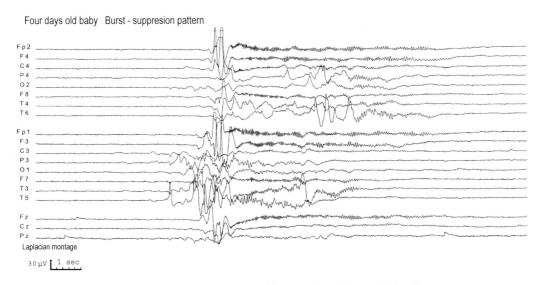

Figure 2.4 Burst suppression pattern in a neonate with severe hypoxic encephalopathy.

Diagnostic Tips

● Segmental and erratic myoclonias affecting face and limbs, usually restricted in a finger, eyebrows, perioral muscles, that are nearly continuous and often shifting from place to place.

● EEG burst-suppression pattern.

OHTAHARA SYNDROME [98,99]

Ohtahara syndrome is a rare and devastating form of severe epileptic encephalopathy of very early life.

Demographic data: Onset is mainly around the first days of life, sometimes intra-uterinely or up to 3 months of age. There may be a slight male predominance. The prevalence and incidence of Ohtahara syndrome are not known. There are approximately 100 cases reported but this may be an underestimation as many newborn babies with such a severe disease and early death may escape clinico-EEG diagnosis. According to one report 'attacks of cerebral spasms occur in 1.5 to 5 per thousand new-born post partum'.[100]

Clinical manifestations: The syndrome manifests clinico-EEG features of mainly tonic spasms and suppression-burst EEG patterns that consistently occur in sleep and awake states.

Tonic seizures usually consist of a forwards tonic flexion lasting 1–10 seconds that are singular or in long clusters, 10–300 times every 24 hours. They may be generalised and symmetrical or lateralised. Less often, one third of the neonates may have erratic focal motor clonic seizures or hemiconvulsions. Alternating hemiconvulsions or generalised tonic-clonic seizures are exceptional.

Diagnostic procedures: These are the same as those for neonatal seizures, attempting to detect an aetiological cause and possible treatment. Metabolic screening and brain imaging are mandatory. Brain imaging usually shows severe abnormalities and malformations of brain development.

Electroencephalography: The EEG suppression-burst pattern comprises bursts of high amplitude abnormal EEG rhythms alternating with almost flat EEG that has a pseudo-rhythmic periodicity. The suppression period lasts for 3–5 seconds. The burst to burst ranges from 5 to 10 seconds. This pattern occurs during both awake and sleep states.

Ictal EEG of tonic spasms is characterised by:

● Diffuse desynchronisation with disappearance of suppression-bursts when tonic spasms cluster in 5–10 second intervals.

● A pattern in which the suppression-burst becomes more frequent, more diffuse and of higher amplitude compared with the interictal pattern.

Aetiology: Symptomatic or possibly symptomatic. The most common cause is malformations of cerebral development but other lesional brain disorders may also be responsible.

Pathophysiology: Ohtahara syndrome is likely to be the earliest age-related specific epileptic reaction of the developing brain to heterogeneous insults, similar to those of West and Lennox-Gastaut syndrome which occur at a later brain maturity age.

Differential diagnosis: The main differential diagnosis of Ohtahara syndrome is from early myoclonic encephalopathy[101] but this may not be of any practical significance.

Prognosis: This is a devastating syndrome associated with high mortality and morbidity. Half the patients die weeks or months from onset and the others soon develop permanent severe mental and neurological deficit. Psychomotor development relentlessly deteriorates. The babies become inactive with spastic diplegia, hemiplegia, tetraplegia, ataxia, or dystonia. If not arrested by death, clinical and EEG patterns change to those of West syndrome within a few months from onset and may also change to Lennox-Gastaut features if patients survive to reach 2–3 years of age.

Management: There is no effective treatment. Adrenocorticotropic hormone therapy and antiepileptic medication of any type are of no benefit. Vigabatrin was recently reported as having a beneficial effect but this is usually short-lived. Neurosurgery in focal cerebral dysplasia is sometimes therapeutic.[102]

APPENDIX 1: NON-EPILEPTIC MOVEMENT DISORDERS IMITATING SEIZURES IN NEONATES AND INFANTS

BENIGN NEONATAL SLEEP MYOCLONUS [103–106]

Benign neonatal sleep myoclonus is a non-epileptic condition of unknown aetiology that occurs only during non-active sleep in otherwise normal neonates. It is entirely benign and remits spontaneously by the age of 2–7 months.

Onset is from the first day to 3 weeks of life with a peak at the seventh day. Boys and girls are equally affected.

The myoclonus mainly affects the distal parts of the upper extremities but may also less often involve the lower limbs and axial muscles. The myoclonic

Table 2.3 Early myoclonic encephalopathy versus Ohtahara syndrome

	Ohtahara syndrome	**Early myoclonic encephalopathy**
Main seizures	Tonic spasms	Erratic myoclonias, focal seizures, clusters of spasms
Main causes	Malformations of cerebral development	Genetic and metabolic
Suppression-burst	Sleep and awake	Probably accentuated by sleep
	Shorter lifespan	Longer lifespan
Paroxysmal bursts	Longer	Shorter
Suppression	Shorter	Longer
Transformation to West syndrome	As a rule	Common but transient

jerks, synchronous or asynchronous, unilateral or bilateral, mild or violent, usually last for 10–20 seconds. Occasionally they may occur in repetitive clusters of 2–3 seconds for 30 minutes or longer, imitating myoclonic status epilepticus or a series of epileptic fits. They may get worse with gentle restraint. Sleep is not disturbed, treatment is not needed and antiepileptic drugs may make it worse.

There are no other clinical manifestations like those accompanying neonatal seizures such as apnoea, autonomic disturbances, automatisms, eye deviation, oral movement or crying.

Neurological and mental state and development are normal.

All relevant laboratory studies including sleep and awake EEG during myoclonus are normal.

There is no beneficial treatment. Anticonvulsants are contraindicated.

Benign neonatal sleep myoclonus is a common non-epileptic condition that can be misdiagnosed as epileptic and even as infantile spasms.

BENIGN NON-EPILEPTIC MYOCLONUS OF EARLY INFANCY [107–110]

Benign non-epileptic myoclonus of early infancy is probably the same disease as 'shuddering attacks'.[111]

Benign non-epileptic myoclonus of early infancy, described by Fejerman and Lombroso,[107] is a paroxysmal, non-epileptic, movement disorder of otherwise healthy infants who have normal EEG and development.

Onset is from around 4–12 months of age and both sexes are probably equally affected.

The attacks are sudden and brief symmetrical axial flexor spasms mainly of the trunk and often the head. Less frequently, there may be flexion, abduction or adduction of the elbows and knees, extension or elevation of the arms. They do not involve localised muscle groups, there are no focal or lateralising seizures. Clinically, the spasm lasts for 1–2 seconds.

The attacks are more likely to occur in clusters, sometimes recurring at frequent and brief intervals several times a day. The intensity of the spasms varies. They are usually mild and inconspicuous but may at times become severe and imitate infantile spasms. They occur in wake states and are also elicited by excitement, fear, anger, frustration or the need to move the bowels or to void.

Benign non-epileptic myoclonus of early infancy has a good prognosis with spontaneous remission in the first 5 years of life, usually by age 2–3. There is no convincing evidence of any beneficial treatment.

The main differential diagnosis of benign non-epileptic myoclonus of early infancy is from infantile spasms. The manifestations of the spasms in both disorders may be similar but a normal EEG is often re-assuring.

HYPEREKPLEXIA OR STARTLE DISEASE [112–117]

Hyperekplexia or startle disease[112–117] is a rare autosomal dominant or recessive neurological disorder mapped to chromosome 5q33-35 from mutations within a neurotransmitter gene.[116,117] Clinically it is characterised by pathological startle responses to unexpected stimulus and generalised stiffness. Clinical symptoms are usually apparent from birth. Clinical phenotypic expression varies from mild to very severe forms that may be fatal.[118]

The minor forms manifest with excessive startle responses only that are often mild and inconsistent. In infancy these are facilitated by febrile illness and in adults by emotional stress.

In the major forms startle responses appear like generalised myoclonus resulting in falls that may be traumatic. There is no impairment of consciousness but the patient remains temporarily stiff after the attack. Sleep episodic shaking of the limbs resembling generalised clonus or repetitive myoclonus is often prominent, lasting for minutes with no impairment of consciousness. The jerks are spontaneous arousal reactions.[119] Neurologically, there is generalised muscle hypertonia–stiffness (**stiff baby syndrome**) that usually improves after the age of 2 years. Gait is unstable, insecure and puppet-like. Tendon reflexes are exaggerated.

In neonates, during the first 24 hours of life, spontaneous apnoea and sluggish feeding efforts occur. After the first 24 hours, surviving infants exhibit the hyperekplexic startle response to nose tapping which is a useful diagnostic test. This startle response is characterised by sudden muscular rigidity, feeding-induced oropharyngeal incoordination, and poor air exchange often with apnoea, persisting with repetitive nose tapping. Untreated infants experience recurring apnoea until 1 year of age.

EEG of startle responses in hyperekplexia is normal.

There is a dramatic response to clonazepam (0.1–0.2 mg/kg/day).[120]

EPILEPTIC SYNDROMES IN INFANCY AND EARLY CHILDHOOD

3

The new diagnostic scheme[10] recognises the following epileptic syndromes starting mainly in the infantile (or very early childhood) period (Tables 1.2 and 1.3).

I. CONDITIONS WITH EPILEPTIC SEIZURES THAT DO NOT REQUIRE A DIAGNOSIS OF EPILEPSY

Febrile seizures
Benign familial infantile seizures*
Benign infantile seizures (non-familial)*

II. IDIOPATHIC EPILEPTIC SYNDROMES

Benign myoclonic epilepsy in infancy

III. EPILEPTIC ENCEPHALOPATHIES (IN WHICH THE EPILEPTIFORM ABNORMALITIES MAY CONTRIBUTE TO PROGRESSIVE DYSFUNCTION)

West syndrome
Dravet syndrome

IV. OTHER SEVERE EPILEPTIC SYNDROMES

Hemiconvulsion-hemiplegia syndrome
Migrating focal seizures of infancy**
Myoclonic status in non-progressive encephalopathies**

FEBRILE SEIZURES [121–133]

Febrile seizures are due to an age-related, predominantly genetic benign susceptibility to convulsive seizures precipitated by fever at a height of at least 38°C, without evidence of intracranial infection or other cause. Children who have suffered a previous afebrile seizure are excluded.

Demographic data: Age at onset is from 6 months to 5 years with a peak at 18–22 months. Boys (60%) are slightly more affected than girls. Prevalence is ~3% of children. Annual incidence rate is 460/100,000 in the age group 0–4 years. Certain ethnic groups have a higher prevalence of febrile seizures (e.g. 7% for Japanese).

---

*Although not specified by the ILAE Task Force, the syndromes of benign infantile seizures (familial and non-familial) are classified by name (seizures) in this group.

**Syndromes in development.

50

Clinical manifestations

> "One minute, he was a little boy with a cold and slight fever, lying on
> the sofa feeling miserable and the next his body was madly convulsing ...
>
> It was very scary"   (From an Internet description by a father)

Generalised tonic-clonic seizures are by far the commonest seizure type (80%).
Tonic (13%), atonic (3%), unilateral or with focal onset tonic-clonic seizures
(4%) may occur in the other one fifth. Ninety-two percent of seizures last for
3–6 minutes. In the others they may be prolonged and may develop into
febrile status epilepticus.

Post-ictal symptoms other than drowsiness are exceptional and should raise
the suspicion of another diagnosis. Todd's paralysis is exceptional (0.4%).

Repetitive seizures in the same febrile illness occur in 16%.

Two fifths (40%) of children will have recurrences, particularly if the first
febrile seizure occurred in the first year of life, during a short and low-grade
febrile illness and there is a family history of febrile seizures. Half of those with
a second febrile convulsion will suffer at least one additional recurrence.

Because of different prognostic implications, febrile seizures are categorised
into simple and complex febrile seizures.

Simple febrile seizures (70% of all) are generalised tonic-clonic
convulsions of <15 minutes duration, and without recurrence within the next
24 hours (or within the same febrile illness).

Complex febrile seizures (30% of all) may last >15 minutes (8%),[134] have
two or more recurrences within 24 hours (16%) or show focal or unilateral
features (6%). The same child may have one, two or all three of these complex
factors.

Aetiology: Genetic predisposition is important, as febrile seizures are often
familial. Children with siblings or parents with febrile seizures have a 4–5-fold
higher risk than the general population. Concordance rates in monozygotic
twins are as high as 70% and in dizygotic twins up to 20%. The mode of
inheritance is unknown. Several genetic models have been proposed including
autosomal dominant, autosomal recessive and polygenic or multifactorial.

Large autosomal dominant kindreds of febrile seizures made it possible to
identify at least four different gene loci[135–139] in chromosome 8q13-21,[135,140]
chromosome 19p13.3 and 19q13.1,[136,137] chromosome 2q23-24[139] and
chromosome 5q14-q15.[138]

Risk factors for a first febrile convulsion: The risk of a first febrile seizure is
about 30% if a child has two or more of the following independent risk factors:

- a first or second degree relative with febrile seizures,

- delayed neonatal discharge of greater than 28 days of age,

- parental report of slow development, and

- day-care attendance.

The risk for younger siblings of affected children is around 10–20% and this is
higher if a parent is also affected. Males are more susceptible than females.
High temperature may be a risk factor for febrile seizures.

The pathophysiology of febrile seizures is unknown. They are a specific response to fever irrespective of cause, although viral illnesses are commoner. A specific association between acute human herpesvirus-6 infection and febrile seizures has been postulated.

Diagnostic procedures: Febrile seizures do not need any investigations if the diagnosis is secure. EEG and brain imaging are unhelpful. However, it is important to distinguish 'febrile convulsions' from 'convulsions with fever' such as in meningitis, encephalitis, cerebral palsy with intercurrent infection, and metabolic or neurodegenerative disease. Lumbar puncture may be mandatory in children who have a convulsion with fever in their first year of life (although this is still debated).

Prognosis: Overall, children with febrile seizures have a six-fold excess (3%) of subsequent afebrile seizures and epilepsy than controls. The risk is 2% after a simple and 5–10% after a complex febrile seizure. Afebrile seizures usually start within 4 years.

Risk factors for later epilepsy are (1) abnormal neurological or developmental status before the first febrile seizure, (2) family history of afebrile seizures, and (3) complex febrile seizures. Simple febrile seizures without any of these risk factors (60%) have only a two-fold excess (0.9%) of unprovoked seizures than controls. The risk after complex febrile seizures increases from 6–8% when a single complex feature is present to 49% if all three elements are present.

The subsequent psychomotor development of children who were normal before the onset of febrile seizures is normal.

MANAGEMENT: [129,130,132,141]

Acute management of a child with a febrile seizure
Control of the seizure is paramount. Treatment of the fever and mainly of the underlying illness is also important. Long-lasting convulsions should be vigorously treated as for status epilepticus. Antipyretic treatment during febrile illnesses does not reduce the recurrence rate.

Prophylactic management
Simple febrile convulsions do not need prophylactic treatment
The consensus for simple febrile seizures is that anticonvulsant therapy is not needed. The risks are small and the potential side-effects of drugs appear to outweigh the benefits.

However, prophylactic treatment may be desired if a child has one or mainly a combination of (1) complex febrile seizures, (2) neurological abnormalities, (3) age less than 1 year, (4) frequent recurrences.

Prophylactic treatment may be continuous with daily medication of mainly phenobarbitone and less often sodium valproate (these may soon change with the introduction of new antiepileptic drugs). Intermittent treatment at the time of a febrile illness (mainly with rectal diazepam) is another alternative (again a debated issue). *Neither of these may be needed for the majority of children with febrile seizures that almost invariably do well.*

Parents of young children should have general information provided by the family doctor about fever and febrile convulsions. Parents who have watched their child during a fit need specific information in order to avoid long-term reactions.

Supportive family management includes education about febrile convulsions, specific instructions about antipyretic and anticonvulsive prophylaxis, and emergency procedures for possible subsequent seizures.

BENIGN INFANTILE SEIZURES (FAMILIAL AND NON-FAMILIAL)

WATANABE-VIGEVANO SYNDROME [142–151]

Benign infantile (familial and non-familial) seizures constitute a benign age and localisation related idiopathic syndrome of infancy. Infants are otherwise entirely normal.

Demographic data: Age at onset is from 3 months to 20 months with a peak at 5–6 months; the familial form mostly starts between 4 and 7 months. Boys and girls are equally affected in the non-familial form but more girls are reported in the familial cases. Only small numbers, around 100 of all types, have been reported so far but this may increase with improved awareness of the condition.

Clinical manifestations: Seizures are mainly diurnal and occur in clusters of 5–10 per day for 1–3 days and may recur after 1–3 months. They are focal seizures manifesting with motion arrest, decreased responsiveness, staring, eye and head deviation and mild clonic movements. Simple automatisms are common. They may or may not progress to generalised convulsions. Alternating from one to the other side is common. Duration is usually short (for half to 3 minutes) but may be longer (3–6 minutes) in the familial cases.

Diagnostic procedures: All relevant tests applied for infantile seizures are normal but these are needed particularly for the sporadic cases.

Considerations on classification

The new ILAE diagnostic scheme recognises two types of benign infantile focal seizures (familial and non-familial).[10]

Three types of benign infantile focal seizures have been described:

a. Benign infantile familial convulsions[144]
b. Benign infantile epilepsy with complex focal seizures[142,143]
c. Benign focal epilepsy with secondarily generalised seizures in infancy.[152]

These have more common than dividing features, as the main protagonists of their description, Watanabe and Vigevano, state in a joint review.[145] Thus, all these are idiopathic seizures, in otherwise normal infants and they

1. are focal with or without secondarily generalised convulsions
2. appear in clusters at the age of around 5–6 months
3. have an entirely benign course.

In the dividing line is the familial or sporadic occurrence. Age at onset may be after the first year of life in the sporadic forms while it is strictly limited to this age group in the familial forms.

Electroencephalography: Interictal EEG is normal. Ictal EEG demonstrates focal discharges that usually spread to neighbour areas or the whole brain (Figure 3.1).

Aetiology: The familial form is most likely autosomal dominant and has recently been linked to chromosome 19q in one study, but not in three other studies.[147] The sporadic cases may be identical to the familial ones, with reduced expressivity.[150]

Differential diagnosis: This may be difficult in the sporadic form which requires long follow-up before such a diagnosis can be established.[149]

Management: In the active seizure period, drug treatment is usually effective. Complete seizure control is achieved in nearly all cases. Recurrences after 1–2 months may occur in one third but these are also easily controlled by drug dose adjustments. Antiepileptic treatment is usually withdrawn after 1–3 years with no relapses.

Watanabe used mainly carbamazepine while Vigevano used sodium valproate or phenobarbitone.

BENIGN MYOCLONIC EPILEPSY IN INFANCY [145,153–158]

Benign myoclonic epilepsy in infancy is a rare early form of idiopathic generalised epilepsy. It may be genetically determined.

Demographic data: Onset is between 6 months and 2 years but in a few infants may start earlier (4 months) or later (2–4 years). Boys are twice as likely

Ictal EEG of a boy 8 weeks old with 3 right sided hemiconvulsions Later (aged 7) had Rolandic seizures and CSWS

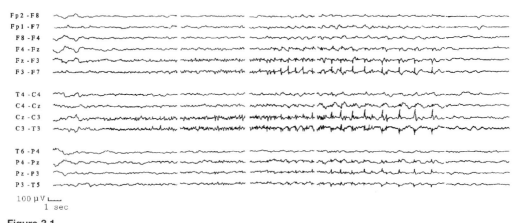

Figure 3.1

Ictal EEG discharge of an 8-week-old baby with three focal seizures of right-sided convulsions involving face and upper limbs. Subsequent EEGs were normal and treatment stopped at age 10 months. He was well until age 7 years when he started having Rolandic seizures and later developed ECSWS (see Figure 4.8; page 85). Brain MRI was normal. (This is case 17.2 in ref [25].)

From Panayiotopoulos (1999)[25] with the permission of the Publisher John Libbey.

to be affected as girls. Prevalence may be around 1–2% of epilepsies starting before the age of 3 years. This syndrome is based on retrospective studies and single case reports of around 80 patients, sometimes heterogeneous.

Girl aged 3 with a 6 weeks history of frequent massive jerks of head and shoulders

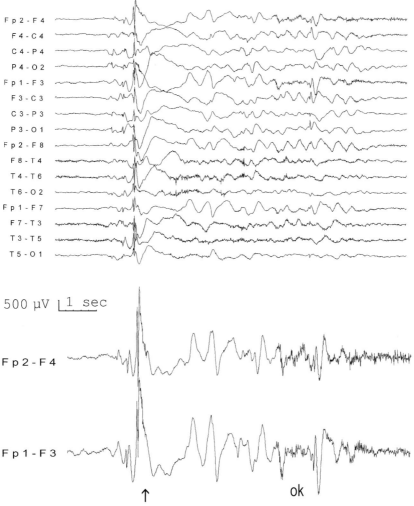

500 µV ⌊1 sec

150 µV ⌊1 sec   Massive jerk of head/shoulders backwards with vocalisation (grunt)

Figure 3.2

A video EEG sample of a 2-year-old girl with frequent myoclonic jerks of mainly head and shoulders with grunting noises. During this video-EEG recording (which was purposely extended to record clinical events), she had two electroclinical seizures. Clinically, the first symptom is a sudden jerk backwards associated with a giant (around 1 mv) spike or multiple spike and slow wave. This is followed by rhythmic slow activity at around 3–5 Hz together with some random spikes and slow waves. The whole discharges lasted for approximately 5–7 seconds. All seizures stopped with sodium valproate and clonazepam and she remained free of seizures with normal serial EEG until the last follow-up at age 5 years.

Clinical manifestations: Myoclonic seizures are the only type of fits allowed in benign myoclonic epilepsy in infancy, although one fifth of the patients may later develop infrequent GTCS.

Myoclonic jerks mainly of the head, eyeballs, upper extremities and the diaphragm are the only type of seizures (Figure 3.2); they rarely affect the lower limbs, causing occasional falls. They clinically manifest with head nodding and more rarely flexion or extension of the body. Upper limbs usually fling upwards and outwards. Eyeballs may roll upwards. A brief yell, probably a result of contraction of the diaphragm, sometimes accompanies other jerks. Consciousness is intact but a cluster of jerks may be associated with mild clouding.

Jerks are brief, singular or clusters that vary in frequency and violence. Myoclonic seizures are usually spontaneous, occurring randomly in alert stages and exaggerated by drowsiness and slow sleep. In some patients, they tend to cluster on awakening or during the first hours of sleep.

One fifth of patients have clinical and EEG photosensitivity. In 10% the myoclonic jerks are predominantly or exclusively elicited by unexpected acoustic or tactile stimuli and these may have a better prognosis.

Aetiology: Benign myoclonic epilepsy in infancy is probably the earliest form of idiopathic generalised epilepsy. There is no evidence that it is linked with any other syndromes of idiopathic generalised epilepsy.

Ten percent of the children may have infrequent simple febrile convulsions and 30% have a family history of epilepsies or febrile convulsions.

Diagnostic procedures: All tests, other than EEG, are normal.

Electroencephalography: Interictal EEG is normal. If myoclonic jerks occur, these are associated with generalised polyspike or spike and slow wave discharges (Figure 3.2). Sleep EEG exaggerates the discharges that occur with or without jerks. EEG generalised discharges of mainly multiple spikes frequently with jerks are often elicited by photic stimulation and in others by unexpected acoustic or tactile stimuli on awake or sleep stage.

Differential diagnosis: Benign myoclonic epilepsy in infancy should first be differentiated from non-epileptic conditions such as hypnagogic jerks and benign non-epileptic myoclonus. Hypnagogic jerks do not occur in awake states and EEG is normal. Benign non-epileptic myoclonus resembles epileptic (infantile) spasms rather than the jerks of benign myoclonic epilepsy in infancy.

It should not be difficult to differentiate benign myoclonic epilepsy in infancy from West syndrome where the epileptic spasms are the main seizure type, which are incompatible with benign myoclonic epilepsy in infancy. Furthermore, interictal hypsarrhythmic EEG and ictal EEG of mainly flattening are also entirely different.

Diagnostic Tips

● Myoclonic jerks of head and upper limbs in alert normal infants that are more pronounced during drowsiness and early stages of sleep. No other type of seizures.

● Myoclonic jerks provoked by unexpected acoustic and tactile stimuli in normal infants.

● Normal awake EEG if jerks do not occur during the recording.

Dravet syndrome of severe myoclonic epilepsy in infancy may be difficult to exclude in the initial stages, although myoclonic jerks start later and they are by rule preceded by severe and recurrent febrile clonic seizures.

Prognosis: Remission usually occurs between 6 months and 5 years from onset; 10–20% of children later develop infrequent GTCS in their early teens. Psychomotor development is often normal but 10–20% of children, if untreated, may later develop usually mild cognitive, behavioural or motor deficits.

Management: Response to treatment with sodium valproate is usually excellent. Patients with photosensitivity are more difficult to control and EEG photosensitivity may persist several years after remission of seizures. Gradual and slow withdrawal of drug treatment over 6 months to a year can be initiated 3–5 years from onset. Patients with acoustic and somatosensory evoked myoclonus may not need treatment or drug withdrawal may be initiated after a year.

WEST SYNDROME

INFANTILE SPASMS [159–179]

West syndrome is an age-related specific epileptic encephalopathy with multiple and diverse causes. It is characterised by a unique type of seizures, epileptic (infantile) spasms (Figure 3.3) and gross EEG abnormalities of hypsarrhythmia (Figure 3.4). Frequently, psychomotor impairment precedes but usually follows the onset of infantile spasms.

Demographic data: Onset is between 4 and 6 months of life, rarely before 3 or after 12 months. Boys are probably more affected than girls. Incidence is 3–5/10,000 live births.

Definition of seizures

ATONIC: Sudden loss or diminution of muscle tone without apparent preceding myoclonic or tonic event lasting ~1–2 seconds, involving head, trunk, jaw, or limb musculature.[11]

ASTATIC (synonym = drop attack): Loss of erect posture that results from an atonic, myoclonic, or tonic mechanism.[11,180]

MYOCLONIC (adjective); MYOCLONUS (noun): Sudden, brief (<100 ms) involuntary single or multiple contraction(s) of muscle(s) or muscle groups of variable topography (axial, proximal limb, distal).[11,181]

NEGATIVE MYOCLONIC: Interruption of tonic muscular activity for <500 ms without evidence of preceding myoclonia.[11,182,183]

MYOCLONIC-ATONIC SEIZURES: Are characterised by myoclonic-atonic sequence. Symmetrical myoclonic jerks of the arms or irregular twitching of the face precede the more or less pronounced loss of tone.[180]

CLONIC (synonym = rhythmic myoclonus): Myoclonus that is regularly repetitive, involves the same muscle groups, at a frequency of ~2–3 Hz, and is prolonged.[11]

TONIC: Sustained increase in muscle contraction lasting a few seconds to minutes.[11,184]

EPILEPTIC SPASM (formerly infantile spasm): A sudden flexion, extension or mixed extension-flexion of predominantly proximal and truncal muscles that is usually more sustained than a myoclonic movement but not so sustained as a tonic seizure (i.e. ~1 s). Limited forms may occur: grimacing, head nodding. Epileptic spasms frequently occur in clusters.[11,185]

Clinical manifestations: Epileptic (infantile) spasms are the defining clinical manifestation of West syndrome. The infant often has signs of psychomotor impairment but may also be normal before the onset of infantile spasms.

Epileptic spasms are sudden, brief, bilateral tonic contractions of the axial and limb muscles that may be symmetrical or asymmetrical. Spasms may be flexor, more often flexor–extensor and less frequently extensor. They may

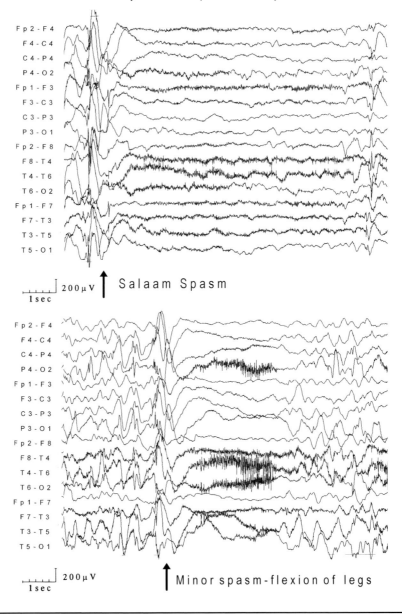

Figure 3.3

From video-EEG of a 7-month-old baby with epileptic spasms and Down syndrome.

There were numerous major (*top*) or minor (*bottom*) epileptic spasms.

involve widespread muscle groups or be segmental. Force is usually violent but may also be mild or intermediate. Spasms often come in clusters of 1–30 per day, each cluster having 20–100 attacks each. They predominantly occur on arousal and alert states, less often during slow sleep (3%) and exceptionally during REM sleep.

Flexor spasms are more typical and well expressed by the eponyms 'salaam spasms', 'jack-knife spasms', 'spasmes en flexion', 'Grusse krampfe' and 'Blitz, nick and salaamkrampfe' (lightning, nodding and salaam spasms). There is abrupt flexion of the neck and the trunk, arms raise forwards or sideways sometimes with flexion at the elbows, legs elevated with flexion at the hips and knees. This sudden, myoclonic-like contraction, lasts for 0.5–2 seconds followed by a tonic-like phase for up to 10 seconds. The spasm is slower than myoclonic jerks and faster than tonic seizures. A cry may follow the end of the attack.

> 'these *bobbings* ... they come on whether sitting or lying; just before they come on he is all alive and in motion ... and then all of a sudden down goes his head and upwards his knees; he then appears frightened and screams out'　　　　　　　　　　　　　　　　　　　(WJ West, 1841)[179a]

Each infant has more than one type of spasm, which may also be influenced by body positions.

Asymmetrical, lateralised or unilateral spasms are highly correlated with contralateral cerebral lesions of symptomatic West syndrome. Infantile spasms may also be combined with focal seizures in symptomatic cases.

Developmental delay, mild or severe, pre-dates onset of spasms in around two thirds of the cases.

Hypsarrhythmia - Infantile spasms

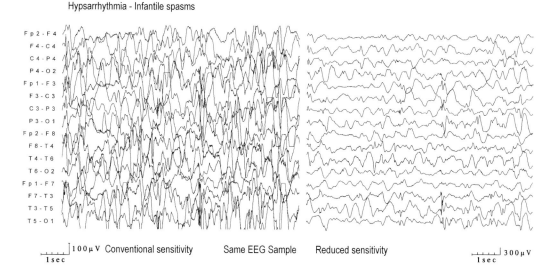

100 μV Conventional sensitivity   Same EEG Sample   Reduced sensitivity   300 μV
1 sec   1 sec

Figure 3.4 Typical hypsarrhythmic pattern seen at routine (left) and reduced (right) sensitivity.

Aetiology: This is extensive and diverse, from severe fatal or mild brain disorders of any type to idiopathic causes or exceptionally reversible exogenous factors (Table 3.1). Severe causes predominate.

Aetiologically, West syndrome is classified as idiopathic without demonstrable lesional causes, possible symptomatic and symptomatic due to discernible organic insults. The description by West (1841)[179a] is probably the best typical case of a symptomatic cause. Unless the aetiology is a specific genetic disorder, such as tuberous sclerosis or twin pregnancy, familial recurrence is rare. Exceptionally, X-linked recessive inheritance, seen exclusively in male offspring from asymptomatic mothers, is described.

Table 3.1   Main causes of epileptic spasms

Prenatal disorders
   Neurocutaneous disorders
      Tuberous sclerosis
      Sturge-Weber disease
      Incontinentia pigmenti (Bloch-Sulzberger syndrome)
      Neurofibromatosis
   Chromosomal abnormalities
      Down syndrome
      Miller-Dieker syndrome (17p13 chromosomal deletion)
   Malformations of cerebral development
      Aicardi syndrome
      Agyria (lissencephaly), pachygyria, polymicrogyria, schizencephaly, laminar
         heterotopia and other diffuse cortical dysplasias
   Hypoxic-ischaemic encephalopathies
   Congenital infections
   Trauma

Perinatal disorders
   Hypoxic-ischaemic encephalopathies
   Infections (meningitis, encephalitis)
   Trauma
   Intracranial haemorrhage

Postnatal disorders
   Metabolic
      Pyridoxine dependency
      Non-ketotic hyperglycinaemia
      Phenylketonuria
      Maple syrup urine disease
      Mitochondrial encephalopathies
   Infections (meningitis, encephalitis)
   Trauma
   Degenerative diseases
   Intracranial haemorrhage
   Drugs (theophylline and anti-allergic agents of histamine H1 antagonists such as ketotifen)

Important points

Drugs such as theophylline[186] or anti-allergic agents of histamine H1 antagonists and particularly ketotifen[187] may induce epileptic spasms and hypsarrhythmia that are entirely reversible upon drug withdrawal.

Also, pyridoxine dependency can present with epileptic spasms.

Previously, there was significant concern that immunisation with various vaccines may cause infantile spasms but this is coincidental because the peak age at onset of infantile spasms corresponds with the immunisation programme for children.

Diagnostic procedures: A thorough clinical neurodevelopment assessment, ophthalmologic and ultraviolet skin examination may reveal the underlying cause, particularly in symptomatic cases, including tuberous sclerosis and Aicardi syndrome. Laboratory screening for electrolyte, metabolic or other disturbances is usually normal. Infectious diseases may be apparent by clinical presentation; suspected infants should have the appropriate investigations including CSF examination. Infants with frequent vomiting, lethargy, failure to thrive, peculiar odours and unexplained neurological findings should have urine amino acid screening, serum ammonia and liver function tests. Most paediatricians rightly recommend these neurometabolic tests in all cases unless an alternative cause is clear. Chromosomal analysis may lead to a specific diagnosis in infants with unexplained West syndrome.

Brain computed tomographic (CT) scan and more specifically magnetic resonance imaging (MRI) are indicated. These should be performed before steroid treatment, which may lead to apparent atrophy on the CT or MRI. Positron emission tomography (PET) of brain glucose utilisation is highly sensitive in detecting focal cortical abnormalities in patients with West syndrome even when CT scan or MRI are normal. Bilateral hypometabolism of the temporal lobes even in the absence of abnormal CT and MRI scans has a poor prognostic significance.[173]

Electroencephalography:[159,165] Hypsarrhythmia is the archetypal interictal pattern and occurs in two thirds of patients (Figure 3.4). This EEG pattern is anarchy, a chaotic mixture of giant abnormal, arrhythmic and asynchronous biological brain electrical activity of slow and sharp waves, multifocal spikes and polyspikes. Because of their high amplitude, individual components and localisation are impossible at routine sensitivity recordings of 100 µV/1 cm (Figure 3.4). There are no recognisable normal rhythms.

Asymmetrical and other patterns of modified hypsarrhythmia occur in one third of cases.

In slow sleep, hypsarrhythmia becomes fragmented and presents with discontinuous repetitive high amplitude discharges of spikes/polyspikes and slow waves, which are more synchronous than in the awake EEG. These are separated by low amplitude traces that may contain sleep spindles. This sleep EEG pattern may be seen in some infants with a relatively normal awake EEG, mainly at onset of infantile spasms. REM sleep shows relative EEG normalisation.

Ictal EEG: Patterns are variable with at least 11 different types lasting for 0.5 seconds to 2 minutes. The commonest and more characteristic pattern in 72% of the attacks is brief (1–5 seconds) (Figure 3.4) and consists of:
- a high–voltage, generalised, slow wave,
- episodic low amplitude fast activity and
- marked diffuse attenuation of EEG electrical activity.

Certain interictal EEG patterns may contribute to an aetiological diagnosis

Symmetrical hypsarrhythmia is most likely to occur in idiopathic and cryptogenic cases. Asymmetrical and unilateral hypsarrhythmia almost always indicates ipsilateral brain structural lesions. Consistently focal slow waves in hypsarrhythmia indicate localised lesions. The slow wave focus becomes more apparent with intravenous diazepam when it reduces the amount of hypsarrhythmia.

Lissencephaly and Aicardi syndrome may have relatively specific EEG patterns with frequent suppression-bursts. West syndrome of tuberous sclerosis rarely has typical hypsarrhythmic appearance while spike foci with secondary generalisation in sleep are frequent.

Progress of hypsarrhythmic EEG pattern with age

The chaotic hypsarrhythmic pattern of West syndrome gradually becomes more organised, fragmented and disappears with age. By age 2–4 years, it may be replaced by the generalised slow sharp and slow wave pattern of Lennox-Gastaut syndrome.

Differential diagnosis: West syndrome should be easy to diagnose because of the unique characteristic features of each attack and because of their serial and unprovoked clustering. However, parents and physicians often miss this. The erroneous diagnosis of exaggerated startle responses or 'colic, abdominal pain' is common.

Benign myoclonus of early infancy (benign non-epileptic infantile spasms) described by Lombroso and Fejerman[107,109,188] is not an epileptic condition but may cause diagnostic problems because of a similar age at onset and similar spasms (page 48). Benign neonatal sleep myoclonus (page 47),[104,105,189] another non-epileptic condition, may also be mistaken for infantile spasms although myoclonic jerks and not spasms is the main symptom which occurs only during sleep. EEG is normal.

Of the non-epileptic conditions, Sandifer's syndrome of gastro-oesophageal reflux may also be confused with infantile spasms. Head cocking, torticollis, abnormal dystonic posturing of the body and mainly opisthotonus may imitate infantile spasms. However, these spells often occur in relation to feeds and the babies often have a history of vomiting, failure to thrive and respiratory symptoms. EEG is normal. Barium oesophagogram, oesophagoscopy, or pH probe may demonstrate the reflux. Hiatus hernia is common.

Diagnostic Tips

● Recognising epileptic (infantile) spasms is easy by the characteristics of the individual attacks and mainly by their clustering, often on arousal.

● It is practically necessary to ask the parents to physically demonstrate and imitate the attacks rather than merely to describe them. If in doubt, demonstrating or showing a video with typical attacks is often conclusive.

● Benign phenomena such as a Moro reflex, attacks of colic or even attempts to sit up may be a cause of confusion that can be avoided by remembering that infantile spasms occur in clusters; singular events are exceptional.

West syndrome is also differentiated from other benign or severe forms or epilepsies of this age group because of the unique presentation of epileptic spasms that differ significantly from myoclonic jerks and tonic seizures.

The frequency at which epileptic spasms are misdiagnosed has been documented by Donat and Wright (1992).[166] In 53 infants who by clinical history were thought to have infantile spasms, video-EEG showed that these were imitators, not genuine, infantile spasms. Nine patients had other types of seizures. Forty-five patients had episodic symptoms that were not seizures: 11 patients had spasticity, 4 had gastro-oesophageal reflux and the other patients had non-epileptic myoclonus, including 19 patients with benign neonatal sleep myoclonus. Three patients had more than one type of symptom. Infantile spasm imitators occurred in neurologically normal or abnormal infants, in patients with normal or abnormal interictal EEG and in patients who also had previous or current infantile spasms.

Prognosis: This reflects the immensely diverse aetiology: 5% die, 65% develop usually intractable epileptic fits of different types and severity such as Lennox-Gastaut or complex focal seizures. Half of the patients have permanent motor disabilities and two thirds have usually severe cognitive and psychological impairment. Only about 5–12% of patients have normal mental and motor development. However, 15–30% of idiopathic or possibly symptomatic (cryptogenic) patients may achieve normality.

Management: Vigabatrin or adrenocorticotropic hormone (corticosteroids are often used in the UK instead of adrenocorticotropic hormone) are the drugs of choice, controlling the infantile spasms in two thirds within days, but the final outcome may not be influenced by treatment. Lamotrigine, levetiracetam, nitrazepam, pyridoxine, sodium valproate, zonisamide and topiramate are also used.

Resective neurosurgery may be the desperate solution in selected medically intractable cases with localised structural lesions. Recently, this has been increasingly recognised as an effective management method.

DRAVET SYNDROME [190–197]

SEVERE MYOCLONIC EPILEPSY IN INFANCY

Dravet syndrome is a rare form of progressive epileptic encephalopathy that may be genetically determined.

Demographic data: Onset is in the first year of life at a peak age of 5 months affecting previously normal children. Boys are twice as likely to be affected as girls. There are about 200 cases reported with Dravet syndrome. Prevalence is ~ 6% of epilepsies starting before the age of 3 years. Incidence is ~1 per 30,000.

Clinical manifestations: Dravet syndrome is characterised by a tetrad of seizures
1. early infantile clonic febrile convulsions,
2. myoclonic jerks,
3. atypical absences and
4. complex focal seizures.

Convulsive, myoclonic or absence status epilepticus are frequent. Neither myoclonic jerks nor absences are a prerequisite for diagnosis. However, the sequence of the seizures, their resistance to treatment and the progression to mental and neurological deterioration are characteristic.

THERE ARE THREE PERIODS OF EVOLUTION:

The first is a relatively mild (pre-seismic) period with seizures usually occurring during febrile illnesses and consisting of clonic convulsions that are either unilateral or generalised, brief or prolonged. They are frequent and often progress to convulsive status epilepticus. Video–EEG reveals a mixture of clonic and tonic components, initially predominating in the head and the face progressing to unilateral or bilateral mainly clonic convulsions with loss of consciousness.

The second is a relentlessly aggressive (seismic) period with the children developing other type of fits such as myoclonic, atypical absence and complex focal seizures. Myoclonic seizures may be limited to the head or a limb, occur many times per day and often constitute myoclonic status epilepticus without loss of consciousness. Atypical absences are brief but may also appear as absence status epilepticus together with erratic small myoclonic jerks. Complex focal seizures manifest with impairment of consciousness, automatisms, atonic or adversive and autonomic symptoms. Secondarily GTCS may occur.

Myoclonic, atypical absence, complex focal and convulsive status epilepticus, alone or together, are common and frequent. They may last for hours or days. They may be re-cycled by photic stimulation, closure of the eyes or fixation on patterns.

The third is a static (post-seismic) period where seizures may improve but serious and residual mental and neurological abnormalities remain forever.

Although this sequence of febrile clonic convulsions, myoclonic jerks, absences and complex focal seizures is seen in more than half of the cases, in others one or another type of seizures may not occur. Myoclonic jerks, initially considered as the defining seizure type, may not be present in one fifth of the patients. In others they may precede the initial febrile clonic convulsions.

Diagnostic Tips

● Prolonged usually unilateral febrile clonic seizures at the age of a few months that recur within 2 months should raise the suspicion of Dravet syndrome.

Although not pathognomonic, onset at this early age, low temperature and prolonged seizures of mainly clonic convulsions may differentiate from febrile convulsions.

● The diagnosis is nearly certain if intractable myoclonic jerks and mental deterioration appear within 1–2 years from onset.

Diagnostic pitfalls in Dravet syndrome

● Not all patients develop myoclonic jerks.

● Not all patients start with febrile convulsions.
● Not all patients develop absence seizures.

Seizure-precipitating factors: Febrile illnesses, raised body temperature and warm environment (hot baths) are frequent precipitants particularly at onset of seizures that are mainly clonic. Photic and pattern stimulation, movements and eye closure mainly precipitate generalised discharges, myoclonic jerks and absence seizures. Self-stimulation is a feature.

Aetiology: Dravet syndrome is probably genetically determined but the mode of inheritance is unknown. One fifth have a family history of various epileptic syndromes or febrile convulsions. Rarely, siblings or twins may suffer from this syndrome.

Diagnostic procedures: The general consensus is that there is no metabolic abnormality and skin and muscle biopsy when performed are normal. There are some recent reports of probably exceptional mitochondrial cytopathy. Other causes of progressive infantile epileptic myoclonic encephalopathies should be excluded. In most of the reported cases with Dravet syndrome, old-fashioned brain imaging techniques including pneumoencephalography were used. These showed some mild cortical or cisterna magna dilatation. In 2 of 11 patients who had MRI there was an increased white matter signal (T2-weighted). Modern high-resolution structural and functioning brain imaging may be more contributory.

Electroencephalography: The EEG is usually normal at onset but later there are frequent and severe paroxysms of generalised polyspikes and slow waves, 2 Hz spike-wave or both. They usually predominate on one side and may be singular or in clusters. These are spontaneous but often are also elicited by photic stimulation and they are facilitated by sleep. Additionally, there are multifocal abnormalities of spike and slow wave. The background EEG is initially normal but progressively deteriorates with excessive amounts of slow activity. Half of the patients (42%) show marked photosensitivity and pattern-sensitivity.

Differential diagnosis: Early diagnosis of Dravet syndrome can be reliably made on clinical criteria from the second or third seizure in the first year of life.

At the initial pre-seismic phase, *febrile convulsions* is the most apparent diagnosis to differentiate (Table 3.2)

Table 3.2   Differentiating Dravet syndrome from febrile convulsions

Paediatricians should maintain a high index of suspicion for Dravet syndrome if febrile seizures are:

- prolonged beyond 15 or 30 minutes
- unilateral
- mainly clonic
- frequent
- precipitated by low fever often below 38°C and
- early onset (before 1 year of age)
- with afebrile seizures

The diagnosis can be certain if other seizure types, particularly myoclonic jerks, and photoparoxysmal discharges occur.

Lennox-Gastaut syndrome is easy to differentiate because of:

- the absence of repeated febrile mainly clonic seizures in the first year of life
- the predominance of drop attacks, axial tonic seizures and specific EEG patterns
- often pre-existing brain lesions.

Tonic seizures in Dravet syndrome are exceptional and again they are different and never repeated in series.[191,197]

Some difficulties may be imposed by the 'epilepsy with myoclonic–astatic seizures' of Doose (page 124) where there may be an early onset with febrile convulsive seizures. However, focal seizures and focal EEG abnormalities do not usually occur in Doose syndrome, which is characterised mainly by myoclonic-atonic seizures.

Benign myoclonic epilepsy in infancy has only brief generalised myoclonic seizures. Febrile convulsions are rare and short. EEG is markedly different without focal abnormalities.

Progressive myoclonic epilepsies due to storage disease[170] may have similar features although at this age they may run a different course.[191,197]

Prognosis: Seizure deterioration and mental and neurological decline are relentless and often fatal. Psychomotor retardation and progressive neurological signs of ataxia and pyramidal symptoms appear within a year from onset. Mortality is high.

Management: Seizures are intractable. Certain drugs may reduce but do not control them and it is doubtful if they can affect outcome. Treatment with sodium valproate, diazepines, melatonin,[198] phenobarbitone (convulsive seizures), ethosuximide (absence and myoclonic seizures) is partially and temporally beneficial. Of the new drugs levetiracetam and topiramate may be beneficial. Carbamazepine and lamotrigine are probably contraindicated.

Long, generalised or unilateral seizures should be prevented by early treatment of infectious diseases and hyperthermia, which are their triggering factors.

HEMICONVULSION-HEMIPLEGIA EPILEPSY SYNDROME [199–205]

Hemiconvulsion–hemiplegia syndrome (HHS) is a rare dramatic sequence of a sudden and prolonged unilateral clonic seizure followed by permanent ipsilateral hemiplegia.[199,205] The event occurs suddenly in an otherwise normal child often during a febrile illness.

Eighty percent of the patients later develop focal epilepsy of the complete hemiconvulsion–hemiplegia–epilepsy syndrome (HHES).

Considerations on classification

The new diagnostic scheme[10] considers hemiconvulsion-hemiplegia (HH) as a syndrome although rightly this was not previously recognised as a separate epileptic syndrome.[9]

Demographic data: Peak age of occurrence is in the first 2 years of life with a range of 5 months to 4 years. This may be an extremely rare condition today with improved emergency care for status epilepticus. There was only one (0.06%) equivocal case in the National Institute of Neurological and Communicative Disorders and Stroke Collaborative Perinatal Project from the USA.[121,122] Although Gastaut initially reported 150 cases,[199] the number of reported cases dramatically decreased in subsequent reports.[201,202,204]

Clinical manifestations: Hemiconvulsions come suddenly out of the blue and consist of unilateral, often asynchronous, clonic jerks lasting for hours or days if not appropriately treated. If very prolonged, they may spread to the other side or more rarely change sides. Deviation of the head and eyes may occur or be the first seizure symptom. Consciousness may be intact.

By definition, severe ipsilateral post-convulsive hemiplegia follows in all cases, which lasts for more than 7 days and is permanent in more than 80% of the cases. The face is always involved and aphasia is present if the dominant side is involved. These signs distinguish acquired post-convulsive from congenital hemiplegia.[170]

Aetiology: The initial hemiconvulsion-hemiplegia event usually occurs in the course of a febrile illness that is often due to a CNS infection such as herpes encephalitis. In a few cases the cause may be traumatic or vascular. However, frequently no cause is found and there may be a high incidence of family history of febrile seizures.

Diagnostic procedures: Diagnostic procedures should include CSF examination, which is probably mandatory in children younger than 18 months in view of the high possibility of a CNS infection. Brain imaging, if possible, should precede lumbar puncture. In the acute stage, there is usually evidence of oedema in the affected hemisphere. Later, a rather characteristic, uniform hemiatrophy follows prolonged episodes. There is hyperperfusion in SPECT during the acute stage followed later by hypoperfusion.[206]

Electroencephalography: EEG is not important at the acute stage. EEG will simply confirm the clinical situation without offering any specific clues to the underlying cause and development.

Ictal EEG consists of a mixture of high amplitude rhythmical 2–3 Hz slow waves intermixed with spikes, sharp waves, spike wave complexes and episodic fast activity (10–12 Hz). Amplitude is higher and spikes predominate in the affected hemisphere with posterior emphasis. There is no consistent relation between clonic convulsions and EEG discharges.

Prognosis: Depends on cause and speed of effective acute management. Focal seizures of temporal, extratemporal, or multifocal origin appear within 1–5 years in 80% of the patients. Most of the patients also have secondarily GTCS and often convulsive status epilepticus. Seizures are usually intractable to antiepileptic medication. Learning difficulties are probably the rule.

Acute management: Immediate control of the seizure is a medical emergency as of status epilepticus. Benzodiazepines, usually diazepam or lorazepam intravenously, are probably the first choice. Treatment of the fever and mainly of the underlying illness is of equal importance. Other than conservative management of residual neurological deficits, little can be done after hemiplegia is established. Hemispherectomy may be very beneficial.

*MIGRATING FOCAL SEIZURES OF INFANCY [193,207,208]

This syndrome in development is based on a few reports of ~20 infants of both sexes with nearly continuous multifocal seizures. Onset is at a mean age of 3 months, without antecedent risk factors. After 1–10 months, the seizures become very frequent. Seizures are focal, usually motor, with variable clinical expression.

Topographically, ictal EEG discharges randomly involve multiple independent sites, moving from one cortical area to another in consecutive seizures. Morphologically they consist of rhythmic alpha or theta activity spreading to involve an increasing area of the cortical surface.

Patients usually regress developmentally and become quadriplegic with severe axial hypotonia. Death may occur soon after or a few years from onset. Control of the seizures and normal development is rare. Treatment with potassium bromide has been successful in two otherwise intractable cases.[208]

Aetiology is unkown. There is no family history. Neuropathological examination of the brain in two cases showed only severe hippocampal neuronal loss and accompanying gliosis.

*MYOCLONIC STATUS IN NON-PROGRESSIVE ENCEPHALOPATHIES [10,209–211]

Myoclonic status in non-progressive encephalopathies is a syndrome in development.

Demographic data: Peak onset is at 12 months (range: 1 day to 5 years). There is two-fold female preponderance. Although its incidence and prevalence are unknown it was found in 0.5–1% of a selected population of children with severe forms of epilepsy.

Clinical manifestations: This syndrome is characterised by repetitive and long (sometimes for days) episodes of atypical myoclonic status that consists of myoclonic jerks and subcontinuous absences. The myoclonic jerks involving eyelids, face and limbs are mostly erratic and asynchronous becoming more rhythmic and synchronous during the absences. The myoclonic jerks are often inconspicuous and the babies may appear just apathetic and ataxic. Myoclonic status may be the first seizure manifestation

---

* Syndromes in development.

but in others the initial seizures are mostly focal motor seizures, myoclonic absences, massive myoclonias, and more rarely generalised or unilateral clonic seizures recurring in some cases only during febrile illness. Tonic seizures are never observed.

Many patients also have frequent and sudden spontaneous massive startle attacks of brief and abrupt loss of postural tone as well as long-lasting bursts of intentional myoclonus or tremor.

Aetiology: Half the cases suffer from a chromosomal disorder (Angelman syndrome, 4p-syndrome). Others have prenatal brain anoxia or migrational disorders. In the remaining one third the aetiology in unknown. A family history of seizure disorders can be found in about one fifth of cases. Metabolic diseases such as non-ketotic hyperglycinaemia may have similar electroclinical patterns.

Diagnostic procedures: Because ictal symptoms may sometimes be mild, confirmation with video-EEG or polygraphic recordings is needed.

Pathophysiology: Considering that patients with Angelman syndrome and some of the patients with 4p-syndrome have a chromosomal deletion eliminating a cluster of GABA-A receptor genes, it has been hypothesised that a loss of GABAergic inhibition plays a role in the pathogenesis of myoclonic status in non-progressive encephalopathies.[210]

Prognosis: This is poor even for those who initially appear only hypotonic. The initial hypotonic state progressively deteriorates to sometimes severe neurological and mental deficits. The myoclonic status improves with age but the patients rarely achieve relatively normal state.

Management: There is no effective treatment other than diazepines, which transiently interrupt the myoclonic status epilepticus.

EPILEPTIC ENCEPHALOPATHIES IN EARLY CHILDHOOD

IN WHICH THE EPILEPTIFORM ABNORMALITIES MAY CONTRIBUTE TO PROGRESSIVE DYSFUNCTION

The new diagnostic scheme considers the following three syndromes among epileptic encephalopathies (with onset in early childhood):[10]

1. **Lennox-Gastaut syndrome**
2. **Landau-Kleffner syndrome**
3. **Epilepsy with continuous spike and waves during slow wave sleep**

LENNOX-GASTAUT SYNDROME [199,212–223]

Lennox–Gastaut syndrome is a childhood epileptic encephalopathy characterised by the triad of:

1. multiple types of intractable seizures that are mainly tonic, atonic and atypical absence seizures
2. cognitive and behavioural abnormalities
3. diffuse slow spike and waves and paroxysms of fast activity on EEG.

Demographic data: Lennox-Gastaut syndrome starts between 1 and 7 years of age with a peak at 3–5 years. Boys (60%) are slightly more often affected than girls. The incidence of Lennox-Gastaut syndrome is low at 2.8/10,000 live births.[231] However, because of its intractable nature prevalence is relatively high at around 5–10% of children with seizures.[219,230,232]

Clinical manifestations: Lennox-Gastaut syndrome is characterised by a cluster of multiform seizures and mental retardation. The most characteristic seizures (in descending order of prevalence) are tonic and atonic fits and atypical absences.

Onset may be insidious with symptoms appearing de novo without conspicuous reason in cryptogenic cases. Previous psychomotor deficits are apparent in symptomatic cases. Cognitive and behavioural abnormalities are present before seizure onset in 20–60% of patients.

Half of the cases of West syndrome and other infantile epileptic encephalopathies progress to Lennox-Gastaut syndrome. Conversely, 10–30% of patients with Lennox-Gastaut syndrome develop from West syndrome or other epileptic encephalopathies, although the transition phase is difficult to evaluate. Focal and generalised seizures are also common predecessors.

Seizures consist of tonic and atonic fits and atypical absences. Falls, often traumatic, are due to tonic and atonic seizures. Myoclonic jerks occur in 11–28% of patients either alone or in combination with other seizures. However, myoclonic jerks do not predominate in the 'pure' Lennox-Gastaut syndrome.

Sleep and inactivity greatly facilitate seizures and EEG abnormalities.

Tonic seizures are the commonest and probably most characteristic seizure type in Lennox-Gastaut syndrome (Figure 4.1). These are usually symmetrical, brief (~10 seconds) and of variable severity from inconspicuous to violent. Descriptively, tonic seizures are:[199]

- **axial** affecting facial, nuchal, trunk, paraspinal, respiratory and abdominal muscles alone or in combination

  Raising the head from the pillow, elevation of the eyebrows, opening of the eyes, upward deviation of the eyeballs, opening of the mouth, stretching of the lips to a fixed smile. An 'epileptic cry' is common at onset of the attacks.

- **axo-rhizomelic**, which are axial seizures also involving proximal (rhizomelic) muscles of upper and less often lower limbs

  Elevation, abduction or adduction of upper limbs and shoulders occur together with the other symptoms of axial tonic seizures.

- **global**, which also involve the distal part of the limbs

  Arms are forced upwards, abducted and semiflexed with clenched fists 'like that of a child defending himself from a facial blow'. The lower limbs are forced in triple flexion at hip, knee and ankle or in extension. Global tonic seizures often cause forceful sudden falls and injuries.

Considerations on classification

There is no consensus of what Lennox-Gastaut syndrome is (see Table 4.1 on inclusion criteria). It is categorised amongst generalised cryptogenic or symptomatic epilepsies (age-related) by the Commission and is defined as follows:[9] 'Lennox-Gastaut syndrome manifests itself in children aged 1–8 years, but appears mainly in pre-school-age children. The most common seizure types are tonic-axial, atonic and absence seizures, but other types such as myoclonic, GTCS or partial are frequently associated with this syndrome. Seizure frequency is high, and status epilepticus is frequent (stuporous states with myoclonias, tonic and atonic seizures). The EEG usually has abnormal background activity, slow spike waves <3 Hz and, often, multifocal abnormalities. During sleep, bursts of fast rhythms (around 10 Hz) appear. In general, there is mental retardation. Seizures are difficult to control, and the development is mostly unfavourable. In 60 per cent of cases, the syndrome occurs in children suffering from a previous encephalopathy, but it is primary in other cases'.

However, Lennox-Gastaut and other syndromes such as epilepsy with myoclonic astatic seizures of Doose (page 124) have undefined boundaries resulting in what appears as 'an overlap of syndromes'.[224,225] There are still significant problems regarding the exact nosological boundaries of Lennox-Gastaut syndrome, as emphasised by Aicardi:[170,220,225] 'The

epilepsies described under the headings of Lennox-Gastaut syndrome and of myoclonic epilepsies raise one of the most controversial problems of childhood epileptology ... There is still considerable confusion surrounding the concept of the Lennox-Gastaut syndrome, so the definition of the syndrome and its relationship to other forms of epilepsy, especially those that feature myoclonic seizures, remains a subject of dispute'. 'Only the more typical syndromes are reasonably well defined, but many patients are impossible to include in a definite category.'[220,225] Doose has similar views:[226–228] 'There is hardly another field in paediatric epileptology presenting such terminological uncertainty and confusion as is to be found in the domain of epileptic syndromes with generalized minor seizures of early childhood ...'.[226–228]

The 'myoclonic variant' of Lennox-Gastaut syndrome is another probably artificial situation as indicated by the fact that this is nearly identical to epilepsy with myoclonic-astatic seizures.[3] Myoclonic seizures are a prominent feature while tonic seizures are few and occur only during sleep. Spike wave complexes may be fast or slow. Most are cryptogenic cases with a similar outcome. Other myoclonic epilepsies with brief seizures reported[216] as intermediate cases between epilepsy with myoclonic-astatic seizures and Lennox-Gastaut syndrome most likely reflect the undefined boundaries of the current definitions.

A series of tonic seizures, reminiscent of epileptic spasms but of longer duration, may occur, especially when Lennox-Gastaut develops from West syndrome.

Concurrent autonomic manifestations may occasionally be the prominent symptom of the attacks.

Tonic seizures occur more often during slow wave sleep than wake states. Some patients may have hundreds of them during sleep. They do not occur during REM sleep. In early onset Lennox-Gastaut syndrome clusters of tonic spasms frequently occur on awakening.

Atypical absence seizures (Figure 4.2) occur in approximately two thirds of patients. There is 'clouding' rather than loss of consciousness with gradual onset and gradual termination. The patients may continue with their activity although more slowly and often with mistakes. Impairment of cognition may be so mild that it is clinically undetectable. Selective impairment of higher cortical functions with maintained responsiveness may occur.

Changes in tone and myoclonic jerks may be very pronounced. Often, there is loss of trunk or head postural tone, facial muscle or neck muscle stiffening, eyelid or perioral myoclonus, random jerks of head or limbs and head nodding.

Atonic seizures of sudden, brief and severe loss of postural tone may involve the whole body or only the head. Attacks are brief (1–4 seconds) frequent and occur in nearly half of the patients. The trunk and head slump forwards and the knees buckle. Atonic seizures are the commonest cause of falls resulting

---

Table 4.1   Inclusion criteria for Lennox-Gastaut syndrome

These are not well defined but most authorities demand the following triad:

1. At least two types among tonic, atonic seizures, atypical absences. Some authors demand atypical absences as being one of the mandatory seizure type. Others prefer tonic seizures. Myoclonic seizures are not a prerequisite criterion for inclusion or exclusion.

2. Generalised slow spike wave discharges. Although all agree with this, episodic fast activity is an additional requested EEG abnormality by others.

3. Impaired intellectual functioning. There are recent reports that this is no longer a prerequisite of Lennox-Gastaut syndrome.

Age at onset, abnormal or normal brain imaging and causative factors are usually not considered important. Accordingly, Lennox-Gastaut syndrome may even start in adult life.

To emphasise this diversity, I take the example of two recent studies from the same country (USA) published in the same journal (*Epilepsia*).[229,230] In one of them[230] inclusion criteria were: 'Onset of multiple seizure types before age 11 years, with at least one seizure type resulting in falls, and an EEG demonstrating slow spike-wave complexes (<2.5 Hz)'. In the other study[229] criteria were 'Multiple seizures (two or more) with one being tonic seizures. Generalised slow spike-wave (at least in one EEG). Age at onset could be at any time.' Mental retardation was not used as a diagnostic criterion in either of them.[229,230]

in severe injuries to the nose or teeth. Generalised loss of postural tone causes a lightning-like fall. The patient collapses on the floor irresistibly without impairment of consciousness and then immediately stands up again. In brief and milder attacks there is only head nodding or sagging at the knees. Longer atonic seizures lasting for 30 seconds to 1 or 2 minutes are rare. The patient remains on the floor unable to stand up.

Atonic seizures always alternate with tonic fits and atypical absences in Lennox-Gastaut syndrome. There may be a predominant tonic component (axial spasm) in these otherwise atonic seizures. Also, myoclonic jerks may precede or less often intersperse with the atonic manifestations.

Myoclonic jerks were initially not included among the seizures of Lennox-Gastaut syndrome but they may occur in 11–28% of patients. Myoclonic attacks are very brief, shock-like muscle contractions that may be isolated or repeated in a saccadic manner, usually for only a few seconds. The jerks are generally bilateral and symmetrical (massive myoclonus) and involve preferentially the axial flexor muscles and the abductors of the arms. They may cause falls.

Epileptic falls (drop attacks) may be the result of various types of seizures such as atonic, tonic, myoclonic-atonic and more rarely myoclonic. These are often difficult to differentiate clinically without polygraphic recording.[233] The falls result in recurrent injury.

Non-convulsive status epilepticus featuring all types of seizures such as atypical absences, tonic and atonic fits and myoclonic jerks occurs in half of the

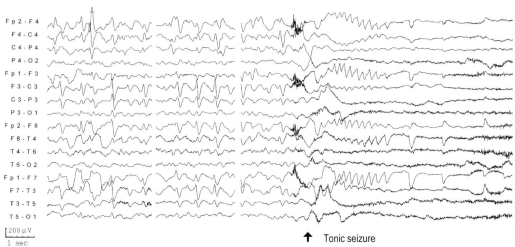

Girl aged 10 years with severe mental and neurological deficits -- Multiform seizures from age 6 months

↑ Tonic seizure

Figure 4.1   Samples from a video-EEG of a 10-year-old girl with Lennox-Gastaut syndrome.

Left: Grossly abnormal interictal EEG.   *Right*: Tonic seizure.

patients. It is often of very long duration (days to weeks), resistant to treatment and repetitive. Depending on the predominant seizure type, status epilepticus in Lennox-Gastaut syndrome may be:

- **absence status epilepticus** of insidious confusional state that can last for days or weeks
- **tonic status epilepticus** which is more often seen in adolescents than in children
- **myoclonic status epilepticus** is rare, occurring when the myoclonic jerks are the dominant seizure type
- **mixed tonic and absence status** is probably the commoner type. It consists of uninterrupted series of brief tonic seizures alternating with atypical absences. There is usually profound obtundation or stupor, intermixed with serial tonic attacks and sometimes with myoclonic–atonic falls.

Aetiology is extensive and diverse. Symptomatic Lennox-Gastaut syndrome due to severe and less often mild brain disorders of any type is by far the commonest, probably 70% of all cases. Prenatal, perinatal and postnatal causes are similar to those responsible for West syndrome (Table 2.1) but Aicardi syndrome and lissencephaly, common in West syndrome, are rare causes in Lennox-Gastaut syndrome. Malformations of cortical development are increasingly identified as a common cause of the Lennox-Gastaut syndrome. Localised malformations of cortical development can produce a typical picture or be associated with incomplete forms of the syndrome.

One third of Lennox-Gastaut syndrome occurs without antecedent history or evidence of brain pathology (idiopathic or possible symptomatic cases). There is no evidence of a genetic predisposition.

Diagnostic procedures: Biochemical, haematological, metabolic and other relevant screening is rarely abnormal depending on cause.

Brain imaging is often abnormal particularly with high–resolution MRI and PET scans.[234–237]

Electroencephalography:[26,238–240] The interictal EEG features at onset may consist of abnormal background with or without generalised slow spike waves. Background abnormalities, found in almost all cases, from onset of seizures, consist of slow and fragmented alpha rhythm, excess of diffuse slow waves, EEG disorganisation. Focal slow waves typically occur in symptomatic cases.

Commonly, EEGs of abnormal background contain paroxysms of fast rhythms characterising tonic seizures (Figures 4.3, 4.4 and 4.5) and slow <2.5 Hz spike-wave generalised discharges characterising atypical absences (Figures 4.1 and 4.2). These EEG patterns may be clinically silent (interictal?) or manifest with inconspicuous or violent seizures (ictal).

Episodic abnormalities are frequent and mainly consist of:

- Slow <2.5 Hz spike and slow wave generalised discharges.

  The slow spike and wave discharges, usually at around 2 Hz, are generalised, bilateral, synchronous, symmetrical and of higher amplitude in the anterior regions. However, they are also often asymmetrical, unilateral and less frequently regional.

- Paroxysms of fast activity or rhythmic rapid spikes at around 10 Hz or much faster.

  These are the most revealing and characteristic features occurring nearly exclusively during slow sleep. Although frequently clinical manifestations are not apparent, brief and inconspicuous tonic seizures mainly of facial muscles often occur (Figures 4.3 and 4.4) but their detection requires video-EEG monitoring. Fast paroxysms often contain rhythms faster than 10 Hz (Figure 4.5).[5]

  Interictal spikes and multifocal spike or sharp slow waves are predominant in the frontal and temporal areas in 75% of the patients. The EEG patterns differ among individuals and change from day to day and even moment to moment.

  Sleep activates additional spike foci, increases the frequency of generalised spike discharges and produces synchronisation of bitemporal and bifrontal spike wave discharges at 1.5–2.5 Hz.[241]

  Ictal EEG: Atypical absences are associated with generalised slow <2.5 Hz spike and slow wave (Figure 4.2). Tonic seizures have accelerating fast paroxysmal activity, which is bilateral and often predominates in the anterior

Slow generalised spike and slow wave discharges

Girl aged 9 with severe mental retardation and multiform seizures of Lennox-Gastaut syndrome

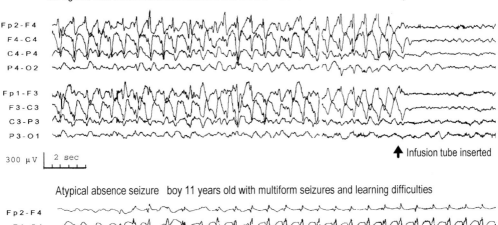

Atypical absence seizure   boy 11 years old with multiform seizures and learning difficulties

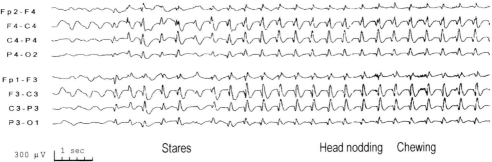

Figure 4.2

Slow spike and wave (<2.5 Hz) discharges in two children with Lennox-Gastaut syndrome. Clinical manifestations may be inconspicuous (*top*) or apparent (*bottom*).

regions and the vertex (Figures 4.3, 4.4 and 4.5). This may be of two types:[199]

1. Very rapid 20 ± 5 Hz initially of low amplitude progressively increasing to 50–100 μV.

2. A more ample and less rapid rhythmic discharge at 10 Hz, identical to that of the tonic phase of the GTCS (epileptic recruiting rhythm) except that it may be of high amplitude from the onset.

Flattening of all EEG activity alone or in combination with fast paroxysms is also common (Figure 4.3). Fast ictal paroxysms may be preceded by generalised spikes/slow wave or EEG suppression.

Atonic attacks occur with generalised spikes and polyspikes, generalised slow spike wave discharges and accelerating fast paroxysms alone or in combination.[199]

Myoclonic attacks show mainly generalised discharges of polyspikes with or without slow waves and fast rhythms.

A combination of clinical manifestations and ictal EEG patterns is common.

Boy aged 7 with Lennox-Gastaut syndrome (agyria, pachygyria and polymicrogyria)   Video EEG during sleep

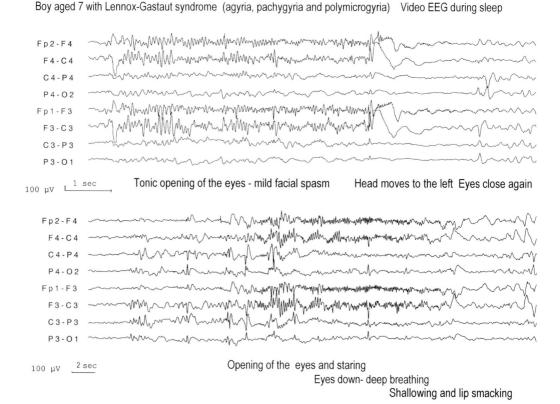

Figure 4.3

From video-EEG of a child with Lennox-Gastaut syndrome due to malformations of cortical development (his older brother also had the same disease).[60] Tonic seizures of varying severity associated with episodic fast or very fast paroxysms. MRI of the two brothers is shown in Figure 1.7.

Man aged 17 years with Lennox-Gastaut syndrome

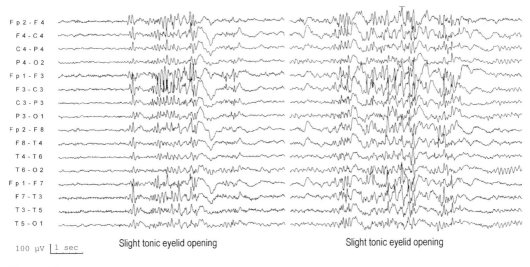

Figure 4.4

From video-EEG of a man aged 17 with Lennox-Gastaut syndrome. EEG fast paroxysms are associated with inconspicuous manifestations of tonic seizures (slight tonic eyelid opening) that would be impossible to detect without video-EEG.

Ictal fast discharges

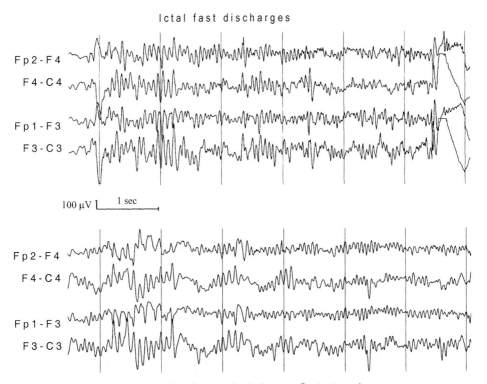

Figure 4.5 Fast ictal paroxysms of various frequencies in Lennox-Gastaut syndrome.

Massive myoclonus, atonic seizures and myoclonic-atonic seizures mainly manifest in EEG with a mixture of slow spike wave, polyspikes and decremental events. Post-ictally, there is diffuse slowing or slow spike wave discharges instead of EEG flattening.

Prognosis: This is appalling:[218,229,231,242–246] 5% die, 80–90% continue having seizures in adult life and nearly all (85–92%) have severely impaired intellectual functioning and behaviour. Many patients are finally institutionalised. Rarely a patient achieves normal mental and motor development.

Cognitive impairment is more likely to develop when onset is before 3 years of age, there are frequent seizures and status epilepticus in symptomatic or West syndrome-related cases.

Differential diagnosis:[225] There are many epileptic and non-epileptic conditions to differentiate from Lennox-Gastaut syndrome (Table 4.2). However, recognising Lennox-Gastaut syndrome in a child is relatively easy because of the characteristic multiform seizure types, pre-existing or developing impairment of cognitive functioning and behaviour and EEG features.

The main differential diagnostic problem is between idiopathic Lennox-Gastaut syndrome and epilepsy with myoclonic-astatic seizures of Doose syndrome (page 124). This is relatively easy in typical presentations (Table 4.3) although these features may not be pathognomonic for a majority of children with overlapping features.[216,225]

Table 4.2 Non-epileptic and epileptic conditions to differentiate from Lennox-Gastaut syndrome

Non-epileptic conditions

Non-epileptic falls, syncope and cataplexy

Nocturnal paroxysmal dystonia

Epileptic syndromes

Late-onset West syndrome

Myoclonic epilepsies of early childhood

Dravet syndrome

Epilepsy with myoclonic absences

Epilepsy with myoclonic-astatic seizures (Doose syndrome)

Myoclonic epilepsy of infancy associated with a fixed encephalopathy

Progressive myoclonic epilepsies and neurodegenerative conditions

Atypical partial benign epilepsy of childhood

Epilepsy with continuous spike and waves during slow wave sleep

Focal epilepsies with secondary bilateral synchrony

Management [223,247,248]

> My 13-year-old daughter has Lennox-Gastaut syndrome. She is on Sabril, Lamictal and Frisium. It seems multiple drug therapies work best for these children. I have found the best control is when the drug level or types are changed. The initial control is good usually reducing the seizures for a month or so but they then start up again. Hence we are always juggling the doses up and down.
>
> (From an Internet description by a mother)

Drug treatments nearly always fail to completely control seizures although a reduction of seizures, usually temporarily, may be achieved. Sodium valproate (all seizures), clonazepam (myoclonic) and phenytoin (tonic) are widely used. Of the new drugs lamotrigine, topiramate[249] and probably levetiracetam may be more effective than old medications. Felbamate reduces drop attacks, absences and other seizure types. However, because of a high incidence of serious, sometimes fatal, side-effects such as aplastic anaemia and hepatic

Table 4.3   Lennox-Gastaut syndrome versus Doose syndrome

	Lennox–Gastaut syndrome	**Doose syndrome**
Main seizures	Tonic, atonic and atypical absences	Myoclonic, atonic and myoclonic–atonic
Tonic seizures	Common and characteristic; diurnal and nocturnal	Probably exclusion criterion (nocturnal tonic seizures are accepted by some authors)
Tonic drop attacks	Common	Incompatible
Atypical absences	Common also occurring independently of other seizures	Uncommon; they usually accompany myoclonic or atonic episodes
Developmental abnormalities before onset of seizures	Common	Exceptional if any
Aetiology	Symptomatic or possibly symptomatic (idiopathic cases are accepted by some authorities)	Idiopathic[10] (although symptomatic or possibly symptomatic cases are included in the ILAE classification of 1989[9])
Genetic predisposition	None	Common
Development from West syndrome	Common	Incompatible
EEG background	Abnormal by rule	Usually normal particularly at onset
EEG episodic fast activity and rapid spikes	Common and often characteristic	Exceptional and mainly in sleep
EEG slow generalised spike wave	Usually <2–2.5 Hz	Usually 2–3 Hz
Prognosis	Commonly bad	Commonly relatively good

failure, it is now licensed only for specific cases (it should be used with caution and for no longer than 2 months if there is no clear response).[250]

Steroid and adrenocorticotropin hormone may be helpful in idiopathic/cryptogenic Lennox-Gastaut syndrome particularly at onset, in status epilepticus, or during periods of marked seizure exaggeration.

Intravenous immunoglobulin gives equivocal results.

Ketogenic diet is undergoing a mini renaissance.

Amantadine, tryptophan, flumazenil, imipramine and many other treatments have had limited success in some patients.[251]

Vagal nerve stimulation (VNS) in childhood epileptic encephalopathies although promising in some studies is probably an ineffective and worthless exercise.[252]

Corpus callosotomy may be considered for intractable drop attacks particularly in cryptogenic cases and provided there is no major diffuse brain malformation.[253,254] Other neurosurgical options are available for children with localised lesions.[254]

One of the aims of treatment is to avoid episodes of status epilepticus, which are often provoked by inter-current illnesses, change in drug regimen and psychological stress. Intravenous benzodiazepines are the most effective drugs, sometimes given with concomitant steroids, and with respiratory assistance if necessary. Intravenous diazepam and lorazepam may induce tonic seizures.

A stimulating but stable environment is important in reducing the number of daily seizures. This may include a strict routine of regular meals, sleep and medication.

Nearly all patients have important educational, behaviouristic and psychological needs, which mandates a multidisciplinary approach to the management of the patient and support for the whole family.

Therapeutic Tips
● With increasing seizures, reducing may be a better option than increasing antiepileptic drugs
● Evaluate the predominant, severe and disabling seizure type for the selection of the next and elimination of the current drug
● Any drug change, adding or deleting, may be temporarily beneficial

---

First line drugs
Sodium valproate – all seizures

Clonazepam and other diazepines – mainly myoclonic jerks

Lamotrigine – probably all but myoclonic seizures particularly small doses as add-on to sodium valproate

Levetiracetam – probably all seizures but needs evaluation

Phenytoin – tonic seizures

Topiramate – probably all seizures

Felbamate – effective but with serious, sometimes fatal, adverse reactions

Ketogenic diet is undergoing a mini renaissance

Second line drugs
Ethosuximide – absences

Vagal nerve stimulation (VNS) – an expensive and probably worthless exercise

Carbamazepine – focal seizures and secondarily GTCS

Corticosteroids and adrenocorticotropic hormone if seizures worsen

LANDAU-KLEFFNER SYNDROME [255–259]

Landau-Kleffner syndrome or acquired epileptic aphasia is a partly reversible, age-related childhood clinical syndrome of mainly linguistic decline and neuropsychological abnormalities as the cardinal clinical symptoms. It is a functional disorder of childhood manifested with acquired verbal auditory agnosia* and other predominantly linguistic deficits that often occur together with other cognitive and neuropsychological–behavioural abnormalities.

Demographic data: Age at onset is mainly before the age of 6 years. Boys are twice as likely to be affected as girls. One or two cases are seen every year in highly specialised centres.

Clinical manifestations: **All childen suffer from linguistic abnormalities; three quarters of them also have seizures.**

Linguistic abnormalities: The first symptom is usually verbal auditory agnosia. The parents notice a gradual inability of the child to respond to their calls despite raising their voices. Verbal auditory agnosia may later progress to non-linguistic sound agnosia such as, for example, the telephone ring. Children with Landau-Kleffner syndrome become incapable of attributing a semantic value to acoustic signals thus making them appear as hypo-acoustic or autistic children. This is why the diagnosis is often delayed, mistaken for acquired deafness or elective mutism. Many of these children have an audiogram, which is normal.

The onset may be subacute progressive or step-wise (stuttering) and gradually worsens and affects other linguistic functions with impairment of expressive speech, paraphasias, stereotypes, perseverations and phonological errors. Probably all types of aphasia can occur. The children express themselves in a telegraphic style or with very simple sentences and some cases may develop fluent aphasia or 'jargon'. Finally, the child may become entirely mute also failing to respond to even non-verbal sounds. One of the most puzzling features of Landau-Kleffner syndrome is the fluctuating course of the linguistic disturbances, characterised by remissions and exacerbations.

Cognitive and behavioural problems occur in more than three quarters of patients with Landau-Kleffner syndrome. Behavioural disorders such as hyperactivity and attention deficit are common and, rarely, there is progression to severe disinhibition and psychosis.

The relative severity of the linguistic, behavioural and cognitive problems can vary over time in the same child and between children. Long-term follow-up studies have shown that Landau-Kleffner syndrome is not always associated with intellectual deterioration.

---

* Although the language disturbance is described as an acquired aphasia, the main deficit is verbal auditory agnosia occurring in an initially normal child who achieved developmental milestones at appropriate ages and has already acquired age-appropriate speech.

The language deficit may be undermined because of other behavioural or cognitive problems.

Seizures: Clinically, seizures may occur in three quarters of the patients but these are usually infrequent and of good prognosis. In one third of them these are single or isolated status epilepticus occurring mainly around 5–10 years. Seizures are often nocturnal, infrequent, respond well to treatment and remit before the age of 13–15 years. Onset is between 4 and 6 years, only 20% of patients continue having seizures after the age of 10 years and in only three cases these persisted after the age of 15.[260] Frequency and severity of seizures

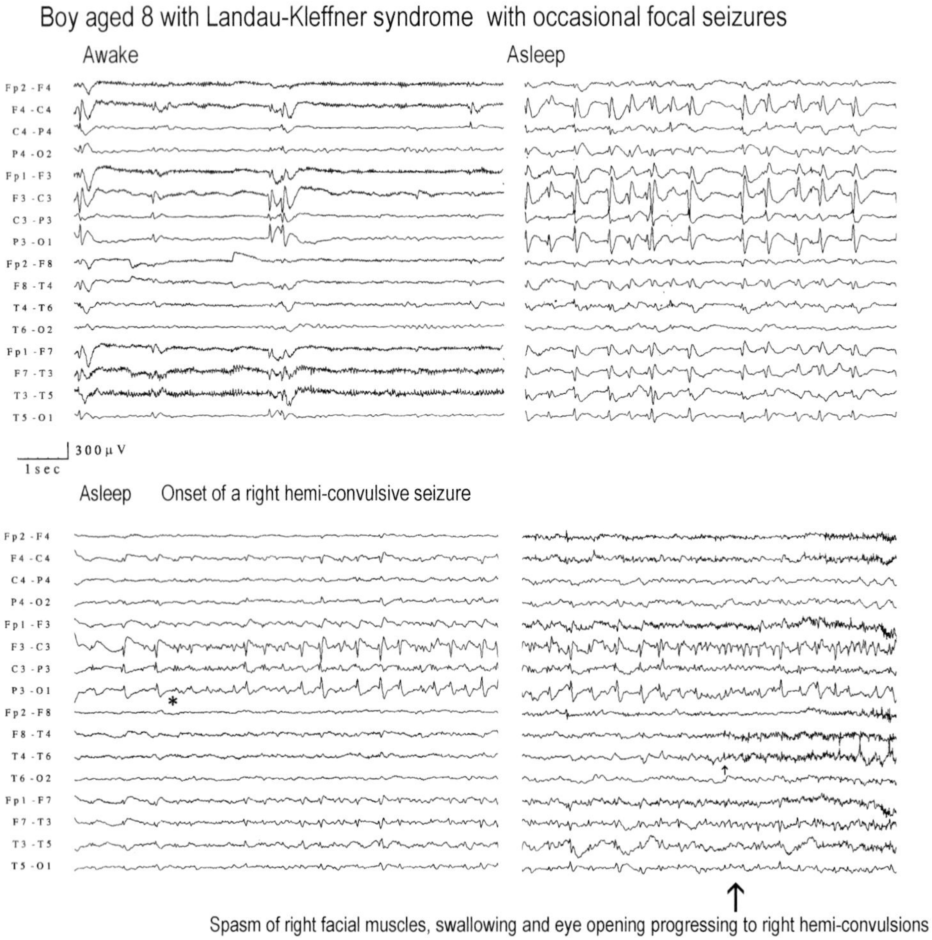

Boy aged 8 with Landau-Kleffner syndrome with occasional focal seizures

Awake   Asleep

Asleep   Onset of a right hemi-convulsive seizure

Spasm of right facial muscles, swallowing and eye opening progressing to right hemi-convulsions

Figure 4.6   From video-EEG of an 8-year-old boy with Landau-Kleffner syndrome before PET scan. He had infrequent seizures, one of which was incidentally captured with video-EEG.

Top: Interictally, there were clusters of sharp and slow wave focal discharges maximum around the left Rolandic regions (left). These became continuous during natural sleep (right).

Bottom: Ictal discharge starts from the left central regions and rapidly spreads to the neighbouring regions. The first clinical signs consisted of right facial spasms (arrow, also note muscle artefacts on the right) progressing to hemiconvulsions.

From Panayiotopoulos (1999)[25] with the permission of the Publisher John Libbey.

are not determined by severity of EEG abnormalities or severity of linguistic and behavioural problems.

Seizure symptoms and seizure type are not well described. They may be heterogeneous. Generalised tonic–clonic seizures (GTCS) and focal motor seizures (Figure 4.6) are emphasised by the Commission.[9] However, atypical absences, atonic seizures with head drop, minor automatisms and secondarily GTCS are reported. Complex focal seizures of temporal lobe origin are very rare and tonic seizures are probably incompatible with Landau–Kleffner syndrome.

Diagnostic procedures: Structural brain imaging is often normal but functional brain imaging demonstrates abnormalities in the temporal lobe.[261]

Electroencephalography is characterised by mainly posterior temporal foci of sharp and slow waves that are often multifocal and bisynchronous, markedly facilitated by slow sleep (Figure 4.7). Continuous spikes and waves during slow sleep occur but this is not a prerequisite for diagnosis.

Prognosis: Seizures and EEG abnormalities are entirely age-dependent and remit by the age of 15 years, although 10–20% of the reported cases continued having infrequent focal motor or GTCS. Language and other neuropsychological disturbances gradually improve at the same age as the

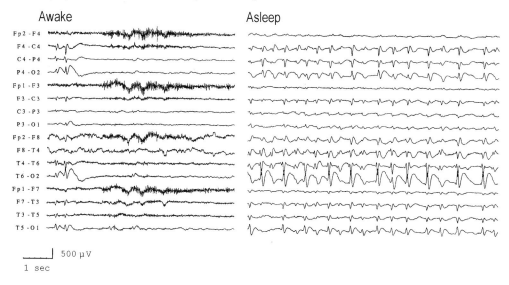

Boy aged 4 with Landau-Kleffner syndrome diagnosed because of this EEG

Awake   Asleep

500 µV
1 sec

Figure 4.7   From video-EEG of a 4-year-old boy referred for possible absence seizures because of 'frequent episodes of inability to understand commands'.

EEG showed clusters of sharp and slow wave focal discharges maximum around the right posterior temporal regions (left).

The technologist allowed time to proceed with sleep EEG during which the paroxysms became continuous (right). The diagnosis of Landau-Kleffner syndrome was made on appropriate clinico-psychological testing.

disappearance of EEG epileptiform activity but although some 10–20% may achieve complete normalisation all others are left with permanent sequelae that may be very severe. There is a consensus that an early onset of Landau-Kleffner syndrome is related with the worst prognosis regarding language recovery. Outcome does not depend on frequency and type of seizures. Only half of patients with Landau-Kleffner syndrome may be able to live a relatively normal social and professional life.

Pathophysiology: Landau-Kleffner syndrome is probably the result of an epileptogenic functional lesion in the speech cortex during a critical period of child development.

Differential diagnosis: The diagnosis of Landau-Kleffner syndrome is clinical, irrespective of EEG and other seizure features. Conversely, the diagnosis of a similarly age-related condition of 'epilepsy with continuous spike and waves during slow wave sleep' (ECSWS) detailed later (page 85), is mainly based on EEG criteria irrespective of clinical manifestations. **Landau-Kleffner syndrome by definition cannot exist without linguistic manifestations, while ECSWS cannot be diagnosed without EEG continuous spikes and wave during sleep.**[262]

Medical treatment: Seizures in Landau-Kleffner syndrome are infrequent, age-limited and often easily controlled with antiepileptic drugs. Therefore, the pharmaceutical attempt is to reduce the epileptiform EEG discharges with the assumption that these are responsible for the linguistic, behavioural and other neuropsychological abnormalities. All traditional antiepileptic drugs, including sleep-modifying drugs such as amitriptyline and amphetamine, have been tried with disappointing results. However, some children responded rather well to high doses of steroids or adrenocorticotropin hormone (ACTH).

The consensus is to first treat Landau-Kleffner syndrome with sodium valproate, ethosuximide and clonazepam or clobazam, alone or in combination. If this fails, which is most likely, ACTH or prednisone should be the treatment of choice, especially in new and younger patients who may respond better, need shorter steroid treatment and are at a high risk for significant residual neuropsychological sequelae. There is an empirical view that the results depend on early treatment and high initial doses of steroids for at least 3 months. Continuation of treatment after this period depends on response and side-effects. Some children with a good response may relapse and this may necessitate lengthy (probably years) continuation of treatment. Steroids are usually used together with valproate or benzodiazepines and these may remain after steroid wean.

The effect of treatment should be monitored with appropriate neuropsychological evaluation and serial awake and sleep EEG.

However, all these approaches are empirical and anecdotal from clinical practice using what was available – old antiepileptic drugs. Naturally, this will now expand to include experience with newer antiepileptic drugs (levetiracetam, lamotrigine, topiramate and zonisamide) that hopefully may offer more successful treatment outcomes.

Neurosurgical treatment: In medically intractable cases of Landau–Kleffner syndrome subpial intracortical transections have been used with relatively good success.[259,263] This ingenious surgical technique has been designed to eliminate the capacity of cortical tissue to generate seizures while preserving the normal cortical physiological function. Success depends on selection of cases with severe epileptogenic abnormality that can be demonstrated to be unilateral in origin despite a bilateral electrographic manifestation.

EPILEPSY WITH CONTINUOUS SPIKE AND WAVES DURING SLOW WAVE SLEEP [256,262,264–267]

Epilepsy with continuous spike and waves during slow wave sleep (ECSWS) or epilepsy with electrical status epilepticus during slow sleep (ESESS) is a partly reversible, age-related childhood clinical syndrome characterised by the triad of:

1. EEG continuous spikes and waves during slow sleep (Figure 4.8)

2. seizures and

3. neuropsychological decline.

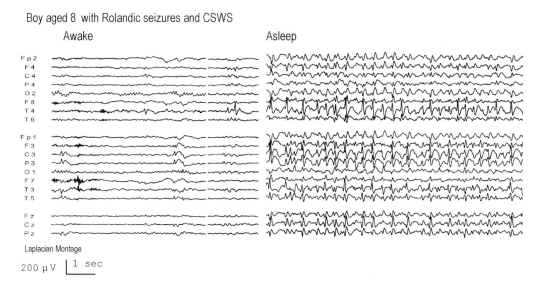

Boy aged 8 with Rolandic seizures and CSWS

Figure 4.8 From video-EEG of an 8-year-old boy who at age 8 weeks had three focal seizures of right-sided convulsions involving face and upper limbs (Figure 3.1; page 54). Subsequent development was excellent but at age 7 years he started having Rolandic seizures and later developed ECSWS associated with impaired scholastic performance (case 17.2 in ref [25]).

When alert, EEG shows infrequent clusters of focal sharp and slow wave discharges (left), which become continuous during sleep (right).

Continuous spikes and waves during slow wave sleep (CSWS) are a prerequisite for the diagnosis of this syndrome.

Demographic data: This syndrome of ECSWS is age-dependent, occurring only in children. Onset of seizures is between 1 and 10 years, with a peak at 4–5 years. The age at onset of CSWS is not certain but may peak at age 8 years with a range from 3 to 14 years, usually starting 1–2 years after the first seizure. There may be a male preponderance (62%).[268] Prevalence is of no more than 0.5% among children with seizures.

Clinical manifestations: More than one third of patients with ECSWS have abnormal neurological signs. Pre- or peri-natal illness, neonatal convulsions, congenital hemiparesis or tetraparesis, psychomotor or language retardation are found in approximately half of the cases. There are three stages of evolution.

The first stage (before the discovery of CSWS) manifests with mainly infrequent nocturnal motor focal seizures, often hemi-clonic status epilepticus and EEG with focal and bi-synchronous generalised discharges.

The second stage (with CSWS) is usually 1–2 years after the first seizure. The discovery of CSWS is usually a result of seizure increase and neuropsychological symptoms that prompt a sleep EEG, which shows continuous spikes and waves during slow sleep.

Seizures become more frequent and complicated with other types of seizures such as typical or more frequent atypical absences, myoclonic absences, absence status, atonic or clonic fits, oro-facial and generalised tonic-clonic convulsions. The general consensus is that tonic seizures do not occur at any stage and are probably incompatible with the diagnosis of ECSWS. The decline of the neuropsychological state and behaviour abnormalities are the most cardinal and disturbing clinical features of ECSWS. Many of these children suffer from complex and severe neuropsychological impairment, mainly of language-related functions, with mental impairment and psychiatric disturbances that may be lifelong, despite some improvement, after an age-related remission of seizures and CSWS. There is a dramatic, sometimes sudden but often insidious decline of the psychomotor development of these children at the time that CSWS is discovered.

Third stage. After a variable period of months to usually 2–7 years this aggressive disorder starts improving and finally all patients remit regarding seizures and EEG gradually improves to normalisation. The neuropsychological state also improves but children rarely reach average normal; more frequently patients are left with significant deficits.

Diagnostic procedures: Brain imaging and particularly MRI is mandatory. More than one third of patients with ECSWS have abnormal brain imaging such as unilateral or diffuse cortical atrophy, porencephaly and developmental brain malformations.

Electroencephalography: ECSWS is mainly an EEG-defined syndrome. Diagnosis can be suspected with brief sleep recordings (Figure 4.8) but all-night sleep recordings are usually needed.

Tassinari described continuous spikes and waves during slow wave sleep as follows:[268]

'As soon as the patient falls asleep continuous bilateral and diffuse slow spike and wave (SW) appear, persisting through all the slow sleep stages. It is not a matter of an "important" or "almost subcontinuous" activation. Indeed, the discharges are continuous and the SW index ranges from 85 to 100 per cent. The SW index was calculated during all-night sleep EEG recordings. It is equal to the total sum of all spike-waves (min) × 100 divided by the total non-REM duration (min). However, other authors also include diseases with a SW index higher than 50 per cent. Thus, they considerably widen the definition of CSWS, from a continuous status of SW, as in our own definition, to a considerable amount of SW during slow sleep. With this method, we have noted that percentage of CSWS is more marked during the first cycle of sleep (95–100%) than in the following cycles (80–70%), but the overall percentage is equal to 85. The physiological sleep patterns (spindles, K complexes or vertex spikes) were seldom distinguishable. In some cases, focal abnormalities, with frontal predominance, can be observed during the rare short periods (seconds) of fragmented diffuse SW discharges in non-REM sleep. During REM sleep the electrical status disappears and the paroxysmal abnormalities consist of rare bursts of diffuse SW, or of focal, predominantly frontal discharges. In four patients, focal, fronto-central rhythmic discharges organized as a subclinical seizure were observed at the end of REM sleep.'

The CSWS consists mainly of spike and wave with no polyspikes or fast episodic activity, which is against this diagnosis. The intradischarge frequency is usually slow (1.5–2 Hz) but faster rates (3–4 Hz) can occur. CSWS is a consistent finding over the active lifespan of this condition.

Physiological slow sleep patterns, the differentiation of non-REM sleep and REM sleep is possible because of the preservation of EEG and polygraphic REM sleep patterns concomitant with the REM-related discontinuation of CSWS. The cyclic organisation of sleep is grossly preserved, 80% of sleep is NREM and there are no apparent sleep disorders. On awakening, EEG abnormalities are similar to those of wakefulness.

Longitudinal sleep EEG studies show a progressive improvement (over approximately 3 years), towards normalisation after an average age of about 11 years.

Differential diagnosis:[267] The main problem is differentiation from patients with Landau-Kleffner syndrome whose EEG shows continuous spikes and waves during slow wave sleep.

However, in Landau-Kleffner syndrome:

- acquired aphasia is the most predominant neuropsychological symptom

- epileptic seizures may not occur and

- interictal EEG foci are mainly temporal while these are mainly frontal in ECSWS.

The second problem in differential diagnosis is with the benign childhood seizure susceptibility syndrome because of the exaggeration of spikes during sleep and atypical evolutions (page 89).

The distinguishing features from Lennox–Gastaut syndrome include:

- the characteristic EEG patterns

- focal motor seizures are rare in Lennox–Gastaut syndrome while tonic seizures are essentially absent in ECSWS and

- overall clinical and seizure improvement over the course of the illness in ECSWS.

Prognosis: Seizures remit in all cases, although they may be initially intractable for months to years. All patients show a global improvement regarding cognitive and behavioural abnormalities after the remission of CSWS and seizures but recovery is always slow and often only partial. Less than one quarter of the patients will resume acceptable social and professional levels and these are more likely among those who had a normal pre-morbid neuropsychological state and a shorter CSWS lifespan.

Management:[267] Seizures may or may not respond to a variety of drugs. The combined use of benzodiazepines and valproate is considered the treatment of choice in this condition. Of the new drugs, lamotrigine, levetiracetam and topiramate may be tried. Carbamazepine may exaggerate continuous spikes and waves during slow sleep.[25]

Only benzodiazepines and adrenocorticotrophic hormone appear to transiently suppress the electrical status and perhaps to improve language function. Short cycles (3–4 weeks) of diazepam (0.5 mg/kg) following a rectal diazepam bolus of 1 mg/kg have been used with some benefit. In cases with severe linguistic impairment subpial intracortical transections have been used with success.[259,263]

BENIGN CHILDHOOD FOCAL SEIZURES AND RELATED SYNDROMES 5

BENIGN CHILDHOOD SEIZURE SUSCEPTIBILITY

Benign childhood focal seizures and related epileptic syndromes are the commonest and probably the most fascinating and rewarding topic in paediatric epileptology.[25] They form a significant part of the everyday practice of paediatricians, neurologists and clinical neurophysiologists who care for children with seizures.

The new diagnostic scheme recognises three syndromes of 'idiopathic childhood focal epilepsy':[10]

1. **Benign childhood epilepsy with centrotemporal spikes (BCECTS)**

2. **Early onset benign childhood occipital epilepsy (Panayiotopoulos type)**

3. **Late onset childhood occipital epilepsy (Gastaut type).**

Considerations on classification

The following should be considered in future revisions of the classification:

1. 'Benign childhood epilepsy with centrotemporal spikes' may (a) occur without centrotemporal spikes; (b) most of the centrotemporal spikes are in fact Rolandic spikes, rarely their location is in the temporal electrodes and (c) similar clinical features may appear in patients with spikes in other than centrotemporal locations. Rolandic seizures/epilepsy may be the most appropriate nomenclature; this is how most paediatricians identify this syndrome and there is no reason why this should change.

2. Early onset benign childhood occipital epilepsy (Panayiotopoulos type) is not 'occipital'. (a) Onset is with autonomic manifestations, which are unlikely to be of occipital origin. Of all other seizure symptoms only eye deviation, which often is not the first ictal symptom, may originate from the occipital lobes. (b) Interictal occipital spikes may never occur and

(c) even ictal EEG has documented anterior or posterior origin. Currently, most authors prefer the eponymic nomenclature 'Panayiotopoulos syndrome' to include all patients with this syndrome irrespective of EEG spikes or topographic terminology.[36,269–271]

3. Other than these three clinico-EEG phenotypes have been documented. All can be unified as 'benign childhood seizure susceptibility syndrome'.

4. Rolandic and Panayiotopoulos syndrome do not fulfil the diagnostic criteria of 'epilepsy' defined as a *'chronic* neurological condition characterised by *recurrent* epileptic seizures.[11] Rolandic and Panayiotopoulos syndrome are age-limited (not 'chronic') and at least one third of patients have a single (not recurrent) seizures. They should be classified among *'Conditions with epileptic seizures that do not require a diagnosis of epilepsy'* which is a new concept of the ILAE proposal to incorporate febrile, benign neonatal, single seizures or isolated clusters of seizures and rarely repeated seizures (oligoepilepsy).[10]

Abbreviations:
BCECTS = benign childhood epilepsy with centrotemporal spikes
BCSSS = benign childhood seizure susceptibility syndrome
COE = childhood occipital epilepsy
CSWS = continuous spike and waves during slow wave sleep

CTS = centrotemporal spikes
ECSWS = epilepsy with continuous spike and waves during slow wave sleep
GTCS = generalised tonic-clonic seizures
OPL = oropharyngolaryngeal
RS = Rolandic seizures

BENIGN CHILDHOOD EPILEPSY WITH CENTRO-TEMPORAL SPIKES (ROLANDIC SEIZURES) [25,272–276]

Benign childhood epilepsy with centrotemporal spikes (BCECTS) or Rolandic seizures/epilepsy (RS) is the commonest manifestation of a childhood seizure susceptibility syndrome that is age-related and genetically determined.

Demographic data: Onset is between 1 and 14 years, three quarters start between 7 and 10 years and there is a peak at 8–9 years. There is a 1.5 male preponderance. Prevalence is around 15% of children with seizures aged 1–15 years. Incidence is 10–20/100,000 children aged 0–15 years.

Clinical manifestations: The cardinal features of BCECTS are infrequent, often single, focal seizures consisting of unilateral facial sensorimotor symptoms, oropharyngolaryngeal (OPL) manifestations, speech arrest and hypersalivation.

Hemifacial sensorimotor seizures, mainly motor, occur in approximately one third of the patients. These may be entirely localised in the lower lip manifesting with sudden, continuous or bursts of clonic contractions, lasting usually seconds to 1 minute. Consciousness is usually preserved. Hemifacial sensorimotor motor seizures may be the only ictal manifestation but often this is associated with inability to speak and hypersalivation. More rarely, ictal symptoms of clonic convulsions may appear nearly simultaneously or spread to the ipsilateral upper extremity. Involvement of the leg is rare.

> The left side of my mouth felt numb and started jerking and pulling to the left and I could not speak to say what was happening to me

Arrest of speech is another common ictal symptom occurring in >40% of RS. The child is inarticulate and attempts to communicate with gestures. A few mainly laryngeal sounds, not words, may be uttered particularly at the beginning. There is no impairment of the cortical language mechanisms.

> My right hand was numb and stiff. My mouth opened and I could not speak. I wanted to say I cannot speak. At the same time it was as if somebody was strangulating me.
>
> She was tryng to speak but only noises came out of her mouth as if her tongue was tied up in her mouth

Oropharyngolaryngeal manifestations are unilateral numbness and dysaesthesia inside the mouth, cheek, teeth and tongue alone or usually with motor phenomena producing strange sounds such as death rattle, gargling, grunting, guttural sounds and their combinations.

Hypersalivation is one of the most characteristic ictal symptoms of RS, probably occurring in as many as one third of them. This is often associated with OPL symptoms but also with pure hemifacial seizures and may be the most pronounced ictal manifestation.

> Suddenly my mouth is full of saliva, it runs out like a river and I cannot speak

Ictal syncope may occur probably as a concurrent symptom of Panayiotopoulos syndrome (page 96).

> She lies there, unconscious with no movements, no convulsions, like a wax, no life

Consciousness is fully retained in more than half (58%) of RS and the patient is able to describe well the events after the fits.

> I felt that air was forced into my mouth, I could not speak and I could not close my mouth. I could understand well everything said to me. Other times I feel that there is food in my mouth and there is also a lot of salivation. I cannot speak.

Duration is usually brief, for 1–2 minutes, but may last longer if seizures progress to convulsions.

Secondarily GTCS are reported in one to two thirds of children with RS. Primarily GTCS are not part of the syndrome of RS.

Circadian distribution: Three quarters of the seizures are nocturnal.

Genetics: Febrile seizures before RS are common (10–20%). Evidence has been reported for linkage of RS to a region on chromosome 15q14.[277]

Diagnostic procedures: All tests except EEG are normal.

Interictal EEG shows centrotemporal spikes (CTS) that are high amplitude sharp and slow wave complexes localised in the 10/20 EEG electrode placement system in the central or mid-temporal electrodes (Figures 5.1, 5.2 and 5.3). These may be unilateral but more often they are bilateral; they are abundant, 4–20 per minute, usually occurring in clusters. They show marked accentuation during sleep by a factor of 2–5 and in 10–20% these may also be evoked by somatosensory stimuli of the fingers or toes. Rarely, children with RS may have CTS only during sleep, the spikes may be very small or the EEG is normal.

The main negative spike component of CTS can usually be modelled by a single and stable tangential dipole source along the rolandic region with the negative pole maximum at the centrotemporal and the positive pole maximum at the frontal regions.

Centrotemporal spikes may occur simultaneously in the same EEG with morphologically similar sharp and slow waves in other locations such as midline, parietal, frontal and occipital. These multi-focal sharp waves are more frequently seen in serial EEG where occipital spikes are usually first to appear.

Frequency, location and persistence of centrotemporal spikes do not determine clinical manifestations, severity and frequency of seizures or prognosis.

Centrotemporal spikes occur in 2–3% of normal school-age children with <10% of them developing Rolandic seizures. They are age-dependent, appearing at a peak age of 7–10 years, often persisting despite clinical remission and usually disappearing before the age of 16 years. They are common among relatives of children with RS. Age-dependent centrotemporal spikes frequently occur in a variety of organic brain diseases with or without seizures.

The combination of a normal child with infrequent seizures and an EEG with disproportionately severe focal epileptogenic activity is highly suggestive of benign childhood seizure susceptibility syndrome.[25]

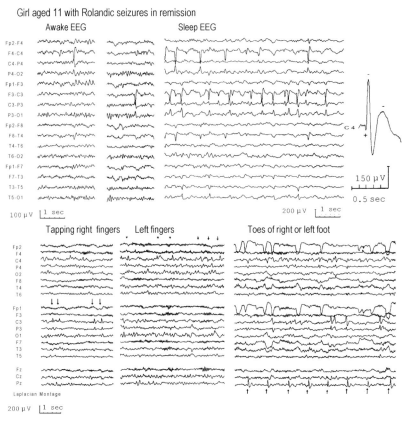

Girl aged 11 with Rolandic seizures in remission

Figure 5.1   From video-EEG of an 11-year-old girl with Rolandic seizures in remission from age 8.

Top: High amplitude centrotemporal spikes (in fact these are central) occur independently right or left and they are markedly exaggerated during natural slow sleep.

Top extreme left: Typical morphology of centrotemporal spikes.

Bottom: Giant somatosensory evoked spikes are evoked by tapping fingers or toes. Note that their location corresponds to the location of the activating stimulus.

From Panayiotopoulos (1999)[25] with permission of the publisher John Libbey.

Facing page **Figure 5.2**   Centrotemporal spikes are mainly Rolandic not temporal spikes.[25,278]

Top, middle and bottom are the same EEG sample at three different montages. This 8-year-old boy was referred for an EEG because of 'a recent GTCS and a 2-year history of unilateral facial spasms. Previously EEG and CT brain scan were normal. No medication. Focal seizures with secondarily generalised convulsions?'

The EEG showed frequent clusters of repetitive centrotemporal spikes on the left. Because the

spikes appeared of higher amplitude in the temporal electrode (T3) (black arrows) the technologist rightly applied additional electrodes at C5 and C6 areas (Rolandic localisation). This showed that the spike is of higher amplitude in the left Rolandic region (C5) (open arrows).

Another EEG 16 months later showed a few small spikes in the right frontal and central midline electrodes.

Clarification

I comply in this book with the nomenclature **'centrotemporal spikes'** although these are rarely temporal; Rolandic spikes would be a more accurate name (see Figure 5.2).

Boy aged 8 with Rolandic seizures- Spikes are Rolandic not Centrotemporal

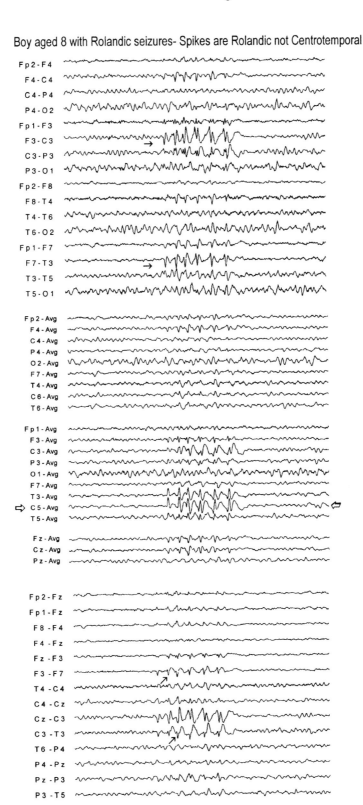

Spikes at C5 electrode

150 µV   1 sec

Evolution and prognosis: Remission occurs within 2–4 years from onset and before the age of 16 years. The total number of seizures is low, 10–20% of patients have a single seizure, most have less than 10 but 10–20% may have frequent seizures that also remit.

Children with RS may develop reversible linguistic abnormalities during the active phase of their disease.[25] Hospital-based studies emphasise learning or behavioural problems that require intervention.[279,280] A few patients (<1%) may derail to atypical evolutions of more severe syndromes of linguistic, behavioural and neuropsychological deficits such as Landau–Kleffner syndrome, atypical focal epilepsy of childhood or epilepsy with continuous spikes and waves during slow sleep.[281,282]

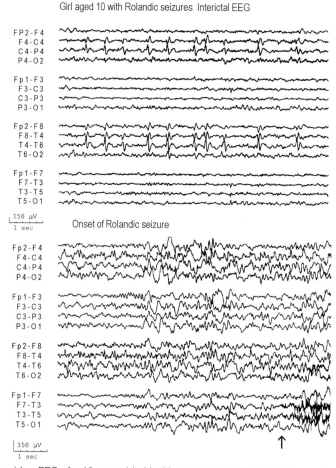

Figure 5.3   From video-EEG of a 10-year-old girl with recent onset Rolandic seizures (case 5.1 in ref [25]).

Top: High amplitude right-sided centrotemporal spikes (C5 and C6 electrodes were not applied). *Bottom:* Onset of ictal discharge in the right centrotemporal regions during sleep. Arrow shows onset of clinical manifestations that started with contractions of the left facial muscles (note muscle artefacts on the left) progressing to a prolonged generalised clonic seizure for 5 minutes.

From Panayiotopoulos (1999)[25] with permission of the publisher John Libbey.

Prognosis is invariably excellent with <2% risk of developing infrequent generalised seizures in adult life.

Management: Children with Rolandic epilepsy may not need antiepileptic medication, particularly if the seizures are infrequent, mild, nocturnal or onset is close to the age of natural remission of this age-limited disorder. See details in 'Management of benign childhood focal seizures' (page 107).

PANAYIOTOPOULOS SYNDROME [36,269,270,283–294]

Panayiotopoulos syndrome is a childhood-related idiopathic benign susceptibility to focal, mainly autonomic seizures and autonomic status epilepticus. The children have normal physical and neuropsychological development.

Demographic data: Age at onset is between 1 and 14 years, with a peak at 4–5 years; 76% start between 3 and 6 years. Boys and girls are equally affected. Children of all races are vulnerable. Prevalence is around 13% of children aged 3–6 years with one or more non-febrile seizures and 6% of the age group 1–15 years; 2–3 per 1000 of the general population of children may be affected. These figures may be higher if cases with currently considered atypical features are included.

Seizure characteristics: Seizures comprise an unusual constellation of autonomic, mainly emetic, symptoms often with unilateral deviation of the

---

Definitions of autonomic seizures and autonomic status epilepticus

Autonomic auras consist of a subjective awareness of a change in the activity of autonomic nervous system function.[295]

Autonomic seizures consist of episodic altered autonomic function of any type at onset or as the sole manifestation of an epileptic event. These may be objective, subjective or both. They must be distinguished from secondary (indirect) effects on the autonomic system by other seizure symptoms.[296]

Pure autonomic seizures are those that solely consist of episodic altered autonomic function from onset to the end.

In the absence of a definition for autonomic status epilepticus, the term I propose is:

Autonomic status epilepticus: is an autonomic seizure that lasts for more than 30 minutes.

Pure autonomic status epilepticus is a pure autonomic seizure that lasts for more than 30 minutes.

Considerations on the classification of autonomic status epilepticus

Childhood autonomic status epilepticus, common and specific, has been ignored in all classifications.[36,297] The new ILAE diagnostic scheme[10] recognises four forms of focal status epilepticus (Table 1.2):[10,298] (a) epilepsia partialis continua of Kozhevnikov, (b) aura continua, (c) limbic status epilepticus (psychomotor status) and (d) hemi-convulsive status with hemi-paresis.

Further, I quote from the relevant ILAE chapter:[298] 'From a clinical point of view aura continua is classified into: (a) somatosensory, i.e. dysaesthesia phenomena that involve the trunk, head and extremities; (b) aura continua that involve the special senses (visual, auditory, vertiginous, gustatory and olfactory). Furthermore aura continua with predominantly (c) autonomic symptoms, and (d) with psychic symptoms can be distinguished'.[298]

It is anticipated that future revisions of the ILAE classifications will recognise this type of autonomic status epilepticus, which also occurs in symptomatic childhood disorders.[36,297]

eyes and other more conventional ictal manifestations. In a typical presentation, a child who is fully conscious, able to speak and understand, complains, 'I feel sick', looks pale and vomits. Two thirds of the seizures start in sleep; the child may wake up with similar complaints while still conscious or else may be found vomiting, conscious, confused or unresponsive.

> Clinically, while asleep, 'he suddenly got up with both eyes open, vomited several times and then showed a prolonged atonic state with cyanosis and irregular respiration for 3 min' (from ictal EEG documentation by Oguni and associates)[286]

The full emetic triad (nausea, retching, vomiting) culminates in vomiting in 74% of the seizures; in others only nausea or retching occurs and in a few, emesis may not be apparent. Other autonomic manifestations may occur concurrently or appear later in the course of the ictus. These include pallor and less often flushing or cyanosis, mydriasis and less often miosis, cardio-respiratory and thermo-regulatory alterations, incontinence of urine and/or faeces and modifications of intestinal motility. Hypersalivation (probably a concurrent Rolandic symptom) may occur. Headache and more often cephalic auras that may be autonomic manifestations may occur particularly at onset. Apnoea and cardiac asystole may be common but only exceptionally are these severe.

More conventional seizure symptoms often ensue. The child gradually or suddenly becomes confused and unresponsive; exceptionally consciousness may be preserved (6%). Eyes and often the head deviate to one side (60%) or eyes gaze widely open (12%). Other symptoms in order of prevalence are speech arrest (8%), hemi-facial spasms (6%), visual hallucinations (6%), oropharyngolaryngeal movements (3%), unilateral drooping of the mouth (3%), eyelid jerks (1%), myoclonic jerks (1%), ictal nystagmus and automatisms (1%). These probably reflect the primary area of the seizure discharge generation. The seizures commonly end with hemiconvulsions often with Jacksonian march (19%) or generalised convulsions (21%).

Ictal syncope is an intriguing and important ictal feature of Panayiotopoulos syndrome. In at least one fifth of the seizures the child becomes unresponsive and flaccid (ictal syncope) before or without convulsions or in isolation.

> Suddenly and without warning she collapsed and became unresponsive while talking to her teacher.
> She complained of 'dizziness' and then her eyes deviated to the left, she fell on the floor and she became totally flaccid and unresponsive for 5 minutes.

Definition

'Ictal syncope' denotes transient loss of consciousness and postural tone that occurs in a seizure before or without convulsions. Ictal syncope is a common and dramatic occurrence in Panayiotopoulos syndrome. The child becomes 'completely unresponsive and flaccid like a rag doll' before and often without convulsions or in isolation.

Hemiconvulsive (2%) or generalised convulsive status (2%) is exceptional. The same child may have seizures with marked autonomic manifestations and seizures where autonomic manifestations may be inconspicuous. The clinical seizure manifestations are roughly the same irrespective of EEG localisations, although there may be slightly less autonomic and slightly more focal motor features at onset in children without occipital spikes.

Duration of seizures: Nearly half (44%) of the seizures last for more than 30 minutes up to 7 hours (mean ~2 hours) constituting autonomic status epilepticus. Of the other half (54%) duration varies from 1 to 30 minutes with a mean of 9 minutes. Lengthy seizures are equally common in sleep and wakefulness. Even after the most severe seizures and status, the patient is normal after a few hours' sleep. There is no record of residual neurological or mental abnormalities. The same child may have brief and lengthy seizures.

Precipitating factors: There are no apparent precipitating factors other than sleep. Fixation-off sensitivity is an EEG phenomenon, which may not be clinically important.

Diagnostic procedures: By definition of an idiopathic syndrome, neurological and mental assessment and high-resolution MRI are normal. The most useful laboratory test is EEG (Figure 5.4). The most important determinant of the neurodiagnostic procedures is the state of the child at the time of first medical attendance.

The child has a typical brief or lengthy seizure of Panayiotopoulos syndrome but fully recovers before arriving in the accident and emergency department or being seen by a physician. A child with the distinctive clinical features of Panayiotopoulos syndrome, particularly ictus emeticus and lengthy seizures, may not need any investigations other than EEG. However, because approximately 10–20% of children with similar seizures may have brain pathology an MRI may be needed.

The child with a typical lengthy seizure of Panayiotopoulos syndrome is partially recovering although still in a post-ictal stage, tired, mildly confused and drowsy on arrival at the accident and emergency department or when seen by a physician. The child should be kept under medical supervision until full recovery, which is the rule after a few hours of sleep. Then guidelines are the same as noted above.

The child is brought to the accident and emergency department or is seen by a physician while ictal symptoms continue. This is the most difficult and challenging situation. There may be dramatic symptoms accumulating in succession, which demand rigorous and experienced evaluation. A history of a previous similar seizure is re-assuring and may prevent further procedures.

Electroencephalography: EEG commonly (90% of cases) reveals functional mainly multifocal high amplitude sharp and slow wave complexes (Figure 5.4). **There is a great EEG variability of functional focal spikes at various electrode locations.** All brain regions are involved although the posterior predominate (Figures 5.4 and 5.5). Two thirds (68%) of patients have at least one EEG with occipital spikes, which are often (64%) concurrent with extra-occipital spikes in at least one EEG. The other third (32%) never show occipital spikes. Instead they have extra-occipital spikes (21%) only, consistently normal EEG (9%) or brief generalised discharges only (2%). EEG with multifocal spikes in more than two and often many brain locations occurs in one third (30%) of the patients; single spike foci are rare (9%). Cloned–like repetitive multifocal spike wave complexes may be characteristic features when they occur (19%).

EEG variability in Panayiotopoulos syndrome in 6 children with autonomic seizures

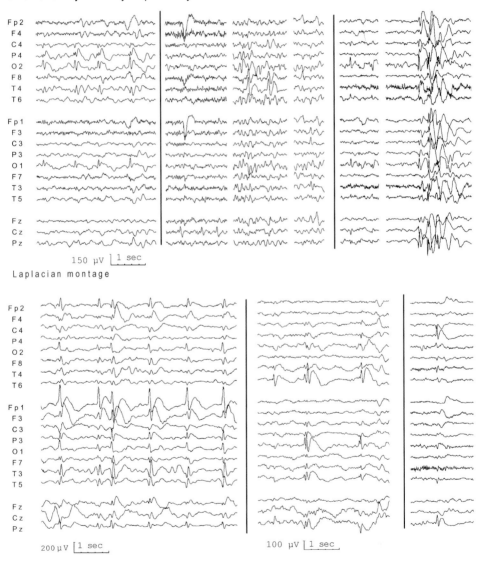

Figure 5.4   EEG variability in Panayiotopoulos syndrome.

Samples from EEGs of six children with typical clinical manifestations of Panayiotopoulos syndrome. Spikes may occur in all electrode locations, they are usually of high amplitude and frequent or repetitive but may also be small and sparse. Brief generalised discharges of small spike and slow wave may be present.

Spikes are usually of high amplitude and morphologically similar to the centro–gyral (Rolandic) spikes. However, small and even inconspicuous spikes may appear in the same or previous EEG of children with giant spikes. Although rare, small positive spikes or other unusual EEG spike configurations may occur.

Brief generalised discharges of slow waves intermixed with small spikes may occur either alone (4%) or more often with focal spikes (15%).

The EEG spikes may be stimulus-sensitive; occipital paroxysms are commonly (47%) activated by the elimination of central vision and fixation while centro–gyral spikes may be elicited by somato–sensory stimuli. Occipital photosensitivity is an exceptional finding.

Functional spikes in any location are accentuated by sleep. If a routine EEG is normal, a sleep EEG should be performed. There is no particular relationship between the likelihood of an abnormal EEG and the interval since the last seizure. EEGs performed soon or some time after a seizure are equally

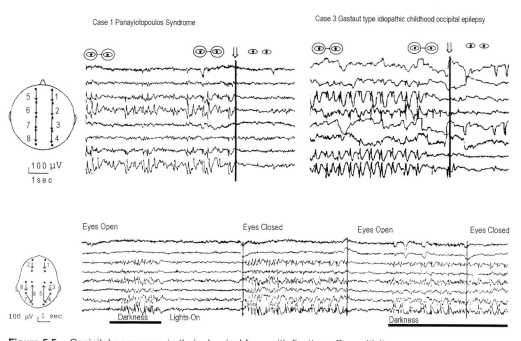

Figure 5.5   Occipital paroxysms in their classical form with fixation-off sensitivity.

Top: EEG of two patients with Panayiotopoulos syndrome and Gastaut-type COE. In routine EEG repetitive high amplitude occipital sharp and slow wave complexes (occipital paroxysms) occur immediately after closing of the eyes and as long as the eyes are closed. The EEG normalises immediately after opening of the eyes and as long as the eyes are open. The activation of the occipital paroxysms is due to the elimination of central vision and fixation (left of the vertical bar, symbol of eyes with glasses) and inhibition by fixation (right of the vertical bar, symbol of eyes without glasses).

Bottom: Effect of darkness on occipital paroxysms: (a) complete darkness activates the occipital paroxysms even when eyes are open; and (b) the occipital paroxysms become continuous in darkness irrespective of whether the eyes are open or closed.

From Panayiotopoulos (1981)[283] with the permission of the Editor of *Neurology.*

likely to manifest with functional spikes which may occur only once in serial routine and sleep EEGs.

Girl aged 8 with Panayiotopoulos syndrome; Ictal EEG of a 9 minutes seizure with ictal vomniting

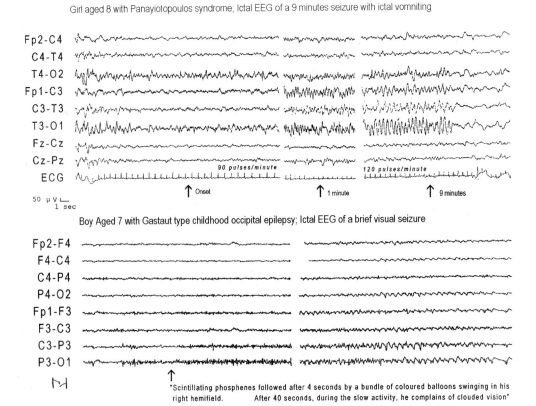

Figure 5.6 (Top) Ictal EEGs in Panayiotopoulos syndrome, (bottom) Gastaut-type childhood occipital epilepsy.

Top: Samples of continuous EEG recording from onset to the end of a 9-minute seizure at sleep stage II of an 8-year-old girl. Clinically this manifested with awakening, eyes opening, frequent vomiting efforts and complaints of frontal headache.[299] The ictal EEG started with remission of the interictal occipital paroxysms and the appearance of occipital sharp rhythms progressing to monomorphic rhythmic theta activity in the bi-occipital regions but mainly involving the right hemisphere in a wider posterior distribution. The slow activity slowed down with the progress of the seizure and ended without post-ictal abnormalities. ECG showed significant tachycardia during the ictus.[299]

Bottom: Ictal EEG during a visual seizure of a boy with Gastaut-type childhood occipital epilepsy. The seizure starts from the left occipital region with fast rhythms associated with visual symptoms. Four seconds later this spreads to the parietal regions and the child sees a bundle of coloured balloons swinging in his right hemifield. This lasted for 40 seconds followed by slow waves, progressively becoming slower and diffuse over the whole brain. At this stage he complained of clouded vision. This boy was normal physically and intellectually and also had a normal CT brain scan. At age 3 years he had a nocturnal left hemi-convulsion. His first EEG showed occipital paroxysms with fixation-off sensitivity. Since the age of 4 years he started having frequent, brief visual seizures (simple coloured visual hallucinations) provoked by sudden darkness.

From Beaumanoir (1993)[299] with permission of the author and the publisher John Libbey.

The background EEG is usually normal but diffuse or localised slow wave abnormality may also occur in at least one EEG of 20% of patients, particularly post-ictally. EEG abnormalities, particularly functional spikes, may persist after clinical remission for many years until mid-teens. Conversely, spikes may appear only once in one of a series of EEGs.

Frequency, location and persistence of functional spikes do not determine clinical manifestations, duration, severity and frequency of seizures or prognosis.

Ictal EEG: Typical cases of Panayiotopoulos syndrome have been documented with ictal EEG (Figure 5.6).[286,290,299] The seizure discharge consists mainly of rhythmic theta or delta activity intermixed with usually small spikes. Onset is unilateral, often posterior but may also be anterior and not strictly localised to one electrode.

Differential diagnosis: Panayiotopoulos syndrome is easy to diagnose because of the characteristic clustering of clinical seizure semiology, which is often supported by interictal EEG findings. The main problem is to recognise emetic and other autonomic manifestations as seizure events and not to dismiss them or erroneously to consider them as unrelated to the ictus and a feature of encephalitis, migraine, syncope or gastro-enteritis. As regards other epileptic conditions the following should be noted. (a) In symptomatic causes of similar autonomic seizures and autonomic status epilepticus in children, there is often abnormal neurological or mental symptomatology, abnormal brain imaging and EEG background abnormalities. (b) Panayiotopoulos syndrome and Gastaut-type idiopathic childhood occipital epilepsy have entirely different clinical manifestations despite common interictal EEG when occipital paroxysms occur (Figure 5.5). (c) Rolandic seizures have different clinical manifestations and emesis has not been reported. However, in some cases of Panayiotopoulos syndrome there are concurrent Rolandic symptoms. This should not be a problem as the management and the prognosis for both syndromes are the same. (d) Cases of Panayiotopoulos syndrome with seizures occurring when the child is febrile may be diagnosed as febrile seizures but this again is of no prognostic significance.

Genetic and other factors: Usually, there is no family history of similar disorders of benign childhood seizure susceptibility, epilepsies or migraine. However, it appears that there is a high prevalence of febrile seizures (~17%). Also, there is a high incidence of abnormal birth deliveries which may be aetiologically linked, these factors need re-evaluation.

Pathophysiology: Clinical and EEG findings indicate that there is a diffuse cortical hyper-excitability, which is maturation-related. This diffuse epileptogenicity may be unequally distributed, predominating in one area, which is often posterior. The preferential involvement of emetic and the autonomic systems in general may be attributed to the activation of vulnerable for children emetic centres and the hypothalamus by epileptic discharges generated at various cortical locations. Children are particularly susceptible to seizures with a striking age-related sequence. Of the commonest idiopathic childhood seizure disorders, febrile seizures appear first at a peak age of 18–22 months followed by Panayiotopoulos syndrome at 4–5 years and Rolandic seizures at 7–10 years. Considering their similarities, it is likely that febrile, Panayiotopoulos and Rolandic seizures are an age-related continuum of this childhood seizure susceptibility (page 102).

Prognosis: Panayiotopoulos syndrome is a remarkably benign condition despite high incidence of autonomic status epilepticus. One third (27%) of patients have a single seizure only; around half (47%) have 2–5 seizures. Only 5% have more than 10 seizures and these sometimes may be very frequent but outcome is again favourable. Furthermore, seizure lifespan is very brief with remission commonly occurring within 1–2 years from onset. The risk of developing epilepsy in adult life is probably no more than that of the general population. However, one fifth (21%) may develop other types of infrequent seizures, usually Rolandic (13%), during childhood and early teens. These are also age-related and remit before the age of 16 years. Atypical evolutions with absences and drop attacks like those occurring in Rolandic epilepsy are exceptional.[300,301]

Improving diagnostic yield through increased awareness, audits and well-publicised practice parameters and guidelines: Despite high prevalence, dramatic and lengthy clinical manifestations and often severe, multifocal EEG spikes, Panayiotopoulos syndrome is practically unknown. Even now both the syndrome and its autonomic seizures and autonomic status epilepticus are conspicuously absent from books on 'epilepsy' and paediatric publications. Yet, Panayiotopoulos syndrome is a frequent occurrence in accident and emergency departments, paediatric consultations and EEG referrals. Paediatricians were receptive and made excellent use of the knowledge that they received regarding febrile and Rolandic seizures. This is thanks to the official panels of experts of paediatric associations, particularly in the USA, Europe and Japan, which are expected to issue similar guidelines for Panayiotopoulos syndrome.

> Paediatricians should be alerted by lengthy autonomic seizures and electroencephalographers by frequent multifocal spikes in a normal child with one or a few seizures. From the EEG point of view it is significant to remember:
>
> an EEG with frequent epileptogenic foci of a normal child with infrequent seizures should raise the possibility of benign childhood focal seizures.

In this respect, EEG with multifocal spikes may be indispensable in the diagnosis of patients with Panayiotopoulos syndrome if clinical information is inadequate or emetic manifestations are inconspicuous.

Management: Current practice parameter guidelines for febrile seizures, if appropriately modified, may be the basis for similar guidelines in Panayiotopoulos syndrome. Based on the risks and benefits of the effective therapies, continuous anticonvulsant therapy is not recommended for children with one or brief seizures. Most clinicians use carbamazepine for recurrent seizures. Lengthy seizures are a medical emergency; rectal diazepam is prescribed for home administration. See details in 'Management of benign childhood focal seizures' (page 107).

GASTAUT-TYPE CHILDHOOD OCCIPITAL EPILEPSY (LATE ONSET) [25,302–305]

Gastaut-type childhood occipital epilepsy (late onset) is a rare manifestation of a childhood seizure susceptibility syndrome with an age-related onset, often age-limited and may be genetically determined.

Demographic data: Age at onset is from 3 to 15 years with a mean age around 8 years. Girls and boys are equally affected. Prevalence is ~2–7% of benign childhood focal seizures.

Clinical manifestations: **Seizures mainly manifest with elementary visual hallucinations, blindness or both.** They are usually frequent and diurnal and mainly last for seconds to less than 3 minutes. **Elementary visual hallucinations** are the commonest and most characteristic ictal symptom, most likely the first and often the only seizure clinical manifestation. Ictal elementary visual hallucinations mainly consist of small multi-coloured circular patterns that often appear in the periphery of a visual field, becoming larger and multiplying in the course of the seizure, frequently moving horizontally towards the other side (Figure 5.7). They develop fast in seconds and last for seconds to 1–3 minutes, rarely longer.

> I see millions of small, very bright, coloured mainly blue and green, circular spots of light which appear on the left side and sometimes move to the right

Elementary visual hallucinations may progress and co-exist with other occipital symptoms such as sensory illusions of ocular movements and ocular pain, tonic deviation of the eyes, eyelid fluttering or repetitive eye closures. Complex visual hallucinations, without the emotional and complicated character of temporal lobe seizures, visual illusions, and other symptoms from more anterior ictal spreading may rarely occur ab initio or from seizure progress. Seizures rarely terminate with hemi-convulsions or generalised convulsions. Ictal blindness, appearing ab initio or less commonly after other occipital seizure manifestations, usually lasts for 3–5 minutes.

> Everything went suddenly black, I could not see and I had to ask other swimmers to show me the direction to the beach

Consciousness is not impaired during the elementary or complex visual hallucinations, blindness and other occipital seizure symptoms (simple focal seizures) but may be disturbed or lost in the course of the seizure, usually prior to convulsions.

Occipital seizures of Gastaut-type COE may rarely progress to other extra-occipital manifestations such as hemiparaesthesia. Spreading to produce symptoms of temporal lobe involvement is exceptional and may indicate a symptomatic cause. Ictal syncope may rarely occur.

Post-ictal headache, mainly diffuse but also severe, unilateral and pulsating or indistinguishable from migraine headache, often occurs in half the patients and in 10% of them it may be associated with nausea and vomiting.[25,306] Headache, mainly orbital, may also be ictal, often preceding the visual or other seizure symptoms in a small number of patients.[25,306]

I then have left sided severe throbbing headache for an hour or so

Diagnostic procedures: By definition all tests other than EEG are normal. However, high-resolution MRI is probably mandatory because of the high incidence of symptomatic occipital epilepsies with the same clinico-EEG manifestations.

Electroencephalography: The EEG shows occipital paroxysms often demonstrating fixation-off sensitivity (Figure 5.8). However, others may have only random occipital spikes, some may have occipital spikes in sleep EEG alone and a few may consistently have normal EEG. Centrotemporal, frontal and giant somatosensory spikes may occur but less often than in Panayiotopoulos syndrome. Whether occipital photosensitivity is part of this syndrome or not is debated (page 104).

Ictal EEG is characterised by regression of occipital paroxysms and the sudden appearance of an occipital discharge that consists of fast rhythms, fast

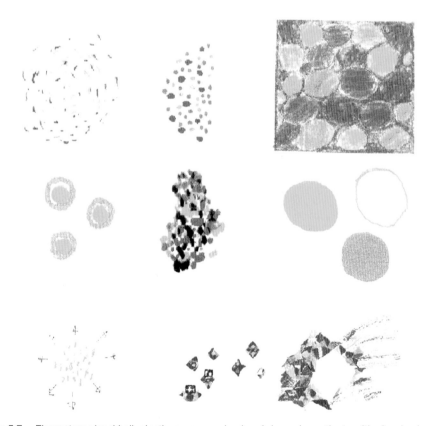

Figure 5.7   Elementary visual hallucinations as perceived and drawn by patients with visual seizures.

From Panayiotopoulos (1999)[306] with the permission of the Editor of *Journal of Neurology, Neurosurgery and Psychiatry.*

spikes or both (Figure 5.6). This is of much lower amplitude than of the occipital paroxysms.

Prognosis is relatively good with remission often occurring within 2–4 years from onset for approximately 50–60% of cases and a dramatically good response to treatment, mainly with carbamazepine, in >90%. However, 40–50% of patients may continue to have visual seizures and infrequent secondarily generalised tonic-clonic convulsions, particularly if not appropriately treated with carbamazepine.

Differential diagnosis: The differential diagnosis from migraine should be easy (Table 8.1). Symptomatic occipital epilepsy often manifests with similar seizures and therefore all patients require high-resolution MRI. Coeliac disease is also associated with similar clinico-EEG manifestations.[307]

Management: In contrast to other phenotypes of the benign childhood seizure susceptibility syndrome, patients with Gastaut-type childhood occipital epilepsy often suffer from frequent seizures and therefore medical treatment – mainly with carbamazepine – is probably mandatory.[25,306]

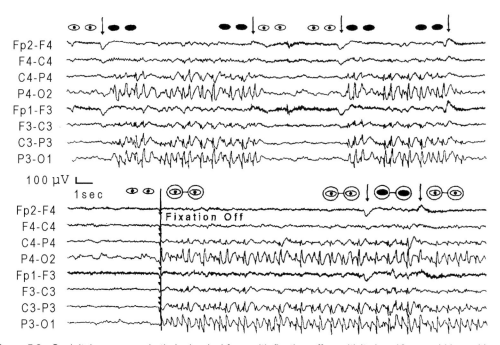

Figure 5.8 Occipital paroxysms in their classical form with fixation-off sensitivity in a 10-year-old boy with Gastaut-type childhood occipital epilepsy (case 26 in ref [25]).

Occipital paroxysms occur as long as fixation and central vision are eliminated by any means (eyes closed, darkness, plus 10 spherical lenses, Ganzfeld stimulation). Under these conditions eyes opening is not capable of inhibiting the spikes. Symbols of eyes open or closed without glasses denote that the recording is with lights on and whenever fixation is possible. Symbols of eyes open or closed with glasses denote that the recording is when fixation and central vision are eliminated by any of the above means.

From Panayiotopoulos (1999)[25] with the permission of the publisher John Libbey.

IDIOPATHIC PHOTOSENSITIVE OCCIPITAL LOBE EPILEPSY

Idiopathic photosensitive occipital lobe epilepsy has been recognised as a new syndrome of reflex epilepsy with age-related onset.[10,25,308,309] However, its boundaries are uncertain as detailed in pages 226-229. Photosensitive occipital seizures may even start in adulthood. Gastaut considered it as part of Gastaut-type COE, children with Rolandic seizures may later develop photosensitive occipital seizures and EEG occipital photosensitivity may also rarely occur in Panayiotopoulos syndrome.[25,36]

OTHER PHENOTYPES OF BENIGN CHILDHOOD SEIZURE SUSCEPTIBILITY SYNDROME [25]

Benign childhood seizures with affective symptoms[310] is probably a rare clinical phenotype of the benign childhood seizure susceptibility syndrome (BCSSS). It manifests with multiple, brief seizures of terror and screaming, autonomic disturbances (pallor, sweating, abdominal pain, salivation), chewing and other automatisms, arrest of speech and mild impairment of consciousness. Generalised seizures do not occur, response to treatment is excellent and remission is reported to occur within 1–2 years.

At the active stage of the disease, behavioural problems may be prominent but these subside with the seizures.

The interictal EEG shows high amplitude sharp and slow wave complexes, morphologically similar to CTS, which are located around the frontotemporal and parietotemporal electrodes. In common with the other benign childhood focal seizures, EEG abnormalities are exaggerated by sleep and may be associated with generalised discharges.

Benign childhood epilepsy with parietal spikes and frequent somatosensory evoked potential[25,311,312] may also be another clinical phenotype of BCSSS. Versive seizures of the head and body, often without impairment of consciousness, are mainly diurnal and infrequent. Multiple daily seizures and focal status epilepticus have been described.

EEG shows parietal spikes with or without somatosensory evoked spikes. Somatosensory evoked potentials are not specific for any syndrome as they also occur in 10–20% of children with Rolandic seizures.[312]

Remission usually occurs within 1 year from seizure onset but EEG abnormalities may persist for longer.

Benign childhood focal seizures associated with frontal[25,313,314] **and midline spikes**[25,315] have been described and long follow-up reports have confirmed a benign course, but no systematic studies have been published. However, it should be remembered that EEG spike foci of various locations are also seen in RS and more commonly in Panayiotopoulos syndrome.

MANAGEMENT OF BENIGN CHILDHOOD FOCAL SEIZURES

Short- and long-term treatment strategies for benign childhood focal seizures are empirical and there is no consensus regarding their management.[25,36] However, current practice parameter guidelines for febrile seizures,[129,130] if appropriately modified, may be the basis for similar guidelines in benign childhood focal seizures and particularly Rolandic epilepsy[25] and Panayiotopoulos syndrome.[36] Based on the risks and benefits of the effective therapies, continuous anticonvulsant therapy is not recommended for children with one or brief seizures. Most clinicians use carbamazepine for recurrent seizures, but this may exceptionally worsen seizures. Lengthy seizures are a medical emergency; rectal diazepam is prescribed for home administration. Recurrent and lengthy seizures create anxiety in parents and patients and, as such, appropriate education and emotional support should be provided.

ACUTE MANAGEMENT OF A CHILD WITH PROLONGED SEIZURES (two thirds of the cases with Panayiotopoulos syndrome)

Control of the seizure is paramount. In the rare occasions that the child is febrile, treatment of possible fever and mainly of the underlying illness is also important.

Long-lasting seizures (>10 minutes) or status epilepticus (>30 minutes to hours) is a feature in two thirds (70%) of children with Panayiotopoulos syndrome. This is a genuine paediatric emergency that demands appropriate and vigorous treatment as for status epilepticus.[132,316] Early treatment, usually parental, is more effective than late emergency treatment.[132]

Parents of children with recurrent seizures should be advised to place the child on its side or stomach on a protected surface and administer a preparation of rectal benzodiazepine.

In an emergency facility, the child's airway should be kept clear, oxygenation maintained, and intravenous or rectal anticonvulsant given to halt the seizure.

Benzodiazepines, usually diazepam intravenously 0.2–0.3 mg/kg or in rectal preparations 0.5 mg/kg/dose, are probably the first choice. Rectal absorption of liquid diazepam is very rapid, reaches the brain within minutes and has a near-intravenous efficacy. A disadvantage of diazepam is its short duration of action. Rectal tubes containing liquid diazepam are the most widely used formulation. Diazepam rectal gel is now available in the USA. Intravenous lorazepam (0.1 mg/kg), less likely to cause respiratory depression and probably with a longer action than diazepam, may be preferred. Bucchal or nasal application of midazolam that may stop status epilepticus and prevent the development of GTCS may be another alternative for home administration.[317–319]

PROPHYLACTIC MANAGEMENT OF BENIGN CHILDHOOD FOCAL SEIZURES

Continuous anticonvulsant treatment is not recommended. Although there are effective therapies that could prevent the occurrence of additional seizures, the potential adverse effects of such therapy are not commensurate with the benefit. The great majority of children with benign focal seizures do not need anticonvulsant treatment even if they suffer lengthy seizures or have more than two recurrences. The risks are small and the potential side-effects of drugs appear to outweigh the benefits.

In situations of recurrent seizures and/or when parental anxiety associated with seizures is severe, small doses of antiepileptic medication may be effective in preventing recurrence. There is no convincing evidence, however, that any therapy will alleviate the possibility of recurrences. In deciding management for a child with benign childhood focal seizures the following should be considered:

- Most children have an excellent prognosis: 10–30% of patients may have only a single seizure and in another 60–70% seizures may be infrequent, usually 2–10. However, 10–20% of patients may have frequent seizures and sometimes the seizures may be resistant to treatment.

- Remission of benign childhood focal seizures is expected in all patients.

- The possibility of future epilepsy is a most unlikely event and probably not higher than of the general population.

- There is no evidence that untreated children have a worse long-term prognosis, although they may be unprotected for seizure recurrences.

- Some children become frightened even by simple focal seizures and despite firm re-assurances some parents are unable to cope with the possibility of another fit.

- Persistence and frequency of EEG functional spikes are not predictive of clinical severity, frequency and degree of liability to seizures.

Continuous prophylaxis consists of daily medication using any antiepileptic drug with proven efficacy in focal seizures – mainly carbamazepine.

PARENTAL ATTITUDE AND EDUCATION

Despite their excellent prognosis, benign childhood focal seizures (like febrile convulsions) are a dramatic experience for parents who are usually young and inexperienced and who often think that their child is dead or dying.

The lesson again comes from the study of parental reactions to a child's first febrile convulsion.[320] Most of the parents knew little about febrile convulsions before the fit and most of them thought the child was dying (77%), suffocating or had meningitis (15%). Afterwards, parental behaviour altered with restless sleep (60%), dyspepsia (29%), watching the child overnight (6%) or when feverish (8%). Parents with previous knowledge of febrile convulsions took more appropriate measures but only 21% positioned the child correctly during the seizure.

Parents of young children should have general information provided by the family doctor regarding Rolandic epilepsy and Panayiotopoulos syndrome. Parents who have watched their child during a fit need specific information in order to avoid long-term reactions.

Supportive family management includes education about these conditions and specific instructions about emergency procedures for possible subsequent seizures.

Stopping medication: Withdrawal of medication practices differ amongst experts, although they all agree that there is no need to continue medication after 1–3 years from the last seizure and certainly by the age of 14 years when benign childhood focal seizures remit in the majority or 16 when they are practically non-existent. My practice is to start gradual withdrawal of medication 2 years after the last seizure, making sure that the child does not have any minor seizures. However, I do not adhere to fixed rules and may continue medication until the age of 13–15 years, depending on the severity, frequency and age at onset of seizures. Thus, in a child that had frequent, severe and difficult to control fits in early childhood, I would not stop medication if there were a seizure-free period of 2–3 years by age 7 years. Conversely, for a child who had three or four nocturnal seizures at age 11 and 12 years I would certainly discontinue medication slowly after a 2-year seizure-free period. I advise very slow withdrawal at monthly steps of reduction so that the drug is completely discontinued approximately 6 months later. The reason for this is that I expect that possible seizure recurrence during the process of very slow drug discontinuation would manifest with mild, brief and simple focal seizures without secondarily generalised convulsions. In the case of barbiturates and diazepines slowly stopping medication is mandatory to avoid risking a possible withdrawal seizure.

UNIFIED CONCEPT FOR THE BENIGN CHILDHOOD FOCAL SEIZURES

BENIGN CHILDHOOD SEIZURE SUSCEPTIBILITY SYNDROME [25,36,321]

Benign childhood epilepsies with focal seizures and focal EEG sharp slow wave complexes are a group of syndromes of probably one disease, which, in my opinion, share common clinical and EEG characteristics. Seizures are infrequent, usually nocturnal and remit within 1–3 years from onset. Brief or prolonged seizures, even status epilepticus, may be the only clinical event of the patient's lifetime. Ictal autonomic manifestations such as hypersalivation, vomiting, headache, pallor or sweating, ictal syncope – unusual in other epileptic syndromes – are frequent and may occasionally appear in isolation. Children with the clinical and EEG characteristics of one may evolve into or simultaneously develop features of another form of benign childhood focal seizures. Febrile seizures are common. Neurological examination and intellect are normal, but some children may experience mild and reversible neuropsychological problems at the active stage of the disorder. Brain imaging is normal. There are usually severe EEG abnormalities, which are disproportionate to the severity of seizures. Epileptogenic foci, irrespective of their location, manifest abundant, high amplitude sharp slow wave complexes, mainly in clusters. They are often bilateral, independent or synchronous, frequently combined with foci from other cortical areas or brief generalised discharges, and are exaggerated in stages I–IV of sleep. A normal EEG is rare and should provoke a sleep EEG study. Similar EEG features resolving with age are frequently found in normal school-age children (2–4%) and children having an EEG for reasons other than seizures.

There is no reason to believe that all these syndromes differ from each other merely because an 'epileptogenic' focus is a little anterior or posterior, lateral or medial to the centrotemporal regions. A unified concept of benign childhood focal seizures is also suggested by the frequency of more than one type of benign childhood focal seizures in an affected child, siblings or both.

It is likely and I propose that all these conditions are linked together due to a common, genetically determined, mild and reversible, functional derangement of the brain cortical maturational process. This is often clinically silent, manifested in more than 90% with EEG sharp and slow waves with an age-related localisation. In the remaining minority, there are infrequent focal seizures and their symptoms are also localisation- and age-related and - dependent. It is possible that a few of these children, with or without seizures, also have usually minor and fully reversible neuropsychological symptoms that are rarely clinically overt, requiring special neuropsychological testing for their detection. Finally, there may be a very small number of patients (<1%) in whom this derangement of the brain maturation process may be derailed, resulting in a more aggressive condition of seizures, neuropsychological manifestations and EEG abnormalities of various combinations and varying degrees of severity, as in for example, atypical benign focal epilepsy of childhood, Landau-Kleffner syndrome, epilepsy with continuous spike and slow wave during sleep.

My overall impression is that the whole aspect of benign childhood focal seizures, their clinical and EEG manifestations and evolution, need appropriate prospective studies like those performed for febrile seizures.

FEBRILE SEIZURES AND BENIGN CHILDHOOD SEIZURE SUSCEPTIBILITY SYNDROME

One of the most stimulating aspects of benign childhood focal seizures is their striking age-related sequence. Common benign seizure disorders are specific to children and these do not occur in adults.

There are three main periods of age-related childhood susceptibility to seizures. The fact that children are particularly susceptible to seizures is well documented. Febrile mainly *generalised* convulsions appear first in early childhood at a peak age of 18–22 months, Rolandic *focal* seizures occur in late childhood at a peak of 7–10 years; Panayiotopoulos syndrome covers the intermediate period between them at a peak of 4–5 years and manifests with mainly autonomic seizures (Figure 5.9). Let me analyse this further as this is likely to be highly significant in our understanding of the disordered age-related maturational processes. The first early period (febrile seizures) consists of a brain vulnerability to seizures that are triggered by fever and mainly manifest with *convulsions* that are commonly *generalised*. The second intermediate period (Panayiotopoulos syndrome) consists of spontaneous seizures that are often *prolonged* for hours and manifest principally with *autonomic* and mainly *emetic* symptoms. The third late period (Rolandic syndrome) consists of spontaneous focal, motor or sensorimotor, seizures. These clinical seizure susceptibility periods also have peculiar EEG accompaniments; the EEG is practically normal in the first period of febrile seizures, shows mainly posterior and multifocal spikes in the intermediate period of Panayiotopoulos syndrome and centro-gyral spikes in the late period of Rolandic seizures. These indicate that the brain in early childhood has a low threshold to generalised convulsions provoked by fever with a relatively silent EEG spike capacity. Subsequently, the autonomic system and particularly the emetic centres become vulnerable, the seizure discharges may be self-sustained and the cortex exhibits a diffuse epileptogenicity, which is unequally distributed and mainly affects the posterior regions. Finally, in the third period of late childhood, brain epileptogenicity shrinks to around the Rolandic regions to produce the distinctive clinical and EEG manifestations of the Rolandic syndrome. These are incontrovertible facts and indicate something

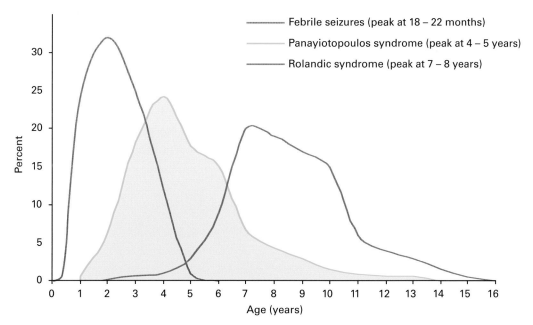

Figure 5.9 Diagrammatic age-related presentation at onset of febrile, Rolandic and Panayiotopoulos syndromes.

very important, but currently they serve only as challenges to our understanding of the developing brain. We should also consider the neonatal and the early infantile period because they also have their own peculiarities, as indicated by the benign neonatal seizures (around the fifth day) and the benign infantile partial seizures (familial and non-familial) of the Watanabe-Vigevano Syndrome.[145,146] This point is exemplified by an otherwise normal boy reported by Lada et al.[271] He first had benign neonatal seizures, then two febrile seizures occurred at the ages of 18 months and 3 years. A brief autonomic seizure with ictal vomiting and deviation of the eyes happened during sleep at age 6 years. EEG showed occipital paroxysms. I have also described a boy who at 8 weeks old had three focal seizures of right-sided convulsions involving face and upper limbs (benign neonatal non-familial seizures of Watanabe-Vigevano syndrome). Subsequent EEGs were normal and treatment stopped at age 10 months. He was well until age 7 years when he started having Rolandic seizures and later developed ECSWS (see Figures 3.1 and 4.8). Brain MRI was normal (case 17.2 of Panayiotopoulos[25]).

Benign focal seizures of adolescence are presented in the following section.

BENIGN (ISOLATED) FOCAL SEIZURES OF ADOLESCENCE [322–328]

Benign (isolated) focal seizures of adolescence constitute an idiopathic, short-lived and transient period of seizure susceptibility of the second decade of life. Around 200 cases have been described.[323,326–330]

Demographic data: This is a seizure susceptibility of the second decade of life with a peak at 13–15 years of age. There is a 71.2% male preponderance. According to Loiseau and Louiset (1992)[323] one quarter of focal seizures with onset between 12 and 18 years of age have a benign course, i.e. they are single or occur in a cluster of up to five seizures during 36 hours, never to occur again. Prevalence may be around 7.5%[324] to 22%[326] of patients having simple focal seizures in the second decade of life.

Clinical manifestations: The syndrome manifests with a single or a cluster of two to five focal, mainly motor and sensory, seizures which in half of the cases progress to secondarily generalised tonic-clonic convulsions. There are no epileptic events preceding or following this limited seizure period, which lasts no more than 36 hours. The seizures by definition are focal but the temporal lobes are rarely involved. Most of the seizures are diurnal (87%). The teenager is fully aware and can give a reliable account of the onset of the clinical manifestations (simple focal seizures) in the majority of episodes (88%).

Consideration on classification

Benign (isolated) focal seizures of adolescence is not a recognised syndrome in the new diagnostic scheme.[10] Its best position should be among the 'Conditions with epileptic seizures that do not require a diagnosis of epilepsy'.[10] Loiseau and Jallon (2002)[328] consider that this is a syndrome of 'isolated focal seizures of adolescence'.

However, consciousness rarely remains intact throughout the whole episode; the seizures usually evolve to impaired cognition and/or to secondarily generalised tonic-clonic convulsions, which occur in half of the cases. The commonest ictal clinical manifestations are motor, usually without Jacksonian marching, and somatosensory. Visual, vertiginous and autonomic symptoms are reported in one fifth of the cases. Experiential phenomena like those in temporal lobe seizures practically never occur.

The physical and mental states of the patients are normal.

Laboratory tests and brain imaging are normal. MRI is normal. The EEG may show some minor, non-specific abnormalities without spikes or focal slowing. In a recent report 9 of 37 cases had functional spikes,[327] which is incompatible with this syndrome; they probably suffered from benign childhood focal seizures detailed in this chapter.

Prognosis: Prognosis is excellent; in 80% of the patients there is a single, isolated seizure event and in the remaining a cluster of two to five seizures all occurring within 36 hours.

Management: This is an interesting seizure susceptibility of adolescence manifesting with one or a cluster of two to five focal seizures. They should not be treated with drugs. However, these patients are difficult to diagnose, as there are no specific features at onset to differentiate them from others with similar clinical manifestations, but of different aetiology – particularly symptomatic or cryptogenic focal epilepsies. My practice is to investigate all adolescents with onset of focal seizures with MRI and EEG, which, if normal, would make the diagnosis of benign focal seizures of adolescence more likely. A definitive diagnosis cannot be made before 1–5 years of freedom from seizures.[323,326]

IDIOPATHIC GENERALISED EPILEPSIES

6

Idiopathic generalised epilepsies (IGE) constitute one third of all epilepsies.[7,9,10,331,332] They are genetically determined, affecting otherwise normal people. They manifest with typical absences, myoclonic jerks and generalised tonic-clonic seizures (GTCS) alone or in varying combinations and severity. Absence status epilepticus is common. Most syndromes of IGE are lifelong. Interictal EEG shows generalised discharges of spike/polyspike and slow wave, which are often precipitated by hyperventilation and sleep deprivation. These discharges are frequently associated with inconspicuous clinical manifestations that become apparent on video-EEG and breath counting during hyperventilation. Normal EEG is unlikely in untreated patients and should generate a new EEG during sleep and awakening. Molecular genetic studies indicate that certain syndromes of IGE are linked to different chromosomes.[333,334] Genetic heterogeneity is common. Treatment is demanding; drugs beneficial in focal epilepsies may be deleterious in IGEs.[7] Most of the IGEs respond well to appropriate drug treatment but this is often lifelong.

SEIZURES OF IDIOPATHIC GENERALISED EPILEPSIES

TYPICAL ABSENCE SEIZURES

Typical absences (previously known as petit mal) are brief (for seconds) generalised epileptic seizures of abrupt onset and abrupt termination. They manifest clinically mainly with impairment of consciousness (absence) and EEG with generalised 3–4 Hz spike and slow wave discharges (Figure 6.1).[7,9,331,332,335,336] They are fundamentally different and pharmacologically unique as compared with any other type of seizures, which also makes their treatment different.[7,336,337]

The clinico-EEG manifestations of absences are syndrome-related.[7,9,331,332,335,336,338]

Abbreviations:

CAE = childhood absence epilepsy
EGTCSA = epilepsy with generalised tonic-clonic seizures on awakening
EMA = eyelid myoclonia with absences (Jeavons syndrome)
EMAS = epilepsy with myoclonic astatic seizures (Doose syndrome)

FS+ = febrile seizures plus
GEFS+ = generalised epilepsies with febrile seizures plus
GTCS = generalised tonic-clonic seizures
JAE = juvenile absence epilepsy
JME = juvenile myoclonic epilepsy (Janz syndrome)
IGE = idiopathic generalised epilepsy
MAE = epilepsy with myoclonic absences
PMA = perioral myoclonia with absences

Impairment of consciousness may be severe, moderate or mild. Automatisms, localised or widespread jerks and autonomic disturbances are common concurrent symptoms. Typical absences are easily precipitated by hyperventilation in around 90% of untreated patients.

DIAGNOSING ABSENCES

The brief duration of absence seizures with abrupt onset and abrupt termination, daily frequency and nearly invariable provocation with hyperventilation makes their diagnosis easy.[7,336,338]

Patients suspected of experiencing absences should be asked to overbreathe for 3 minutes while standing, counting their breaths and with hands extended in front of them. This will provoke an absence in nearly all untreated patients. Documentation with camcorders should be recommended. The differentiation of typical absences from complex focal seizures, detailed in Table 6.1, may be more difficult in adults, where absences are often misdiagnosed as temporal lobe seizures.[339] Absences occur in 10% of adult patients with epileptic seizures.[339]

Table 6.1 Differential diagnosis of typical absences from complex focal seizures

	Typical absences	Complex focal seizures
Clinical criteria		
Duration for less than 30 seconds	As a rule	Exceptional
Duration for more than 1 minute	Exceptional	As a rule
Non-convulsive status epilepticus	Frequent	Rare
Daily in frequency	As a rule	Rare
Simple automatisms	Frequent	Frequent
Complex behavioural automatisms	Exceptional	Frequent
Simple and complex hallucinations or illusions	Exceptional	Frequent
Bilateral facial myoclonic jerks or eyelid closures	Frequent	Exceptional
Evolving to other focal seizure manifestations	Never	Frequent
Sudden onset and termination	As a rule	Frequent
Post-ictal symptoms	Never	Frequent
Reproduced by hyperventilation	As a rule	Exceptional
Elicited by photic stimulation	Frequent	Exceptional
EEG criteria		
Ictal generalised 3–4 Hz spike and wave	Exclusive	Never
Interictal generalised discharges	Frequent	Exceptional
Interictal focal abnormalities of slow waves	Exceptional	Frequent
Normal EEG in untreated state	Exceptional	Frequent

The primary differences are shown in red.

From Panayiotopoulos (2002)[336] with the permission of the Editor of *Medlink*.

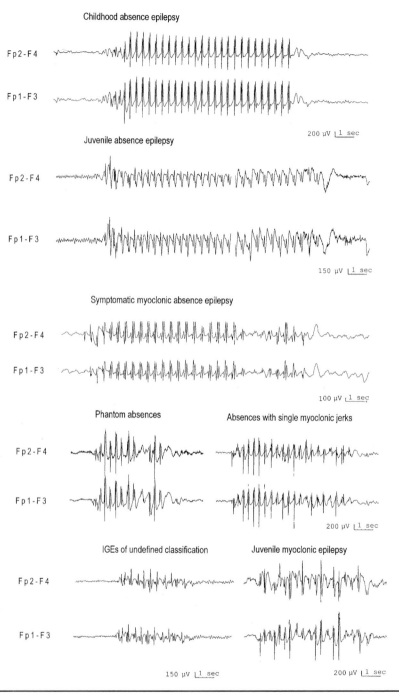

Figure 6.1

Examples from video-EEG of generalised discharges of 3 Hz spike or multiple spike and slow wave of typical absence seizures. These seven patients had different syndromes of idiopathic and symptomatic absence epilepsies. Note that the discharges may be brief or prolonged, with or without polyspikes, of regular or irregular sequence. Also, note that the intra-discharge frequency of the spike wave complexes may show significant variations. Although there are significant variations between various syndromes, the discharge itself is not pathognomonic of any syndrome. The syndromic diagnosis requires homogeneous clustering of symptoms and signs.

Generalised 3–4 Hz spikes/polyspikes slow waves are the EEG accompaniment of typical absence seizures (Figure 6.1).

The EEG, ideally video-EEG, would confirm the diagnosis of typical absence seizures in more than 90% of untreated patients mainly during hyperventilation.[336] If not, the diagnosis of absences should be questioned. Focal spike abnormalities and asymmetrical onset of the ictal 3–4 Hz spike wave discharges are common and may be a cause of misdiagnosis particularly in resistant cases.[335]

MYOCLONIC JERKS

Myoclonic jerks are shock-like, irregular and often arrhythmic, clonic-twitching movements that may be singular or repetitive.[8,340,341] They are of variable amplitude and force, ranging from mild and inconspicuous to violent – they may make the patient fall on the ground, drop or throw things or kick. Commonly, the same patient experiences both mild and violent jerks. Myoclonic jerks predominantly affect eyelids, facial and neck muscles, upper more than lower limbs and body. Myoclonic jerks of IGE mainly occur on awakening. Precipitating factors are sleep deprivation, fatigue, excitement or distress and often photic stimulation. The patient is fully aware of myoclonic jerks except when these occur during absence seizures. The location and extent of myoclonic jerks varies between syndromes of IGE.

Polyspikes are the EEG accompaniment of myoclonic jerks (Figures 6.2, 6.3 and 6.4).

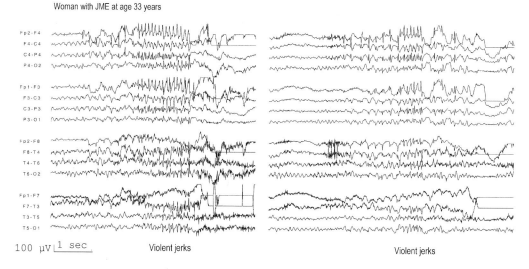

Woman with JME at age 33 years

100 μV | 1 sec

Violent jerks   Violent jerks

Figure 6.2 From video-EEG. Generalised multiple spike discharges occur concurrently with violent myoclonic jerks.

DIAGNOSING MYOCLONIC JERKS

Elicitation of the characteristic history of myoclonic jerks is something of an art. It is often necessary to physically demonstrate mild myoclonic jerks of the fingers and hands, and to inquire about morning clumsiness and tremors.[342] Questions like 'do you spill your morning tea?', 'do you drop things in the morning?', with simultaneous demonstration of how myoclonic jerks produce this effect, may be answered positively by patients who denied myoclonic jerks on direct questioning. Further elaboration is required to confirm that clumsiness was due to genuine myoclonic jerks. If the patient reports normal hypnagogic jactitations, it is reassuring that the concept of myoclonic jerks has been understood. Diagnostic yield may be improved by emphasising the close relation of jerks to fatigue, alcohol and sleep deprivation. Some patients do not report their jerks, erroneously assuming that this is a self-inflicted normal phenomenon related to excess of alcohol and lack of sleep.

GENERALISED TONIC-CLONIC SEIZURES

GTCS are primary in the sense that they are generalised from onset without warning other than a series of myoclonic jerks or absences that often herald GTCS. This contrasts with secondary GTCS of focal epilepsies that are often preceded by an aura or focal sensorimotor symptoms. Overall GTCS occur on awakening (17–53% of patients), diffusely whilst awake (23–36%) or during sleep (27–44%) or randomly (13–26%).[343] It is undetermined what proportion of these patients also have other generalised seizures (jerks or absences).

STATUS EPILEPTICUS IN IGE

The new ILAE diagnostic scheme[10] considers status epilepticus as a 'continuous seizure' with two main categories (Table 1.2):

a. Generalised status epilepticus.

b. Focal status epilepticus.

The sub-categories of generalised status epilepticus are relevant to this chapter:

1. Generalised tonic-clonic status epilepticus

2. Clonic status epilepticus

3. Absence status epilepticus

4. Tonic status epilepticus

5. Myoclonic status epilepticus

IGEs manifest with all these types of generalised status epilepticus. Absence status epilepticus is probably the commonest of all and the most likely to escape diagnosis or to be misdiagnosed.[9,10,335,344–347]

ABSENCE STATUS EPILEPTICUS IN IGE

Absence status epilepticus in IGE (typical) is defined as a prolonged, more than half an hour, generalised non-convulsive seizure of impairment of the content of consciousness (absence) and EEG generalised spike-polyspike and slow wave discharges.

Impairment of consciousness may be mild or severe and associated with other mainly motor disturbances such as:

● mild clonic jerks of eyelids, corner of the mouth, or other muscles

● atonic components leading to drooping of the head, slumping of the trunk, dropping of the arms and relaxation of the grip

● tonic muscular contraction causing head retropulsion or arching of the trunk

● automatisms ranging from lip-licking and swallowing to clothes fumbling or aimless walking and

● autonomic components such as pallor and less frequently flushing, sweating, dilatation of pupils and incontinence of urine.

The above symptoms may be continuous or repetitive but the patient does not fully recover in between before cessation of the seizure.

The ictal EEG is characteristic with usually regular and symmetrical generalised discharges of 1–4 Hz spike or multiple spike and slow wave complexes. The background interictal EEG may be normal or abnormal, often associated with brief or long runs of paroxysmal generalised 1–4 Hz spike/multiple spike activity, polyspike discharges and focal spike or slow wave abnormalities characterising the underlying epileptic syndrome.

With the possible exception of childhood absence epilepsy, all IGEs with typical absences may manifest with typical absence status either as a spontaneous expression of their natural course or provoked by external factors or inappropriate treatment manoeuvres.

Considerations on classification:

Absence seizures are broadly divided into:

a. typical absences of mainly IGE with generalised >2.5 Hz spike or polyspike and slow wave

b. atypical absences of symptomatic/cryptogenic epilepsies with slower <2.5 Hz generalised discharges.

Similarly, absence status epilepticus is divided into:

a. typical absence status epilepticus of mainly IGE

b. atypical absence status epilepticus of symptomatic and cryptogenic generalised epilepsies.

Furthermore, to comply with seizure and syndrome classification, absence status epilepticus may be 'situation related'[9] 'not requiring the diagnosis of epilepsy'[10] caused by the introduction or withdrawal of certain drugs, intoxication, electrolyte or metabolic disturbances. Symptomatic absence status may also be caused by severe brain anoxia or other brain damage

It should be emphasised that absence status epilepticus, like the absence, is not one but many types of a prolonged seizure. Although the shared symptom of all types of absence status epilepticus is impairment of cognition this is often associated with other clinical manifestations such as myoclonic jerks, eyelid or perioral myoclonia, which may be syndrome-related.

Impairment of consciousness, memory and higher cognitive functions: The cardinal symptom shared by all cases of typical absence status is altered content of consciousness of usually a fully alert patient. Memory and higher cognitive intellectual functions such as abstract thinking, computation and personal awareness are the main areas of disturbance. This varies from very mild to very severe with intermediate states of severity occurring more often.

Mild is experienced as a state of slow reaction, behaviour and mental functioning:

> My mind slows down, able to understand but takes longer to formulate answers
>
> I become slow but can communicate verbally with others
>
> Slow down in my behaviour, muddling with words
>
> Like in a trance, missing pieces of conversation

Moderate and severe impairment of consciousness manifest with varying degrees of confusion, global disorientation and inappropriate behaviour:

> Confused, cannot recognise people other than close relatives, disorientated in time and place, very quiet
>
> Disturbed, vague, uncooperative, confused
>
> Markedly confused, goes into a dreamy state, able to formulate some monolectic answers to simple questions, puts trousers over pyjamas
>
> Confused, makes coffee twice, fades away mentally and physically, disoriented in time and place

Usually, the patient is alert, attentive and cooperative. Verbal functioning is relatively well preserved but this is often slow with stereotypic and usually monosyllabic or monolectic answers. Movement and coordination are intact. Rarely the patient may become completely unresponsive.

Behavioural abnormalities and experiential phenomena: Although the most common behavioural changes refer to daily activities disturbed by the impairment of consciousness, some patients become depressed, agitated and occasionally hostile and aggressive. More commonly than usually appreciated there are experiential and sensational phenomena such as:

> Sensation of viewing the word through a different medium and a feeling of not being in the same world as everyone else. Uncontrollable rush of thoughts. A feeling of fear of losing control of my mind
>
> A feeling of closeness
>
> A funny feeling that I cannot elaborate
>
> A strange feeling of not being myself
>
> Edgy, worried and uncomfortable
>
> My character changes completely, I become extremely snappy, have a severe headache
>
> Weird

Simple gestural and ambulatory automatisms, autonomic behaviour and fugue-like states may occur in 20% of the patients who also have severe impairment of consciousness:

Replies yes to any question and fumbles with his clothes

Myoclonic jerks in absence status epilepticus: Segmental, usually eyelid or perioral and less often limb, myoclonic jerks frequently occur during typical absence status varying in degree and severity. They are most likely to occur in syndromes manifesting with similar myoclonic phenomena during brief absences (see descriptions in the relevant sections of individual IGE syndromes).

Generalised tonic-clonic seizures associated with idiopathic typical absence status: Ending with a GTCS is probably the rule irrespective of syndrome. However, absence status epilepticus always ends with GTCS if untreated in only one third of patients. In the rest, it may also terminate spontaneously without GTCS. It is exceptional for GTCS to precede or intersperse with typical absence status. It is also exceptional for more than one GTCS to occur following absence status epilepticus.

Duration and frequency of idiopathic absence status: This usually lasts for an average of 3–4 hours, rarely a minimum of half an hour, often exceeding 6–10 hours and occasionally enduring for 2–10 days. Frequency also varies from one in a lifetime to an average of 10–20 or catamenial. This depends on treatment strategies and syndromic classification.

Post-ictal state: Amnesia of the event is exceptional. Usually the patient is aware of what happens during the absence status, some are able to write down their experiences even when in status, others have a patchy recollection of the events – usually missing the last part prior to GTCS. Following a GTCS the patient feels tired, has headache and is confused for a varying duration of time.

Age at onset and sex: It is rare for absence status epilepticus in IGE to start before the first decade. Other types of seizures such as absences, myoclonic jerks and GTCS may pre-date for many years the first occurrence of absence status epilepticus. Mean age at onset of absence status epilepticus is 29 years with a range of 9–56. Absence status epilepticus may be the first overt type of seizure.

Precipitating factors: Inappropriate or discontinuation of anti-absence medication is the commonest precipitant of idiopathic absence status epilepticus. Sleep deprivation, stress and excess of alcohol consumption, alone or usually combined, are common precipitating factors. Some patients may have catamenial precipitation. In others this mainly starts on awakening.

Differential diagnosis: Idiopathic absence status epilepticus is often unrecognised or misdiagnosed. It is surprising how often physicians are deceived by the general good appearance, alertness and cooperation of the patient who also may be aware of the impaired mental state during absence status epilepticus. Basic testing of memory and higher cognitive functions is essential for diagnosis.

It is important to remember that more than half of the patients are aware of the situation when entering or during absence status epilepticus, which is of great practical significance regarding termination of this state and prevention of the impending GTCS by appropriate self-administered medication.

Idiopathic absence status is easy to diagnose provided that the associated IGE with typical absences (often combined with myoclonic jerks and GTCS) is correctly identified. The commonest misdiagnosis occurs because absences are not recognised or are misdiagnosed as complex focal seizures (Table 6.1). A previous or a new EEG invariably shows generalised discharges in IGE. It may be normal or may show specific focal spikes in partial epilepsies, mainly temporal lobe epilepsy.

The differentiation of typical (idiopathic) absence status from atypical (usually symptomatic or possibly symptomatic) absence status is also easy. The main distinction of the atypical absence status is that it occurs mainly in children with symptomatic or cryptogenic generalised epilepsies who also have a plethora of other types of frequent seizures such as atypical absences, tonic and atonic seizures, myoclonic jerks and GTCS. Most of them also have moderate or severe learning and physical handicaps. In addition, interictal EEG is often very abnormal with slow background and frequent brief or long runs of slow generalised spike and slow wave, paroxysmal fast activity and paroxysms of polyspikes. It is often difficult to define the boundaries, onset and termination, of atypical absence status epilepticus because these children frequently have alterations of behaviour and alertness as well as long interictal slow spike and slow wave discharges.

Atypical absence status is clinically characterised by fluctuating impairment of consciousness, often with other ictal symptoms such as repeated serial tonic or atonic seizures and segmental or generalised jerks. The ictal EEG pattern is of slow <2.5 Hz spike and slow wave generalised activity. Both the clinical patterns and the EEG abnormalities are more variable than those of the typical absence status epilepticus.

Additional discriminating features of atypical absence status epilepticus are:

a. gradual onset and offset

b. level of consciousness and other co-existent type of seizures tend to fluctuate, sometimes for weeks, with little distinction between ictal and interictal phases

c. initiation or termination with a GTCS is exceptional

d. incontinence is common.

Absence status epilepticus may be induced by drugs, or electrolyte and metabolic disturbances in patients who do not suffer from an epilepsy disorder.[348,349] The most well-documented example is from diazepine withdrawal. De novo absence status epilepticus is often misdiagnosed as psychotic state or dementia.

SYNDROMES OF IGE RECOGNISED IN THE NEW ILAE DIAGNOSTIC SCHEME [10]

Idiopathic generalised epilepsies as listed in the new ILAE Classification Scheme[10] are shown in Tables 1.4 and 6.2 in accordance with age at onset. Benign myoclonic epilepsy in infancy is detailed on page 54.

Table 6.2 Idiopathic generalised epilepsies in the new ILAE Classification Scheme[10]

Benign myoclonic epilepsy in infancy

Epilepsy with myoclonic-astatic seizures

Childhood absence epilepsy

Epilepsy with myoclonic absences

Idiopathic generalised epilepsies with variable phenotypes

        Juvenile absence epilepsy

        Juvenile myoclonic epilepsy

        Epilepsy with generalised tonic–clonic seizures only

Generalised epilepsy with febrile seizures plus (syndrome in development)

Considerations on classification:

The classification of IGE is probably one of the most significant and debated issues. There are two schools of thought with diversely opposing views:[331]

a. IGE is one disease

b. IGE comprises a large group of many distinct syndromes.

The evidence so far is not conclusive in favour of one or the other and any new classification should not take sides without firm evidence.

In practical terms the view that 'IGE is one disease' would be an overall easy clinical diagnostic approach but this would discourage the diagnostic precision required for genetic studies, prognostic and therapeutic implications. The view that 'IGE comprises a large group of many distinct syndromes' would be more demanding diagnostically, requiring sometimes exhaustive clinical and video-EEG data, but this is often a price that we have to pay as physicians in pursuing the fact that 'accurate diagnosis is the golden rule in medicine'. This view also (a) satisfies 'maximum practical application to differential diagnosis'[350] which is a main reason for re-organising the classification of epileptic syndromes in the forthcoming revisions and (b) takes advantage of 'significant advances in our understanding'[351] of IGEs which constitute one third of 'epilepsy'.

Along these lines there is no justification for the unification of 'IGEs with onset in adolescence' in a single syndrome as proposed recently.[352] The major conceptual problem in this proposition is that it takes *'age at onset-adolescence'* as the most significant almost defining factor, which is at variance with the definition of a syndrome.[9] Further, the same IGE syndrome may start in childhood, adolescence and occasionally adult life.[9] On the surface, syndromes of IGEs may look alike if their clinico-EEG manifestations are not properly analysed and synthesised. For example, JME and JAE both manifest with absences, myoclonic jerks and GTCS. However, severe absences are the main and the most disturbing seizure type in JAE, myoclonic jerks may not occur or may be randomly distributed.[336,336] Conversely, myoclonic jerks on awakening is the defining symptom of JME; absences are mild and occur in only one third of patients. The clinico-EEG features of typical absence seizures that may be syndrome-related are well described in video-EEG studies.[336,336,338] Unifying all typical absence seizures as a single type is of no benefit to any cause.

In genetic terms, animal studies document numerous syndromes of IGEs[337] and this is likely to be the case in humans.[331]

EPILEPSY WITH MYOCLONIC ASTATIC SEIZURES [224,353–357]

DOOSE SYNDROME

Epilepsy with myoclonic astatic seizures* (of Doose)[224,353,354] is considered an *idiopathic generalised epilepsy* in the new diagnostic sceme.[10] The diagnosis of this syndrome requires careful application of inclusion and exclusion criteria. Its characteristic symptom, myoclonic-astatic seizures, is shared by many other childhood syndromes and particularly epileptic encephalopathies.

  Demographic data: Prevalence may be ~1–2% of all childhood epilepsies; two thirds are boys. Onset is between 7 months and 6 years and there is a peak at 2–4 years.

Useful seizure definitions

Astatic is not synonymous with atonic seizures.
ATONIC: Sudden loss or diminution of muscle tone without apparent preceding myoclonic or tonic events, lasting ~1–2 seconds, involving head, trunk, jaw, or limb musculature.[11]

ASTATIC (synonym = drop attack): Loss of erect posture that results from an atonic, myoclonic or tonic mechanism.[11,180]
The new diagnostic scheme uses only the terms 'atonic' or 'myoclonic atonic' seizures.[10]

Considerations on classification:

The new ILAE diagnostic scheme considers 'Epilepsy with myoclonic astatic seizures'* as IGE,[10] a view which is similar to that of Doose:[226]
'Myoclonic astatic epilepsy belongs to the epilepsies with primarily generalized seizures and thus stands in one line with absence epilepsies, juvenile myoclonic epilepsy, as well as the infantile and juvenile idiopathic epilepsy with generalized tonic clonic seizures. Like these types of epilepsy, myoclonic astatic epilepsy is polygenically determined with little nongenetic variability. The disease is characterized by the following criteria: genetic predisposition (high incidence of seizures and/or genetic EEG patterns in relatives); mostly normal development and no neurological deficits before onset; primarily generalized myoclonic, astatic or myoclonic astatic seizures, short absences and mostly generalized tonic clonic seizures; no tonic seizures or tonic drop attacks during daytime (except for some rare cases with a most unfavourable course); generalized EEG patterns (spikes and waves, photosensitivity, 4–7 Hz rhythms), no multifocal EEG-abnormalities (but often pseudofoci).'[226]
This contrasts markedly with the previous classification of 1989 where 'myoclonic astatic epilepsy' was listed as 'cryptogenic/symptomatic' generalised epilepsy in the same group of disorders as that of the Lennox-Gastaut syndrome.[9]

The problem may reflect lack of specific diagnostic criteria and undefined boundaries of certain epileptic syndromes and particularly epileptic encephalopathies, which may manifest with myoclonic-astatic seizures. This particularly refers to Dravet syndrome, Lennox-Gastaut syndrome and atypical benign epilepsy of childhood. Cases of benign and severe myoclonic epilepsy in infants may have been included in epilepsy with myoclonic-astatic seizures.[224] Other myoclonic epilepsies with brief seizures reported as intermediate cases between epilepsy with myoclonic-astatic seizures and Lennox-Gastaut syndrome probably prove this point.[216] However, it is generally accepted that some children with myoclonic astatic seizures are otherwise normal with no discernible causes other than a strong genetic epileptic background and these probably represent the genuine, idiopathic syndrome of 'epilepsy with myoclonic astatic seizures'. This point is exemplified in the study of Kaminska et al. (1999)[358] who found evidence that 'epilepsy with myoclonic astatic seizures' is distinct from Lennox-Gastaut syndrome, and the distinction appears from the first year of the disorder.
A further exciting development is that myoclonic-astatic seizures frequently occur in patients with 'generalised epilepsy with febrile seizures plus' (page 147).[196]

Clinical manifestations: Doose syndrome is characterised by myoclonic-astatic seizures that often occur together with atonic, myoclonic and absence seizures; myoclonic-astatic status epilepticus is common.

Children are normal before the onset of seizures. In two thirds, febrile and afebrile generalised tonic-clonic seizures appear first, several months before the onset of myoclonic–astatic seizures.

Myoclonic-astatic (in fact myoclonic-atonic) seizures are the defining symptoms (100% of the cases).[224] These manifest with symmetrical myoclonic jerks immediately followed by loss of muscle tone (post-myoclonic atonia) (Figure 6.3).

In addition, **atonic and absence seizures** occur frequently, sometimes many per day in the active period of the disease.

Boy aged 6 with myoclonic-astatic epilepsy

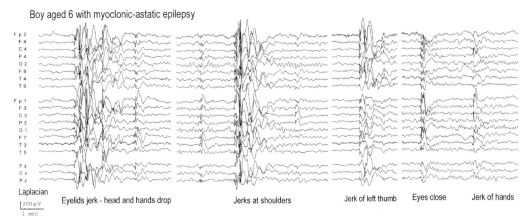

Eyelids jerk - head and hands drop   Jerks at shoulders   Jerk of left thumb   Eyes close   Jerk of hands

Figure 6.3

Samples from video-EEG of an 8-year-old normal boy with Doose syndrome. The background activity was normal but there were frequent (at least every 10 seconds) generalised discharges of high voltage spike/polyspikes and slow wave complexes at 3–6Hz with anterior maximum. They were brief for 1–4 seconds. These were frequently associated with single jerks of mainly the shoulders but on other occasions of the thumb, eyelids or elsewhere. The jerks occurred simultaneously with the first or the second polyspike wave complex of the discharges.

Some jerks were followed by atonic attacks. The EEG also showed brief (<0.5 seconds) abortive generalised discharges of polyspikes at around 15 Hz with anterior maximum and an alternating but not consistent side emphasis. There were no clinical manifestations.

The paroxysmal discharges occurred with eyes opened and closed, spontaneously and during overbreathing. IPS did not evoke photoparoxysmal responses.

Diagnostic criteria of idiopathic epilepsy with myoclonic–astatic seizures [356]

Inclusion criteria

1. Normal development before the onset of seizures and normal MRI

2. Onset of myoclonic, myoclonic-atonic or atonic seizures between 7 months and 6 years of age

3. Normal background EEG with generalised 2–3 Hz spike, polyspike slow wave discharges without focal spike discharges

Exclusion criteria

1. Dravet syndrome, Lennox-Gastaut syndrome, benign myoclonic epilepsy in infancy or other epileptic syndromes manifesting with myoclonic-astatic seizures

2. Tonic seizures

Atonic seizures of sudden, brief and severe loss of postural tone may involve the whole body or only the head. Attacks are brief, 1–4 seconds, and frequent. Generalised loss of postural tone causes a lightning-like fall. The patient collapses on the floor irresistibly. In brief and milder attacks there is only head nodding or bending of the knees.

Myoclonic jerks may precede or less often intersperse with the atonic manifestations (Figure 6.3).

More than half of the cases have brief **absence seizures** often together with myoclonic jerks, facial myoclonias and atonic manifestations. Absence seizures alone without other than impairment of consciousness clinical symptoms are exceptional.

Tonic seizures are an exclusion criterion.

Non-convulsive status epilepticus lasting for hours or even days (Figure 6.4) is common, affecting one third of the patients. This manifests with varying degrees of usually severe cognitive impairment or cloudiness of consciousness interspersed with repetitive myoclonic and atonic fits. Facial myoclonus of eyelids and mouth may be continuous together with irregular jerks of the limbs and atonic seizures of head nodding or falls. Non-convulsive status epilepticus may occur several times during a period of 1–2 years.

Aetiology: Epilepsy with myoclonic astatic seizures may be genetically determined in multifactorial polygenic fashion with variable penetrance.[224,353,354] One third have familial seizure disorders and idiopathic generalised epilepsy.[224,353,354] Of significant interest are the clinical and molecular studies of generalised epilepsy with febrile seizures plus (page 147) where myoclonic–atonic seizures are common.[196]

Diagnostic procedures: By definition all tests other than EEG are normal.

Electroencephalography: Interictal EEG may be normal at the stage of febrile or afebrile generalised convulsions. Rhythmic theta activity in the parasagittal montage may be the only significant abnormality. Subsequently, when myoclonic-atonic seizures appear, there are frequent generalised discharges of 2–3 Hz spikes and waves in clusters interrupted by high amplitude slow waves in cases with predominant atonic or myoclonic-atonic seizures. In children with predominantly myoclonic seizures, these are paroxysms of irregular spikes or polyspikes-waves.

The ictal EEG of myoclonic and atonic seizures associates with discharges of irregular spike waves or polyspike waves at a frequency of 2.5–3 Hz or more (Figure 6.3). Atonia is usually associated with the slow wave of a single or multiple spike wave complex and the intensity of the atonia is proportional to the amplitude of slow wave. Drop attacks are associated with diffuse EMG paucity, indicating their true atonic nature.[356]

In non-convulsive status, the EEG shows continuous or discontinuous and repetitive 2–3 Hz spikes and waves (Figure 6.4).

Differential diagnosis: The differential diagnosis of epilepsy with myoclonic astatic seizures is mainly between benign myoclonic epilepsy in infants (see page 54), Dravet syndrome (see page 63), Lennox-Gastaut syndrome (see page 70)

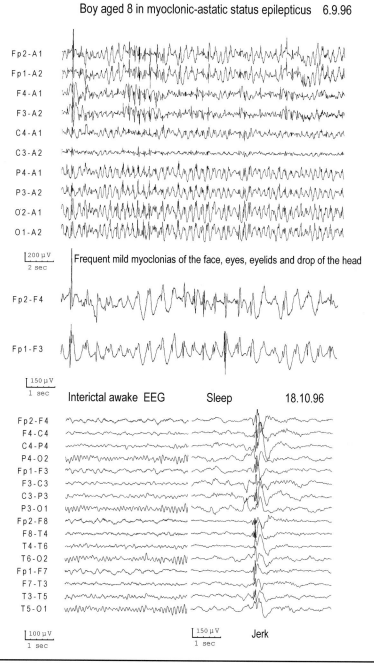

Boy aged 8 in myoclonic-astatic status epilepticus   6.9.96

Figure 6.4

Top: Samples of video-EEG of a boy in myoclonic-astatic status epilepticus. The EEG showed electrical status epilepticus during wakefulness and sleep. This consisted of nearly continuous generalised discharges of spike (or double spikes) and slow wave complexes at 2.5–3Hz. This pattern occasionally alternated with relatively normal background lasting <30 seconds. The main clinical manifestations were frequent facial subtle myoclonias (eyelid fluttering,

upper deviation of the eyes with spontaneous eye opening associated with fast eyelid fluttering, subtle facial twitches) and few massive myoclonic jerks occasionally with some atonic components. Clinically there was no apparent impairment of consciousness. *Middle:* Detail of the EEG in the top of the figure. *Bottom:* Video-EEG 1 year later had normal background with a few myoclonic jerks during sleep only.

and late onset West syndrome (see page 57). In general, children with the idiopathic form of epilepsy with myoclonic astatic seizures are normal before the development of seizures, have a strong family of IGEs, and background EEG and brain imaging are normal.

Progressive myoclonic epilepsies such as myoclonic epilepsy with ragged-red fibres, Lafora or Unverricht–Lundborg disease may initially imitate Doose syndrome. However, the associated relevant neurological abnormalities and sometimes the relentless progress and deterioration will establish the diagnosis.

Atypical benign partial epilepsy of childhood may also imitate Doose syndrome because of repeated falls, absences and diffuse slow spike wave activity mainly in sleep EEG.[25,170,359] This is a rare condition of children with normal neurological and intellectual state and a good final outcome. The main differentiating point is that these children also have nocturnal focal seizures similar to the Rolandic seizures that are often the initial seizure type. Also EEG shows centrotemporal and other functional spikes in various locations. Atonic seizures occur in clusters lasting for one to several weeks, usually separated by free intervals of several weeks or months. They may involve the whole axial musculature and/or both lower limbs with multiple daily falls that can produce severe injuries. On other occasions, they may be localised – manifested with brief (1–2 seconds) sudden head drop or hand focal atonia. Brief focal atonia may manifest as a transient dropping of one arm lasting from 100 to 150 ms when patients are asked to keep both arms outstretched in front of the body. The brief focal atonia of the arm occasionally would progress to atonic seizures or atonic-absence seizures. Some patients may additionally have GTCS, brief absences and occasionally jerks. Focal sensorimotor fits are exceptional. Atonic attacks are associated with the slow wave component of spike wave complexes, and the location of the EEG discharges corresponds to that of the atonic episodes.

Similar clinico-EEG features may occur in atypical evolutions of Rolandic epilepsy[282,360] and Panayiotopoulos syndrome[300,301] but these are preceded by typical presentations of these syndromes (see Chapter 5). A similar but reversible clinico-EEG condition may be induced by carbamazepine in a few children with Rolandic epilepsy.[25] This possibility should be considered in children with Rolandic seizures and dramatic deterioration after treatment with carbamazepine or other drugs such as vigabatrin.

Children with 'epilepsy with continuous spike and waves during slow wave sleep' (page 85) may also have drop attacks due to atypical absences or negative myoclonus.

Diagnostic Tips

● The diagnosis is probably secured if myoclonic-atonic seizures start in a previously normal child with pre-existing febrile or afebrile convulsions and familial seizure disorders (however, see page 147 for generalised epilepsy with febrile seizures plus[196]).

● Differential diagnostic problems with Lennox-Gastaut syndrome probably reflect ill-defined inclusion and exclusion criteria (page 70).

Non-epileptic myoclonus of many neurological disorders rarely raises a diagnostic problem with Doose syndrome, unless it is a part of a degenerative disease with associated epileptic features.[355]

Prognosis: This is unclear, probably because of different selection criteria.

Half of the patients may achieve a seizure-free state and normal or near normal development. These may correspond to the idiopathic form of epilepsy with myoclonic astatic seizures. Spontaneous remission with normal development has been observed in a few untreated cases but these may belong to benign myoclonic epilepsy in infancy (see page 54).

The others, probably belonging to symptomatic or possibly symptomatic cases or other syndromes, may continue with seizures, severe impairment of cognitive functions and behavioural abnormalities. Ataxia, poor motor function, dysarthria and poor language development may emerge.

Management: Drugs are dictated by seizure type. Sodium valproate – effective in myoclonic jerks, atonic seizures and absences – is the most efficacious. In resistant cases, small doses of lamotrigine have a beneficial pharmacodynamic interaction with sodium valproate. Ethosuximide, benzodiazepines, acetazolamide, sulthiame and even bromides are used in resistant cases. Topiramate may reduce the frequency of drop attacks and tonic-clonic seizures. Levetiracetam because of its broad effectiveness in all these seizures, may become the first choice..

Carbamazepine, phenytoin and vigabatrin are contraindicated.

In non-convulsive status epilepticus intravenous benzodiazepines are often efficacious, although rarely they may precipitate tonic status.

CHILDHOOD ABSENCE EPILEPSY

Childhood absence epilepsy (CAE) is the prototype IGE of typical absence seizures.[335,336,338,361,362] It is genetically determined, age-related and affects otherwise normal children. Table 6.3 lists inclusion and exclusion criteria.

Demographic data: Age of onset is between 2 and 10 years of age, with a peak at 5–6 years. Two thirds are girls. Prevalence is ~10% and annual incidence rate is ~7/100,000 of children with epileptic seizures younger than 15–16 years of age.

Clinical manifestations: CAE manifests with the most characteristic and classical example of typical absence seizures. Absences are severe and frequent, tens or hundreds per day, for which CAE is also known as pyknolepsy.[18] They are of abrupt onset and abrupt termination (Figure 6.5). Their duration varies from 4 to 20 seconds, although most of them last around 10 seconds. Clinically, the hallmark of the absence is abrupt, brief and severe impairment of consciousness with unresponsiveness and interruption of the ongoing voluntary activity, which is not restored during the ictus. The eyes spontaneously open, overbreathing, speech and other voluntary activity stops within the first 3 seconds from the onset of the discharge. Automatisms occur in two thirds of the seizures but are not stereotyped. The eyes stare or move slowly. Mild myoclonic elements of the eyes, eyebrows and eyelids may feature in childhood absence epilepsy but these are usually mild, occurring at the onset of the absence. However, more severe and sustained myoclonic jerks of facial muscles may indicate other idiopathic generalised epilepsies with absences.

The attack ends as abruptly as it began. The seizure ends with sudden resumption of the pre-absence activity as if it was not interrupted.

Typical absence seizures are nearly invariably provoked by hyperventilation.

Seizures other than typical absences are not compatible with childhood absence epilepsy. The only exception is solitary or infrequent GTCS long after the onset of TAS (usually in adolescence after absences have remitted) and febrile convulsions.

Aetiology: Childhood absence epilepsy is a syndrome of idiopathic generalised epilepsy, which is genetically determined. The mode of transmission is unknown and may be multifactorial. In monozygotic twins, 84% had 3 Hz spike wave and only 75% of pairs had clinical absence seizures. These figures were 16 times less frequent in dizygotic twins.[363]

'Two separate loci also are present for pyknoleptic CAE, namely, CAE that evolves to JME in chromosome 1p and CAE with grand mal in chromosome 8q24.'[333] However, according to the criteria proposed in this chapter neither of these groups is childhood absence epilepsy. There are also reports implicating chromosome 5q31.1 and 19p13.2 (see an excellent recent review in ref [362]).

Acquired factors may play a facilitating role.

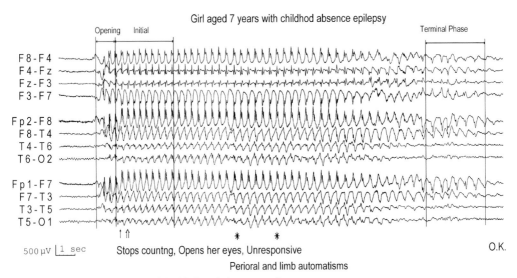

Girl aged 7 years with childhod absence epilepsy

Figure 6.5   Girl aged 7 years with childhood absence epilepsy.

The seizure occurred during hyperventilation with breath counting. She stopped counting (black arrow), opened her eyes (open arrow) and became unresponsive. Marked perioral automatisms occurred later (*). She abruptly recovered at the end of the discharge (O.K.). Note the regular spike wave of the discharge, which in the initial phase is 3 Hz, gradually slowing down to 2 Hz in the terminal phase. The opening phase (1 second of the discharge) is usually asymmetrical and asynchronous with faster or irregular frequencies. (See also Figures 1.3 and 6.1.)

Diagnostic procedures: In typical cases only EEG is needed.

Electroencephalography: The EEG in childhood absence epilepsy has normal background, with frequent rhythmic posterior delta activity. Ictal discharges consist of generalised high-amplitude spike and double or occasionally triple spike and slow wave complexes (Figure 6.5). They are rhythmic at around 3 Hz (2.5–4 Hz) with a gradual and regular slowdown of the frequency by 0.5–1 Hz from the initial to the terminal phase of the discharge. The opening phase of the discharge, 1 second from the onset, is usually fast and unreliable for these measurements. There are no marked variations in the relation of spike to the slow wave, no fluctuations in the intradischarge frequency and certainly no fragmentations of the ictal discharges (Figure 6.5).

Table 6.3   Criteria for childhood absence epilepsy

Inclusion criteria

1. Age at onset between 4 and 10 years and a peak at 5–7 years.
2. Normal neurological state and development.
3. Brief (4–20 seconds, exceptionally longer) and frequent (tens per day) absence seizures with abrupt and severe impairment (loss) of consciousness. Automatisms are frequent but have no significance in the diagnosis.
4. EEG ictal discharges of generalised high-amplitude spike and double (maximum occasional three spikes are allowed) spike and slow wave complexes. Spike-wave is rhythmic at around 3 Hz with a gradual and regular slowdown from the initial to the terminal phase of the discharge. The duration of the discharges varies from 4 to 20 seconds.

Exclusion criteria

The following may be incompatible with childhood absence epilepsy:

1. Other than typical absence seizures such as GTCS, or myoclonic jerks before or during the active stage of absences.
2. Eyelid myoclonia, perioral myoclonia, rhythmic massive limb jerking, and single or arrhythmic myoclonic jerks of the head, trunk or limbs. However, mild myoclonic elements of the eyes, eyebrows, and eyelids may be featured – particularly in the first 3 seconds of the absence seizure.
3. Mild or no impairment of consciousness during the 3–4 Hz discharges.
4. Brief EEG 3–4 Hz spike wave paroxysms of <4 seconds, multiple spikes (>3) or ictal discharge fragmentations.
5. Visual (photic) and other sensory precipitation of clinical seizures.

From Loiseau and Panayiotopoulos (2002)[361] with the permission of the authors and the Editor of *Medlink*.

Diagnostic Tips

● Typical absence seizures of childhood absence epilepsy are easy to diagnose and reproduce by hyperventilation.

● Any child with sudden, brief and frequent cessation of physical and mental activity should be tested clinically for absences. This is easily performed with the hyperventilation test.

● Ask the child to overbreathe for 3 minutes while counting his/her breaths and holding hands outstretched in front of the body. This will evoke an absence in more than 90% of children with childhood absence epilepsy.

● It is essential that a video-EEG is performed before initiating treatment for appropriate confirmation and documentation of the clinico-EEG characteristics of the absences. If this is not possible the clinical manifestations should be documented with video (camcorders).

Differential diagnosis: CAE should be the easiest type of epileptic syndrome to diagnose because seizures have abrupt onset and termination, daily frequency and are nearly invariably provoked by hyperventilation. In practical terms a child suspected of experiencing typical absences should be asked to overbreathe for 3 minutes while standing, counting his/her breaths and with hands outstretched in front of the body. This will provoke an absence in as many as 90% of those who suffer.

> Childhood absence epilepsy is not synonymous with any type of absence seizures starting in childhood. Therefore, other epilepsy syndromes with absence seizures that may be lifelong and have a worse prognosis should be meticulously differentiated from childhood absence epilepsy.

Diagnosis should improve with heightened awareness and video-EEG studies. Exclusion criteria for childhood absence epilepsy are vital (Table 6.3).

Automatisms have no significance in the diagnosis. They should not be taken as evidence of complex focal seizures (see Table 6.1), which require entirely different management.

Prognosis: By applying strict criteria of diagnosis, an excellent prognosis may be provided. Remission occurs before the age of 12 years. Less than 10% of the patients may develop infrequent or solitary generalised tonic–clonic seizures in adolescence or adult life. It is exceptional for patients to continue having absence seizures as adults. Poor social adjustment of these patients has been reported.

Management: Treatment is mainly with monotherapy of sodium valproate, ethosuximide or lamotrigine, which controls the absences in more than 80% of patients. Adding small doses of lamotrigine to sodium valproate may be the best combination in resistant cases. Of the new drugs levetiracetam and topiramate are promising.

EPILEPSY WITH MYOCLONIC ABSENCES

Epilepsy with myoclonic absences (MAE) is a rare syndrome of childhood which demands scrupulous exclusion of other forms of symptomatic or possibly symptomatic cases manifesting with the same seizure (myoclonic absences).[364–366]

Demographic data: Age at onset varies from the first months of life to early teens with a median at 7 years. Boys predominate. It is a very rare disorder with an approximate prevalence of 0.5–1% amongst selected patients with

---

Considerations on classification:

Myoclonic absences (the seizures) may feature either in normal or neurologically and mentally abnormal children.[336] Epilepsy with myoclonic absences (the syndrome) was previously categorised amongst the 'cryptogenic or symptomatic generalised epilepsies

and syndromes'.[9] The new ILAE diagnostic scheme considers only the idiopathic form (Table 1.2 and 1.3),[10] which probably represents less than one third of the whole spectrum of epileptic disorders manifesting with myoclonic absences. The others are symptomatic or probably symptomatic cases.[9]

epileptic disorders.[366,367] I have seen only three cases over a period of 15 years out of nearly 200 patients with video-EEG recorded typical absence seizures.[7,368]

Clinical manifestations: **The myoclonic absences** are the defining symptom of epilepsy with myoclonic absences. These manifest with impairment of consciousness, which varies from mild to severe and rhythmic myoclonic jerks mainly of the shoulders, arms and legs with a concomitant tonic contraction. Eyelid twitching is practically absent but perioral myoclonias are frequent. The jerks and the tonic contraction may be unilateral or asymmetrical and head/body deviation may be a constant feature in some patients. The tonic contraction mainly affects shoulder and deltoid muscles that may cause elevation of the arms. The duration of the absences varies from 8 to 60 seconds. Myoclonic absences occur many times per day.

Other seizures such as GTCS or atonic fits occur in two thirds of the patients, often predicting an unfavourable prognosis (these are probably symptomatic cases). Absence status is rare.

Aetiology: Myoclonic absences (the seizures, not the syndrome) are due to idiopathic, cryptogenic or symptomatic causes including chromosomal abnormalities.[369] One third are idiopathic and only these belong to this syndrome.

Diagnostic procedures: By definition, in MAE all other tests except EEG should be normal. Brain MRI and chromosomal testing[369] are needed for the detection of the symptomatic cases.

Electroencephalography: Background EEG is usually normal at onset but may deteriorate later or may be abnormal in symptomatic cases. In half the cases interictal EEG shows brief generalised, focal or multifocal spike and slow wave.[366]

Ictal EEG shows generalised rhythmic 3 Hz spike/multiple spike and slow wave discharges even in those with unilateral or asymmetrical clinical manifestations (Figure 6.6). Polygraphic studies revealed that each myoclonic jerk coincides with the spike component of the discharge.[366]

Differential diagnosis: The differential diagnosis of MAE from other types of syndromes with absences is easy because of the characteristic type of myoclonic absences. The difficulty is between idiopathic and symptomatic/cryptogenic cases which manifest with the same seizure type (myoclonic absences). Symptomatic cases often have abnormal neurological state, abnormal background EEG and abnormal brain MRI. Chromosomal abnormalities are common.[369] Additionally, absences with rhythmic myoclonic jerking but <2.5 Hz spike/polyspike slow wave and other characteristics of atypical absences may occur in epileptic encephalopathies[366,367,370] and these may be some of the cases with chromosomal abnormalities.[369]

Prognosis: Nearly half of children with epilepsy with myoclonic absences have impaired cognitive functioning before the onset of absences but these are probably symptomatic cases. However, half of those who were normal before the onset of absences develop cognitive and behavioural impairment. This may mean a deteriorating effect of the EEG discharges on cognition without their early suppression with treatment.

Myoclonic absences are often resistant to treatment. Half of the patients (probably the symptomatic ones) continue having seizures in adult life, developing features of other types of epilepsy such as Lennox–Gastaut syndrome or juvenile myoclonic epilepsy.

Management: Early control of absences may prevent subsequent cognitive deterioration and secure normal development. Treatment often requires high doses of sodium valproate often combined with ethosuximide or lamotrigine. New drugs such as levetiracetam and topiramate or old drugs such as clonazepam and acetazolamide should be tried. The aim is to stop myoclonic absence seizures as early as possible.

Normal boy aged 8 years with idiopathic myoclonic absence epilepsy; at age 19 years he is well and unmedicated

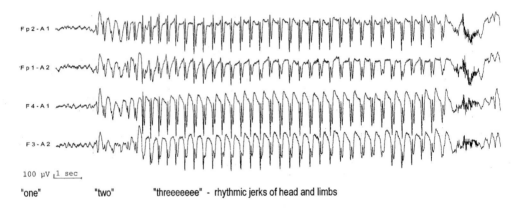

"one" "two" "threeeeeee" - rhythmic jerks of head and limbs

Girl 15 months old with symptomatic myoclonic absence epilepsy; at age 14 she is mentally and physically disabled with intractable seizures

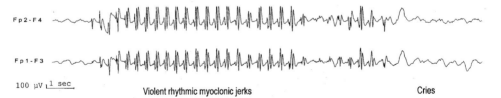

Violent rhythmic myoclonic jerks Cries

Figure 6.6 Samples from video-EEG of idiopathic and symptomatic myoclonic absence seizures.

Top: Boy aged 8 years with myoclonic absences from age 6. These were frequent, hundreds per day, and manifested with rhythmic myoclonic jerks and unresponsiveness. Sodium valproate failed to achieve control but absences ceased completely when ethosuximide was added at age 8. Medication was withdrawn at age 11. No further seizures occurred in the next 6 years of follow-up and he is academically successful.

Bottom: Girl aged 15 months with myoclonic absences due to birth anoxia. Typical absence seizures started at 15 months of age. These were many per day, lasted for 8–10 seconds and were characterised by synchronous and bilateral myoclonic jerks of limbs and head with apparent loss of consciousness. Subsequently, she developed frequent, mainly nocturnal GTCS while myoclonic absences continue. These are intractable to any appropriate medication. At age 8 she has learning difficulties and spastic quadraparesis.

JUVENILE ABSENCE EPILEPSY

Juvenile absence epilepsy (JAE) is a syndrome of IGE[9,10,335] mainly manifested with severe absence seizures; nearly all patients (80%) also suffer from generalised tonic-clonic seizures (GTCS) and one fifth from sporadic myoclonic jerks.[335,336,368,371,372]

Demographic data: Main age at onset is from 9 to 13 years (70% of the patients) but range is from 5 to 20 years.[335,372] Myoclonic jerks and GTCS usually begin 1–10 years after the onset of absences. Rarely GTCS may precede the onset of absences.[335,371]

Both sexes are equally affected. The exact prevalence of JAE is not known because of variable criteria. In adults older than 20 years prevalence of JAE may be around 2–3% of all epilepsies and around 8–10% of IGE.[373,374]

Clinical manifestations: Frequent and severe typical absences are the characteristic and defining seizures of JAE (Figure 6.7). The usual frequency of absences is approximately 1–10 per day but this may be much higher for some patients.[335,371,372] Nearly all patients also develop GTCS and one fifth of them also suffer from mild myoclonic jerks.

Typical absences are the defining seizure type of JAE. These are severe and frequent, often daily, and very much similar to those of CAE although they may be milder. The hallmark of the absence is abrupt, brief and severe impairment of consciousness with total or partial unresponsiveness. Mild or inconspicuous impairment of consciousness is not compatible with JAE. The ongoing voluntary activity usually stops at onset but may be partly restored during the ictus. Automatisms are frequent, usually occurring 6–10 seconds after the onset of the EEG discharge (Figure 6.7). In JAE, mild myoclonic elements of the eyelids are common during the absence. However, more severe and sustained myoclonic jerks of facial muscles may indicate other IGE with absences. Severe eyelid or perioral myoclonus, rhythmic limb jerking and single or arrhythmic myoclonic jerks of the head, trunk or limbs during the absence ictus are probably incompatible with JAE (Table 6.4).

The duration of the absences varies from 4 to 30 seconds but it is usually long (~16 seconds).

Generalised tonic-clonic seizures are probably unavoidable in untreated patients. GTCS occur in 80% of the patients, mainly after awakening,

Considerations on classification:

The ILAE Task Force has not yet reached definite conclusions regarding the definition of JAE although there is a tendency to consider JAE as part of a broader syndrome of IGE in adolescence.[10,352]

The 1989 ILAE Classification broadly defined JAE by frequency of absences (less frequent than those of childhood absence epilepsy) and age at onset (around puberty).[9] These are insufficient criteria for the categorisation of any syndrome.[335] Thus, epidemiology, genetics, age at onset, clinical manifestations, other type of seizures, long-term prognosis and treatment may not accurately reflect the syndrome of JAE. Recently, JAE has been re-defined on a cluster of video-EEG-studied clinical and EEG manifestations (Table 6.4).[335,368]

although nocturnal or diurnal GTCS may also be experienced.[335,371–373,375,376] GTCS are usually infrequent but they may also become severe and intractable.

Myoclonic jerks occurring in 15–25% of the patients are infrequent, mild and of random distribution. They usually occur in the afternoon hours when the patient is tired rather than in the morning after awakening.[335,347]

Absence status epilepticus occur in one fifth of the patients.[346,347]

Seizure-precipitating factors: Mental and psychological arousal are the main precipitating factors for TA. Conversely, sleep deprivation, fatigue, alcohol, excitement, lights alone or usually in combination are the main precipitating factors for GTCS.

Some authors reported that 8% of JAE patients suffer from photosensitivity clinically or EEG.[371] However, clinical photosensitivity that is consistent with provocation of seizures (absences, GTCS or jerks) may be incompatible with JAE. These patients may have other IGE.[335] EEG photosensitivity that is facilitation of absences by IPS may not be uncommon.

Aetiology: JAE is determined by genetic factors but mode of transmission and relation to other forms of IGE and particularly CAE and JME have not yet been established; a single Mendelian mode appears to be unlikely.

There is an increased incidence of epileptic disorders in families of patients with JAE and there are reports of monozygotic twins with JAE.[368,372,377] A proband with JAE was found in 3 of 37 families selected because at least three members were affected by IGE in one or more generations.[378] However, only one sibling also had JAE while other members mainly had GTCS.[378]

JAE still has to pass the test of genetic identification. JAE may be linked to chromosome 8,[379] 21,[380] 18[334] and probably 5.[334] Heterogeneity may be common, as indicated in animal models. Autopsy[381] and studies with new MRI techniques[382] found microdysgenesis and other cerebral structural changes in patients with JAE.

Diagnostic procedures: All except EEG tests are normal.

Electroencephalography: The EEG in untreated patients is abnormal with absences easily elicited by hyperventilation (Figure 6.7). The inter-ictal EEG is normal or shows only mild abnormalities. Focal epileptiform abnormalities and abortive asymmetrical bursts of spike/multiple spike are common.

The ictal EEG shows generalised, spike or multiple spike and slow waves at 3–4 Hz. The frequency at the initial phase of the discharge is usually fast at 3–5 Hz. There is a gradual and smooth decline in frequency from the initial to the terminal phase. The discharge is regular, with well-formed spikes, which retain a constant relation with the slow waves (Figure 6.7).

Differential diagnosis: In general, and particularly in adults, absences are often misdiagnosed as complex partial seizures, although their differentiation is easy (Table 6.1).[373,383]

The differentiation of JAE from other IGEs with absences may be more difficult without appropriate video-EEG evaluation.[7,335,368] In children, it is often difficult to distinguish between CAE and JAE, because their features overlap and manifestations are similar. In JAE absences often start later, usually they are less frequent and impairment of cognition is less severe.[368] Automatisms are equally prominent in both. Limb myoclonic jerks (not during the absences) and/or GTCS in the presence of severe absences indicate JAE.

JAE is distinctly different from Jeavons syndrome of very brief seizures marked with rapid eyelid myoclonia, perioral myoclonia with absences of rhythmic perioral myoclonia during the absence, epilepsy with myoclonic absences of rhythmic myoclonic jerks.

In adolescents, the differential diagnosis between JAE and JME should not be difficult. Severe absences are the major problem in JAE, myoclonic jerks are the main seizure type in JME. Absences in JME are mild and often inconspicuous (page 139).

Prognosis: JAE is a lifelong disorder although seizures can be controlled in 70–80% of the patients. However, there is a tendency for the absences to become less severe in terms of impairment of cognition, duration and frequency with age and particularly after the fourth decade of life.[371,376] GTCS are usually infrequent – often precipitated by sleep deprivation, fatigue and alcohol consumption. Myoclonic jerks if present are not troublesome for the patient. However, one fifth of the patients may have frequent and sometimes intractable absences and GTCS, and this figure may be higher if appropriate treatment is not initiated during the early stages of JAE.

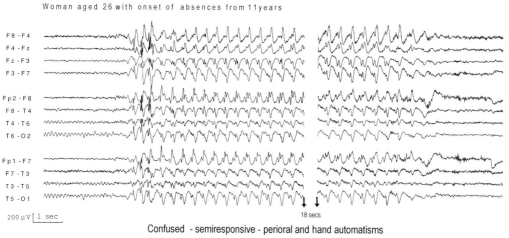

Woman aged 26 with onset of absences from 11 years

200 μV | 1 sec

18 secs

Confused - semiresponsive - perioral and hand automatisms

Figure 6.7

From video-EEG of a 26-year-old normal woman. She started having frequent (tens per day) typical absence seizures with severe impairment of consciousness at age 11 years. At age 14 years she had her first GTCS. Since then long absences of 20–30 seconds have continued daily. Also she has 3–5 GTCS every year mainly in the morning, after awakening. These are preceded by clusters of absences. Occasionally, she also has random, infrequent and mild limb myoclonic jerks, which started at age 20. Treatment with various appropriate anti-absence drugs resulted in minor improvement but compliance varies.

From Panayiotopoulos (2002)[336] with the permission of the Editor of *Medlink*.

Management: The treatment of IGE is detailed on page 156. In JAE, the consensus is that because of the frequent combination of absences and GTCS the drug of choice is sodium valproate, which controls all seizures in 70–80% of the patients. If monotherapy with valproate is partially effective, add-on treatment with lamotrigine (particularly if GTCS is the problem) or ethosuximide (particularly if absences persist) may further improve or control the situation. Control of absences is usually (90%) associated with good control of GTCS and it is adversely affected by the frequency and the duration of GTCS before starting valproate treatment.

All these approaches may need significant re-assessment with the introduction of newer drugs such as levetiracetam and topiramate.

Patients should be warned regarding precipitating factors of GTCS.

Treatment may be lifelong because attempts to withdraw medication nearly invariably lead to relapses even after many years free of seizures.

Table 6.4 Main inclusion and exclusion criteria for juvenile absence epilepsy (JAE)

Inclusion criteria

1. Unequivocal clinical evidence of absence seizures with severe impairment of consciousness. Nearly all patients may have GTCS. More than half have myoclonic jerks but these are mild and do not show the circadian distribution of JME.

2. Documentation of ictal 3–4 Hz generalised discharges of spike or multiple spike and slow wave discharges longer than 4 seconds that are associated with severe impairment of consciousness and often with automatisms. Normal EEGs in treated patients are common.

Exclusion criteria

The following may be incompatible with juvenile absence epilepsy:
Clinical exclusion criteria

1. Absences with marked eyelid or perioral myoclonus or marked single or rhythmic limb and trunk myoclonic jerks.

2. Absences with exclusively mild or clinically undetectable impairment of consciousness.

3. Consistent visual, photosensitive and other sensory precipitation of clinical absences is probably against the diagnosis of JAE. However, on EEG, intermittent photic stimulation often facilitates generalised discharges and absences.

Electroencephalographic exclusion criteria

1. Irregular, arrhythmic spike/multiple spike and slow wave discharges with marked variations of the intra-discharge frequency.

2. Significant variations between the spike/multiple spike and slow wave relations.

3. Predominantly brief discharges (<4 seconds).

JUVENILE MYOCLONIC EPILEPSY

JANZ SYNDROME

Juvenile myoclonic epilepsy (JME) is one of the most important IGEs that is genetically determined.[8,340,341,384–386]

Demographic data: The triad of absences, jerks and GTCS shows a characteristic age-related onset. Absences, when a feature, begin between the ages of 5 and 16 years. Myoclonic jerks follow between 1 and 9 years later, usually around the age of 14–15 years. GTCS usually appear a few months later, occasionally earlier, than the myoclonic jerks. Both sexes are equally affected. Prevalence is 8–10% amongst adult and adolescent patients with epilepsies.

Clinical manifestations: JME is characterised by the triad of:

● myoclonic jerks on awakening,

● GTCS in nearly all patients and

● typical absences in more than one third of the patients.

> Lots of *blanks* and *jerks*; then I had a *grand mal* ... I usually have fits when rushing after getting up; usually does not happen later in the day.
>
> From the diary of a patient with JME[384]

Myoclonic jerks occurring after awakening are the most prominent and pathognomonic seizure type.[340,341,386–389] They are shock-like, irregular and arrhythmic, clonic movements of proximal and distal muscles mainly of the upper extremities. They are often inconspicuous, restricted to the fingers, making the patient prone to drop things or look clumsy. They may be violent enough to cause falls. One fifth of the patients describe their jerks as unilateral but video-EEG shows that the jerks affect both sides (Figure 6.2).[388,390]

Some patients (<10%) with mild forms of JME never develop GTCS.[341]

Typical absence seizures. One third of patients have typical absences, which are brief with subtle impairment of consciousness (Figures 6.8 and 6.9). They are different from the absence seizures of childhood or juvenile absence epilepsy.[341,368,391]

Absences appearing before the age of 10 years may be more severe. They become less frequent and severe with age.[341,368,391]

One tenth of patients do not perceive absences despite generalised spike slow wave EEG discharges lasting more than 3 seconds.[341,391] However, on video-EEG with breath counting during hyperventilation, such EEG discharges often manifest with mild impairment of cognition, eyelid flickering or both (Figures 6.8 and 6.9).[7]

Generalised tonic–clonic seizures usually follow the onset of myoclonic jerks.[340,341,386–389,392] Myoclonic jerks, usually in clusters and often with an accelerating frequency and severity, may precede GTCS, a so-called clonic-tonic-clonic generalised seizure.[388]

Status epilepticus. Myoclonic status epilepticus is probably more common than appreciated.[341,393] This almost invariably starts on awakening,

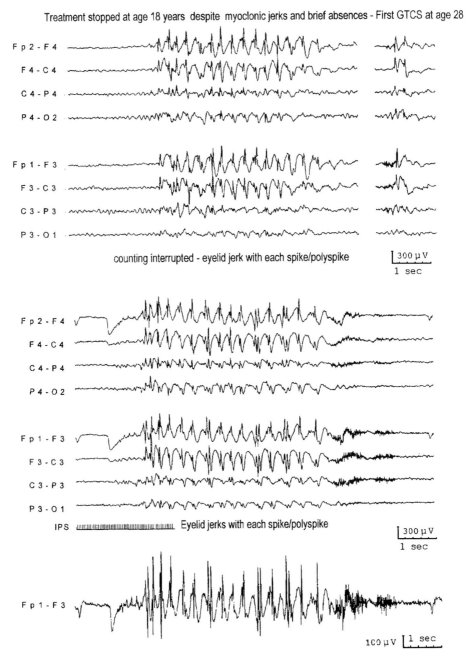

Treatment stopped at age 18 years despite myoclonic jerks and brief absences - First GTCS at age 28

counting interrupted - eyelid jerk with each spike/polyspike

300 μV
1 sec

IPS   Eyelid jerks with each spike/polyspike

300 μV
1 sec

100 μV   1 sec

Figure 6.8   From video-EEG of a woman aged 28 years with JME from age 9.

This woman was referred for a routine EEG as 'probable IGE-absences from age 9 until age 18 years. Myoclonus as a teenager when sleep deprived. Recently suffered her first ever GTCS following sleep deprivation. No absence/myoclonus for 10 years. Treatment with sodium valproate was withdrawn at age 18 years'. Video-EEG documented that she still had brief absences manifested with mild impairment of cognition and eyelid jerks. These were spontaneous, or induced by hyperventilation (*top*) and IPS (*bottom*). Note the multiple spike wave of the discharges and the irregular intra-discharge frequency (magnification on the bottom). Also, note bi-frontal spike and slow wave discharges (*upper right*).

associated with a precipitating factor such as sleep deprivation, or missing medication. Consciousness may not be impaired, although in some patients absences often intersperse with myoclonic jerks (Figure 6.10).

Pure absence status epilepticus is exceptional[346] and generalised tonic-clonic status epilepticus is infrequent.

Circadian distribution. Seizures, principally myoclonic jerks, occurring within half to 1 hour of awakening are characteristic of JME.[340,341,386–389,392] Myoclonic jerks occur rarely at other times unless the patient is tired. GTCS occur mainly on awakening but may also be purely nocturnal or random. Absence seizures rarely show a circadian predilection.

Seizure-precipitating factors: Sleep deprivation and fatigue, particularly after excessive alcohol intake, are the most powerful precipitants of jerks and GTCS in JME.

Sleep deprivation means a late night followed by a brief sleep suddenly interrupted by early awakening in order to go to work or on a trip. A telephone call early in the morning may frequently have disastrous effects.

Photosensitivity is confirmed with EEG in one third of the patients but this may be of no clinical significance. Probably less than one tenth of the patients have seizures induced by photic stimulation in daily life (Figure 6.8).

Other common and prominent precipitants of seizures are mental stress, emotions and particularly excitement, concentration, mental and psychological arousal, failed expectations or frustration.

Aetiology: JME is genetically determined:[340,388,392,394] 50–60% of families of probands with JME report seizures in first or second degree relatives.[392,395] Inheritance is probably complex.[333,396,397] Proposed models of inheritance include polygenic with a lower manifestation threshold for females, autosomal dominant with variable penetrance, a two-locus model with a dominant gene on chromosome 6p and an as-yet unknown recessive gene or, most possibly, that different genotypes with different modes of inheritance underlie the phenotype.[398]

Families with autosomal[394] or dominant[394,396] Mendelian inheritance have been described but these may be rare.

Molecular studies favour a susceptibility locus for JME in chromosome 6p11-12 (EJM1)[333] or 15q14 (EJM2).[399,400] A gene, C6orf33, in the EJM1 region has been identified.[401]

An association of JME with an HLA-DR allele[402,403] was not replicated.[404]

Genetic heterogeneity of JME is a possible explanation for such discordant observations.

Diagnostic procedures: All tests except EEG are normal. With new MRI technologies, abnormalities of cerebral structure in some patients with JME involving mesio-frontal cortical structures have been reported.[405]

Electroencephalography: The EEG in untreated patients is usually abnormal, with generalised discharges of an irregular mixture of 3–6 Hz spike/polyspike and slow wave, with intra-discharge fragmentations and unstable intra-discharge frequency (Figures 1.1, 6.8 and 6.9). One third of the patients show photoparoxysmal responses and one third may also have focal EEG abnormalities.

A normal EEG in a patient suspected of having JME should prompt an EEG on sleep and awakening.

Focal abnormalities are recorded in approximately one third of patients. These are focal single spikes and spike slow wave complexes or focal slow waves.

The typical EEG discharge of a myoclonic jerk is a generalised burst of multiple spikes of 0.5–2 seconds duration (Figures 6.2 and 6.10).

The ictal discharges of absences in JME are distinctly different to those in CAE and JAE. They consist of spike/double/treble or multiple spikes usually preceding or superimposed on the slow waves. Multiple spikes consist of up to 8–10 spikes with a characteristic 'worm-like' or compressed capital W appearance ('Ws'). The number and amplitude of spikes shows considerable inter- and intra-discharge variation. The intra-discharge frequency of the spike/multiple spike slow wave complexes varies from 2 to 10 Hz, mainly 3–5 Hz. The frequency is often higher in the first second from onset. Fragmentations of the discharge are common and characteristic. 'Ws' and fragmentation of discharges are observed in all patients, but vary

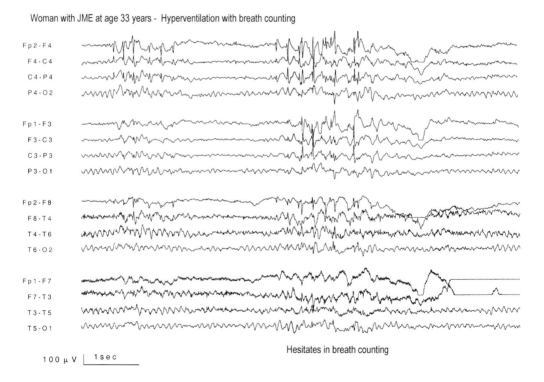

Woman with JME at age 33 years - Hyperventilation with breath counting

100 μV   1 sec

Hesitates in breath counting

Figure 6.9 Focal and asymmetrical generalised discharges in a woman with JME (also illustrated in Figures 6.2 and 6.10).

quantitatively between patients and between discharges (Figures 1.1, 6.1, 6.8, 6.9 and 6.10).

Brief discharges are far more common than long ones and most of the discharges last for 1–4 seconds.

Photoparoxysmal discharges are evoked in 27% of patients.

Differential diagnosis: JME is a typical example of a frequently misdiagnosed common epileptic syndrome resulting in avoidable morbidity.[406,407] Failure to diagnose JME is a serious medical error because JME defies all aspects of general advice regarding 'epilepsy'. Diagnosis should improve with heightened medical awareness. Physicians should be ever alert to the possibility of JME.

> The rate of misdiagnosis of JME is as high as 90%.[406,407] Factors responsible include lack of familiarity with JME, failure to elicit a history of myoclonic jerks, misinterpretation of absences as complex focal seizures, misinterpretation of jerks as focal motor seizures, and high prevalence of focal EEG abnormalities.

JME is easy to diagnose because of a characteristic clustering of myoclonic and other generalised seizures of IGE, circadian distribution, precipitating factors and EEG manifestations. Patients are otherwise normal and there is no mental or physical deterioration if properly diagnosed and treated.

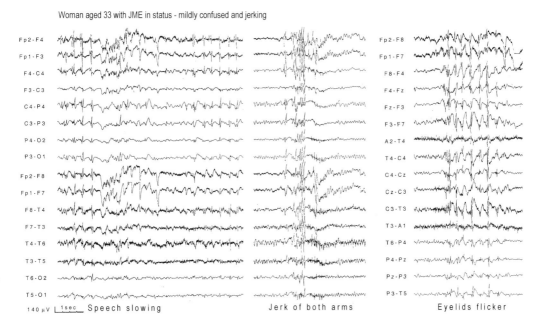

Woman aged 33 with JME in status - mildly confused and jerking

140 µV | 1 sec | Speech slowing   Jerk of both arms   Eyelids flicker

Figure 6.10 Myoclonic-absence status epilepticus in JME.

From video-EEG of a woman with classical JME but on carbamazepine at the time of this recording. The patient was mildly confused, with continuous jerking of hands (*middle*), slowing of speech (left) and eyelid flickering.

As regards other IGEs, juvenile absence epilepsy may be more difficult to differentiate because this syndrome may also manifest with similar clinical and EEG manifestations. The main differentiating factor is that absences with severe impairment of consciousness, not the myoclonic jerks, are the main seizure type in juvenile absence epilepsy. Myoclonic jerks if they occur are mild and random, often lacking the circadian distribution of juvenile myoclonic epilepsy.

Another formidable situation is when juvenile myoclonic epilepsy starts with absences in childhood before the development of myoclonic jerks. There are no prospective video-EEG studies of these patients. Retrospectively examining EEG and clinical manifestations of these patients, I am of the opinion that their absences are distinct from childhood or juvenile absence epilepsy in that they are usually shorter and milder and ictal EEG often contains multiple spike slow waves. Certainly, this situation is not childhood absence epilepsy progressing to juvenile myoclonic epilepsy as some authors reported.[408] It is juvenile myoclonic epilepsy starting with absences before the development of myoclonic jerks.

Prognosis: All seizures are probably lifelong, although improving after the fourth decade of life. Juvenile myoclonic epilepsy may vary in severity from mild myoclonic jerks to frequent and severe falls and GTCS if not appropriately diagnosed and treated.

Seizures are generally well controlled with appropriate medication in up to 90% of the patients.[341,384,388,409] Patients with all three types of seizures are more likely to be resistant to treatment.[410]

Management: Advice regarding lifestyle, avoidance of precipitating factors and long-term medication is essential for a patient with an incontrovertible diagnosis of JME. Avoidance of alcohol indulgence and compensating for sleep deprivation is mandatory. Some patients with mild forms of JME have GTCS or myoclonic jerks only after excessively violating these factors.

Sodium valproate is the most effective anticonvulsant in JME because it prevents absences, myoclonic jerks and GTCS. Sodium valproate dosage depends on severity of JME. An average patient would usually require sodium valproate 500 mg bd. However, sodium valproate is undesirable for some women.

Clonazepam at small doses (0.5–2 mg at night) is probably the most effective drug for myoclonic jerks. However, clonazepam alone may not suppress and may even precipitate GTCS.[341,411] Further, clonazepam may deprive patients of the warning of an impending GTCS provided by the myoclonic jerks.[341,411]

Diagnostic Tips

Generalised tonic–clonic seizures, usually preceded by myoclonic jerks, are nearly pathognomonic of JME if they occur in the morning after:

● A party to celebrate a birthday, end of school-term or New Year's Eve

● Waking up early in the morning to travel for vacations, particularly after a late night

● Replacement of sodium valproate by carbamazepine in women wishing to start a family

● Withdrawal of appropriate medication after many seizure-free years

Phenobarbitone is extensively used as a very effective drug in monotherapy treatment of JME by European neurologists.[340,387,392]

Of the new anticonvulsant drugs, levetiracetam may soon become first choice; in a case-note review of more than 30 patients with resistant JME 62% became seizure free.[414a] Lamotrigine may exaggerate myoclonic jerks but is highly efficacious when combined with sodium valproate.[7,412,413] Lamotrigine monotherapy is still controversial.[7,414]

Contraindicated drugs include vigabatrin, tiagabine and carbamazepine. Carbamazepine is not effective in jerks and absences but its effect in GTCS of IGEs has not been clarified.

IDIOPATHIC GENERALISED EPILEPSY WITH GENERALISED TONIC-CLONIC SEIZURES ONLY

Generalised tonic-clonic seizures (GTCS) are a common feature in IGEs and occur predominantly on awakening. Overall GTCS are reported to occur on awakening (17–53% of patients), diffusely while awake (23–36%) or during sleep (27–44%) or randomly (13–26%).[343] It is undetermined what proportion of these patients also has other generalised seizures (jerks or absences).

GTCS are the most severe forms of epileptic seizures, while absences and myoclonic jerks may be mild and sometimes inconspicuous to the patient and imperceptible to the observer.[339] They are often detected only by meticulous history-taking or video-EEG. A patient with a first GTCS has often suffered from minor seizures (absences, myoclonic jerks or both), sometimes many years before the GTCS.

Demographic data: Age at onset varies from 6 to 47 years with a peak at 16–17 years; 80% of patients have their first GTCS in the second decade of life. Men (55%) slightly predominate probably because of differences in alcohol exposure and sleep habits. The prevalence of 'IGE with GTCS only' is unknown. If strict criteria apply (GTCS only) this may be very small (0.9% of IGEs) but others give a prevalence of 13–15% among IGEs.[415,416]

Clinical manifestations: By definition all patients suffer from GTCS but this syndrome has not been examined in its entirety. Only IGE with GTCS on awakening (EGTCSA) has been extensively studied[417–419] and presented in this chapter.

Sleep deprivation, fatigue and excessive alcohol consumption are main precipitating factors. With age, GTCS tend to increase in frequency and become more unpredictable.

Considerations on classification

'IGE with GTCS *only*' is considered a syndrome in the new ILAE diagnostic scheme[10,352] and incorporates 'epilepsy with GTCS on awakening (EGTCSA)', previously recognised as a separate syndrome.[9]

'IGE with GTCS *only*' has not been precisely defined by the ILAE Task Force.[10] Its name implies that it includes only those patients with GTCS *alone* (i.e. without absences and/or jerks) and that these may occur at any time. However, it is more likely that it is a broader category (rather than a syndrome) of 'IGE with *predominantly* GTCS' (also including patients with mild absences, myoclonic jerks or both).

145

Patients suffer from GTCS, which occur within 1–2 hours after awakening either from nocturnal or diurnal sleep. The seizure may occur while the patient is still in bed or during his breakfast or upon arriving at work. Seizures may also occur during relaxation or leisure.[343,417,418]

Janz described patients with EGTCSA as unreliable, unstable and prone to neglect.[418,419] The sleep patterns of patients with EGTCSA are particularly unstable and modifiable by external factors (i.e. antiepileptic drugs), and the patients may suffer from chronic sleep deficit.[343,417,418]

Precipitating factors: Sleep deprivation, fatigue and excessive alcohol consumption are the main seizure precipitants. Shift work and changes in sleep habits, particularly during holidays and celebrations, predispose to GTCS on awakening. Also, 13% of patients are reported to show photosensitivity on EEG.

Aetiology: There is a high incidence of epileptic disorders in their families[343,418] and a link to the EJM-1 locus has been reported.[420] Conversely, adolescent-onset idiopathic GTCS epilepsy with GTCS at any time whilst awake was not linked to the EJM-1 locus.[420]

Diagnostic procedures: By definition all tests other than EEG are normal.

Man aged 19 years with 2 GTCS at age 14 and 18 on awakening after sleep deprivation

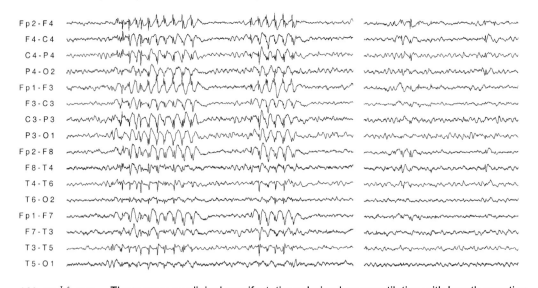

100 µV 1 sec   There were no clinical manifestations during hyperventilation with breath counting

Figure 6.11

Asymptomatic generalised discharges of spikes/multiple spikes and slow waves on video-EEG of a 19-year-old university student who had two GTCS at ages 14 and 18. They both occurred half an hour after awakening from a brief sleep (exam periods). There was no clinical history of any other type of seizures and there were no other symptoms preceding either of the GTCS.
Note that the discharges may start from right or left. Also note focal spikes at various locations.

Electroencephalography: EEG shows generalised discharges of spike/multiple spike slow waves in half of patients with pure EGTCSA (Figure 6.11) and 70% of those with additional absences or myoclonic jerks preceding GTCS.

A normal routine EEG should prompt a video–EEG performed on sleep and on awakening. Myoclonic jerks or, more frequently, brief absences will often be revealed.

Focal EEG abnormalities, in the absence of generalised discharges, are rare. Photoparoxysmal responses are reported in 17% of females and 9% of males with EGTCSA.[343]

Differential diagnosis: The differential diagnosis is mainly from patients with other IGEs that share with EGTCSA the same propensity to seizures after awakening and the same precipitating factors. Juvenile myoclonic epilepsy, juvenile absence epilepsy and eyelid myoclonia with absences are examples of IGE syndromes that may cause diagnostic difficulties. Symptomatic and focal epileptic seizures with secondary generalisation may also occur, predominantly on awakening.

Prognosis: As in all other types of IGEs with onset in the mid-teens, EGTCSA is probably a lifelong disease with a high (83%) incidence of relapse on withdrawal of treatment.[418]   Characteristically, the intervals between seizures become shorter with time, the precipitating factors less obvious, and GTCS may become more random (diurnal and nocturnal), either as a result of the evolution of the disease or drug-induced modifications.[343,417,418]

Management: Patients should be warned of the common seizure precipitants – sleep deprivation with early waking and alcohol consumption – and when possible should avoid occupational night shifts. After adjusting their lifestyles, patients may become seizure-free. Drug treatment is that of IGE with GTCS (page 156).

GENERALISED EPILEPSIES WITH FEBRILE SEIZURES PLUS [421–426]

The new ILAE diagnostic scheme considers 'generalised epilepsies with febrile seizure plus' (GEFS+) as a syndrome in development.[10]

Generalised epilepsy with febrile seizures plus is an extraordinary familial epilepsy syndrome described by Berkovic and his associates.[421]

> 'Febrile seizures plus' is a term to comprise childhood onset of multiple febrile seizures which (unlike the typical febrile seizure) continue beyond the age of 6 years and often afebrile seizures also occur. Febrile seizures usually remit by mid childhood (median 11 years).

GEFS+ is characterised by the presence of febrile and heterogeneous afebrile seizures observed in several members of large pedigree studies. There is a variety of clinical phenotypes including typical febrile seizures, 'febrile seizures plus' (FS+) and other seizure types such as in Dravet syndrome (page 63), absences, myoclonic or atonic seizures and more frequently myoclonic-atonic seizures (page 124).

'Febrile seizures plus' (FS+) is the commonest phenotype. Febrile seizures start earlier (median 1 year) than the typical febrile seizures, they are often multiple and continue beyond 6 years. They usually remit by mid childhood (median 11 years).

Patients express very variable phenotypes combining febrile seizures, generalised seizures often precipitated by fever at age >6 years, and focal seizures, with a variable degree of severity.

To produce the different seizure types observed in families with GEFS+, seizure predisposition determined by the GEFS+ genes could be modified by other genes and/or by environmental factors.

Two genes have been found:

GEFS1, mapped to chromosome 19q and identified as the sodium–channel beta1–subunit.

GEFS2, on chromosome 2q and identified as the sodium–channel alpha1–subunit.

OTHER SYNDROMES OF IGE FOR CONSIDERATION

The following are other main possible syndromes of IGE that remain unrecognised by the ILAE Committees:[9,10]

- **IGE with absences of early childhood**
- **Perioral myoclonia with absences**
- **Idiopathic generalised epilepsy with phantom absences**
- **Jeavons syndrome (eyelid myoclonia with absences).**

IGE WITH ABSENCES OF EARLY CHILDHOOD [375,427–429]

Typical absences starting from early childhood (a few months to 5 years of age) are not a specific expression of a distinct syndrome. This may be the first manifestation of epilepsy with myoclonic absences, perioral myoclonia with absence, eyelid myoclonia with absences, childhood absence epilepsy or more severe forms of generalised epilepsies. By excluding all these, it is realistic to propose that there is a syndrome of IGE that starts in early chidhood primarily manifesting with absences, often combined with GTCS and possibly with myoclonic jerks.

Doose,[428,429] having studied 140 cases with onset of absences in early childhood, rightly concluded that 'this is an heterogeneous subgroup within IGE. There is a distinct overlap with early childhood epilepsy with GTCS and myoclonic astatic epilepsy on the one side and with childhood absence epilepsy on the other. Thus it should not be regarded as a special syndrome'. I am in complete agreement with this statement. Age at onset of absence seizures alone cannot define an epileptic syndrome. However, with improved diagnostic skills, applying inclusion (for example, including absences and GTCS) and exclusion criteria (for example, excluding childhood absence epilepsy and cryptogenic cases) it appears that there is such an idiopathic generalised epilepsy that we have to define more precisely.

This is an IGE (occurring in otherwise normal children)[428,429] with:

1. Onset of absences between 1 and 5 years of age. Absences are markedly different from childhood absence epilepsy. Clinically they are less severe and less frequent. Ictal EEG 3–4 Hz spike or multiple spike wave discharges are very irregular and termination is not abrupt but often fades with slow spike/wave.
2. GTCS are common (two thirds) and often the first seizure type. Boys are more likely to suffer GTCS than girls.
3. Myoclonic jerks and myoclonic–astatic seizures occur in 40% of patients.
4. Absence status may lead to cognitive impairment.
5. Background EEG shows a moderate excess of slow waves.
6. Long-term prognosis is worse than in childhood absence epilepsy.
7. Strong family of IGE and generalised spike/wave discharges in EEG of unaffected members and particularly mothers.

PERIORAL MYOCLONIA WITH ABSENCES [336,430]

Typical absences with motor symptoms of perioral myoclonia are a non-specific symptom. However, this often combines with a clustering of other clinical and EEG features, suggesting that this is an interesting syndrome within the IGEs.

Demographic data: Age at onset is wide, from 2 to 13 years (median 10). Girls are far more frequently affected than boys. The syndrome is uncommon in children (<1% with typical absences) but, because it fails to remit, is relatively common in adults (9.3%) with typical absence seizures.

Clinical manifestations: Typical absence seizures with perioral myoclonia are the defining symptom. The characteristic feature is perioral myoclonia, which consists of rhythmic contractions of the orbicularis oris muscle that cause protrusion of the lips, contractions of the depressor anguli oris resulting in twitching of the corners of the mouth or rarely more widespread involvement, including the muscles of mastication, producing jaw jerking (Figure 6.12).

Considerations on classification:

Perioral myoclonia with absences has been recognised neither as a seizure type nor as a syndrome.[9,10] The fact that absences with perioral myoclonia is a discrete seizure type has been unequivocally documented with video-EEG recordings.[336,430] The symptom of perioral myoclonia may rarely occur in absence seizures of other IGEs and as such perioral myoclonia alone cannot be taken as sole evidence of the syndrome of perioral myoclonia with absences.

However, there is often a non-fortuitous clustering of other symptoms indicating that these may often constitute the main symptom of a syndrome within the broad spectrum of IGE, which we propose to call perioral myoclonia with absences. Other manifestations of this syndrome include GTCS, which often start early (before or together with the absences), frequent occurrence of absence status, resistance to treatment and persistence in adult life.[336,430]

Impairment of consciousness varies from severe to mild. Most patients are usually aware of the perioral myoclonia. Duration is usually brief, lasting a mean of 4 seconds (range 2–9 seconds). Absences of perioral myoclonia may be very frequent, occurring many times per day, 1–2 per week, or may be rare. All patients suffer GTCS, which often start before or soon after the onset of

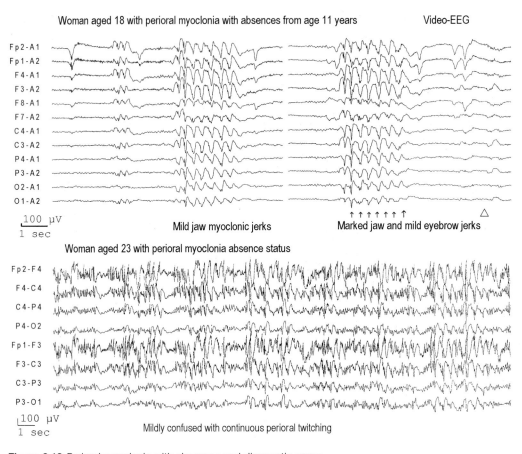

Figure 6.12 Perioral myoclonia with absences and diagnostic errors.

Top: From video-EEG recording of a woman with perioral myoclonia with absences (case 6 in ref [430]). She was referred because of 'focal motor seizures and secondarily GTCS'. She had onset of GTCS and absences at age 11 years, which continue despite treatment with various combinations of sodium valproate, ethosuximide, clonazepam, lamotrigine and acetazolamide. Absences were frequent, often in daily clusters and consisted of brief (~5 seconds) moderate impairment of consciousness with violent rhythmic jerking of the jaw. GTCS occurred 1–10 times per year, usually after awakening, preceded by clusters of absences with the jaw myoclonus spreading to limb jerks prior to generalised convulsions. She was more concerned about the absences because they interfered with her daily life 'everyone notices the jerks of my jaw' and less with the GTCS which usually occurred at home. The initial misdiagnosis of 'focal motor seizures' was because the jaw jerking was described by her mother as unilateral.

Bottom: From EEG of 23-year-old woman while in perioral status epilepticus (case 2 in ref [430]). She was mildly confused with continuous perioral twitching. This ended with a GTCS. Initial presentation at age 11 years was with GTCS. Absences with perioral myoclonia were noted at the same time and were diagnosed as focal motor seizures.

clinically apparent absences. Exceptionally, GTCS may start many years after the onset of absences. GTCS are usually infrequent (ranging from one per lifetime to 12 per year) and are often heralded by clusters of absences or absence status.

Absence status is very common in PMA (57%) and frequently ends with GTCS (Figure 6.12). It is commoner than in any other syndrome of IGE with typical absences.[346] Perioral myoclonia may be more apparent than impairment of consciousness or vice versa.

Aetiology: Half of the patients have first degree relatives and mainly siblings with IGE and absences.[431]

Diagnostic procedures: All except EEG are normal.

Electroencephalography: Interictal EEG frequently shows: (a) abortive bursts or brief <1 second generalised discharges of 3–7 Hz spike or multiple (3–4) spikes and slow wave. These are usually asymmetrical and may give the impression of secondary bilateral synchrony; (b) focal abnormalities, including single spikes, spike wave complexes and theta waves with variable side emphasis.

The ictal EEG consists of generalised discharges of spikes or multiple spike and slow wave at 3–4 Hz with frequent irregularities of the discharges in terms of the number of spikes in the spike wave complex, the fluctuations in spike amplitude and the occurrence of fragmentations.

There is no photosensitivity.

Differential diagnosis: Patients with perioral myoclonia with absences are frequently erroneously diagnosed as having focal motor seizures because of: (a) the prominent motor features of the absences which are often reported and sometimes recorded as unilateral and (b) interictal focal EEG abnormalities.

However, this error is unlikely to happen if EEG is properly obtained and interpreted. Also, patients with focal motor seizures are unlikely to suffer non-convulsive status epilepticus, which is common in perioral myoclonia with absences.

The main differential diagnosis is from childhood absence epilepsy, juvenile absence epilepsy or IGE with phantom absences depending on age at onset. Video-EEG invariably reveals perioral myoclonia that sometimes may be subtle, particularly in treated patients. Onset of GTCS before or at the same age as typical absences, the relatively brief duration of the absence seizures and perioral myoclonia, and the frequent occurrence of absence status epilepticus are useful clinical indicators in favour of perioral myoclonia with absences and against childhood, juvenile or other forms of IGE.

Prognosis: Absences and GTCS may be resistant to medication, unremitting and possibly lifelong.

Management: Treatment is with sodium valproate alone or combined with ethosuximide, small doses of lamotrigine or clonazepam.

Absence status, of which most patients are aware, should be terminated with immediate self-administered medication of oral midazolam or rectal diazepines.

IDIOPATHIC GENERALISED EPILEPSY WITH PHANTOM ABSENCES[339]

The syndrome is characterised by the triad of:

- phantom absences that are inconspicuous, never appreciated before the onset of GTCS
- GTCS which are commonly the first overt clinical manifestation, usually start in adulthood and are infrequent
- absence status which occurs in half of the patients.

Demographic data: The first overt clinical manifestations of GTCS usually appear in adult life, although absences may have started much earlier. Men and women are equally affected. Prevalence was estimated at 15% among IGE with typical absences, 10% of IGE and 3% of 410 consecutive patients older than 16 years with epileptic seizures.[339] Genton et al.[432] reported that among 253 consecutive cases of IGE, 32 (15.4%) patients had rare GTCS with generalised spike wave discharges in the interictal EEG.

Clinical manifestations: This syndrome manifests with phantom absences, late onset GTCS and frequently absence status, absences and myoclonic jerks, alone or in combination. Absence status epilepticus is common.

'Phantom absences' denote typical absence seizures, which are so mild that they are inconspicuous to the patient and imperceptible to the observer.[336,339] They are disclosed by video–EEG recording and breath counting during hyperventilation. The absences manifest with interruption, delays or errors of counting and occasionally with eyelid blinking. Ictal EEG shows brief (usually 3–4 seconds), 3–4 Hz spike/multiple spike and slow wave generalised discharges (Figure 6.13). Phantom absences are common in patients with idiopathic generalised epilepsies but are often unrecognised.

GTCS are usually the first overt clinical manifestation (Figure 6.14).[339] These are of late onset, infrequent and without consistent circadian distribution or specific precipitating factors.

Half of the patients suffer from absence status, which often lasts for many hours alone or before GTCS (Figure 6.14). This manifests with cognitive

---

Considerations on classification:

Phantom absences, mild absence seizures, have not been categorised as such by the ILAE.[9,10] The absences are simple, brief (usually 2–4 seconds) causing only inconspicuous impairment of cognition, which is not clinically disturbing to the patient. Although not classical they fulfil the criteria of typical absences with more than 2.5 Hz generalised discharges of spike wave.[339]

There is reasonable evidence to support that phantom absence is not only a discrete seizure but may also constitute the main symptom of a syndrome within the broad spectrum of IGE. There is non-fortuitous

clustering of other symptoms such as GTCS of usually late onset, frequent occurrence of absence status and persistence in adult life.[339] The fact that these patients have IGE is beyond any doubt as they all are of normal intelligence and physical state, high-resolution MRI is normal, the EEG shows generalised discharges of spike/multiple spike and slow waves and the seizures are generalised.

The syndrome of IGE with phantom absences has not been recognised.[9,10] Accordingly, these cases are probably categorised amongst undefined IGE or other syndromes of IGE.

impairment, which is usually of mild or moderate severity. The patient is poorly communicating, slow, feels strange and confused, makes errors at work, looks depressed but does not become unresponsive. More commonly than usually appreciated there are experiential, mental and sensational symptoms. The patient is often aware of the impending GTCS and tries to find a safe place to have it. There may be some post-ictal recollection of the events.

Aetiology: IGE with phantom absences is probably genetically determined.[339]

Diagnostic procedures: All except EEG are normal.

Electroencephalography: The background activity is normal but half of the patients have EEG focal paroxysmal abnormalities consisting of short transients of localised slow, sharp waves or spikes, or both, occurring either independently or in association with the generalised discharges.[339,433] EEG photosensitivity is exceptional.

Ictal EEG consists of spike/multiple spike and slow wave at 3–4 Hz with occasional fragmentations (Figure 6.13). They are typically brief (2–4 seconds), usually lasting no more than 5 seconds. Mild cognitive impairment manifested with hesitation, discontinuation and errors in breath counting is the only clinical ictal symptom during the generalised discharges. A few patients may also have mild ictal eyelid fluttering.[339,433] Hyperventilation is a major provocative factor.

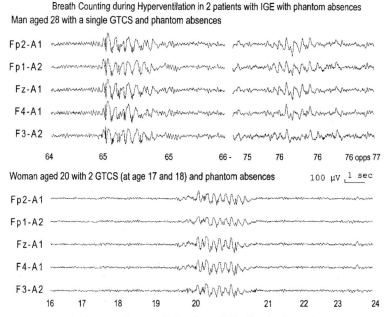

Figure 6.13 From Video-EEG of two patients suffering from IGE with phantom absences.

The numbers denote the actual breath counting during hyperventilation. Note that errors, when they occur, are only related to these brief discharges. Errors consist of hesitation in pronouncing the next consecutive number, repetitions and erroneous counting sequence. These absences are impossible to detect without breath counting and video-EEG.

During absence status epilepticus EEG shows continuous generalised mainly 3 Hz spike/multiple spike slow activity.

Differential diagnosis: The main problems to consider in IGE with phantom absences are:

- the first overt unprovoked GTCS appears in adult life

- absence status epilepticus

- differentiation from other syndromes of IGE.

It is essential to take a careful clinical history and to interpret symptoms correctly, which may be suggestive of typical absences and absence status. A history of altered consciousness preceding GTCS should not be taken as evidence of complex focal seizures (see Figure 6.15 for differentiation), depression or an unspecified seizure prodrome.

Prognosis: IGE with phantom absences may be a lifelong propensity to seizures, which is of undetermined onset and remission. Patients are of normal intelligence, which does not show any signs of deterioration. Further, phantom absences, although frequent, do not appear to affect daily activity. IGE with phantom absences is usually easily controlled with appropriate antiepileptic medication although some cases may be resistant.

Management: There are many unanswered questions as to whether patients with phantom absences need treatment. All patients with IGE with phantom absences had a normal life without medication until their first GTCS – probably many years after the onset of frequent daily mild absence seizures. We do not know how many people in the general population with the same problem will never develop GTCS or absence status. However, for those that

Facing page **Figure 6.14**

From video-EEG of a highly intelligent woman, aged 76 years, with phantom absences, absence status and GTCS (case 1 in ref [339]). She had her first overt seizure at age 30 years. She was moderately confused for 12 hours before a GTCS. Since then she had experienced 1–3 similar episodes every year. She was misdiagnosed as temporal lobe epilepsy and was on primidone and sulthiame for nearly 40 years. Retrospectively she admits brief episodes of mild impairment of cognition: 'The absences lasted a couple of seconds; the other state (absence status) lasts much longer, for 24 hours or more ... They may be linked I suppose'. No further seizures of any type occurred in the next 11 years of follow-up on monotherapy with sodium valproate 1000 mg daily.

Upper: Absence status. There was continuous spike and occasional polyspike and slow wave activity mainly at 3Hz. Note also slower or faster components and some topographic variability of the discharge.

The patient was fully alert, attentive and cooperative. Movements and speech were normal. There were no abnormal ictal symptoms other than severe global memory deficit and global diminution of content of consciousness. She was unable to remember her name, how many children she had, date and location. She could not perform simple calculations but could repeat up to five numbers given to her. She could read text correctly and she wrote her address correctly although she could not remember it on verbal questioning. She did not know where she was but given the choice between various locations she correctly recognised that she was in the hospital. This absence status epilepticus was successfully terminated with intravenous administration of diazepam.

Bottom: Interictal video-EEG. Brief generalised discharges of 3 Hz spike and slow waves lasting 2–3 seconds without apparent clinical manifestations.

will eventually have GTCS treatment may be mandatory. Drugs of choice are the same as those for IGE with absence seizures (see page 156).

IGE with phantom absences

Woman aged 68 in absence status epilepticus - Video EEG 1991

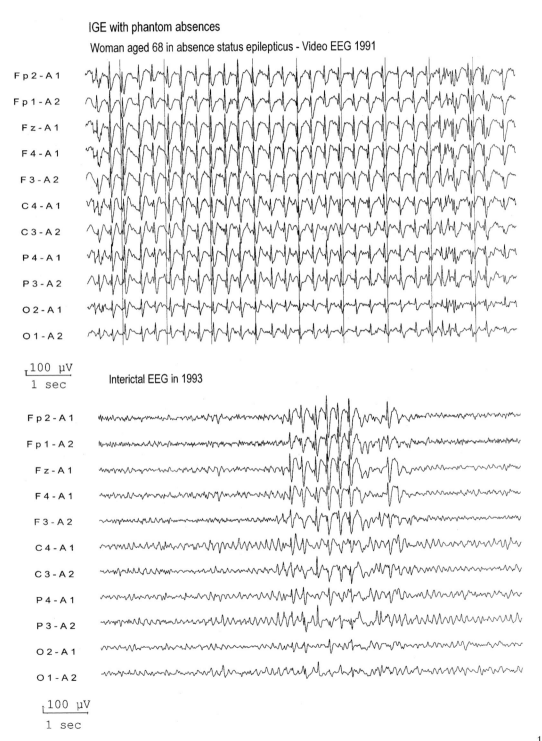

Interictal EEG in 1993

JEAVONS SYNDROME

EYELID MYOCLONIA WITH ABSENCES

Reflex IGE provoked by specific modes of precipitation (photic, pattern, video games, emotional upset and intense thinking) are well described.[434,435] Photosensitive IGE is by far the commonest. Eyelid myoclonia with absences (Jeavons syndrome) is one of the most distinctive reflex IGEs with well-defined clinico-EEG manifestations as detailed in pages 230-233.

TREATMENT OF IDIOPATHIC GENERALISED EPILEPSIES

Idiopathic generalised epilepsies demand different treatment strategies to focal epilepsies.[7] Ignoring this fact results in avoidable morbidity.

1. Certain drugs that are beneficial in focal epilepsies (carbamazepine, tiagabine, vigabatrin, phenytoin) are not only ineffective but even contraindicated in IGE.[7]

2. A drug that is efficacious for one type of generalised seizure may not affect others. Clonazepam, for example, is the best drug for myoclonic jerks but is ineffective in GTCS. Also, ethosuximide is efficacious only in absence seizures and epileptic negative myoclonus. If a drug is found to be efficacious in 'generalised' childhood epileptic encephalopathies, it does not follow that this is also the case in IGEs. A typical example is vigabatrin (West syndrome), which is contraindicated in IGE.

   It should be emphasised that this guide on the treatment of IGEs is based on data available before the introduction of newer antiepileptic drugs. This is likely to change dramatically, particularly with use of levetiracetam, which is the newest and most promising of all (see pages 209-211). Based on clinical experience, levetiracetam is likely to become the first choice drug in IGE. Formal placebo-conrolled trials to establish both the efficacy and safety of levetiracetam in IGEs are currently underway.

MONOTHERAPY

The first line monotherapy treatment is with sodium valproate or lamotrigine.[7] It appears that sodium valproate has superior efficacy to lamotrigine and also affects myoclonic jerks, whereas lamotrigine action is currently unpredictable. However, lamotrigine appears superior to sodium valproate regarding adverse reactions. Sodium valproate – with such adverse reactions as polycystic ovaries, weight gain and teratogenicity – is unacceptable to some women, particularly those of childbearing age.[414,436] Conversely, lamotrigine is associated with a high incidence of idiosyncratic reactions that sometimes may be very serious. Efficacy and adverse reactions have to be carefully balanced in these cases because treatment is often lifelong.

According to a recent review,[7] sodium valproate controls absences in 75% of patients, GTCS in 70% and myoclonic jerks in 75%. Lamotrigine controls absences in possibly 50–60% and GTCS in 50–60% but may worsen myoclonic jerks. Ethosuximide controls 70% of absences but has no effect on GTCS that may worsen.

Monotherapy should not be abandoned before making sure that maximum tolerated dose has been achieved if smaller doses have failed. If monotherapy fails or unacceptable adverse reactions appear then replacement of one by the other is the alternative.

Ethosuximide, with equal efficacy to sodium valproate in absences, is suitable for monotherapy in childhood absence epilepsy.[7] It is ineffective in GTCS and therefore cannot be used as monotherapy in any other syndrome of IGE.

Clonazepam is suitable only in pure myoclonic epilepsies with no other types of seizures, although it is also beneficial for absences.

Of the new antiepileptic drugs, levetiracetam,[7,437] topiramate[7,438] and Zonisamide[439] appear promising. Gabapentin has no effect.[440] Vigabatrin and tiagabine are contraindicated because they are pro-absence drugs and may induce absence status epilepticus.[7]

Leveritacetam (Keppra), the newest antiepileptic drug licensed as an add-on therapy for focal onset seizures,[441] has potential for a much broader application in focal and generalised epilepsies.[437,442,443] This derives from reports that levetiracetam has a significant anti-myoclonic effect,[442] suppresses photosensitivity[437] and has a unique mode of action in animal models of absence seizures.[443] Levetiracetam appears to be well tolerated, relatively void of significant side-effects and has a positive effect on cognition and some aspects of quality of life (pages 209-211).[441,441a]

POLYTHERAPY

For monotherapy failures, the combination of sodium valproate with small doses of lamotrigine (25–50 mg) appears to be the most effective.[7] In resistant

---

First line drugs[7]

Sodium valproate (often unsuitable for some women)

Lamotrigine (may exaggerate myoclonic jerks)

Ethosuximide (only for absences; may exaggerate GTCS)

Clonazepam (only for pure myoclonic syndromes)

Newer drugs that may be potentially effective

Levetiracetam (probably the most promising broad-spectrum drug)

Topiramate

Zonisamide

Second line or adjunctive drugs

Phenobarbitone or phenytoin (for those without absence seizures)

Clonazepam (particularly for myoclonic jerks; may exaggerate GTCS)

Acetazolamide (only for absences)

Contraindicated drugs

Carbamazepine (although it may control GTCS if added to first line drugs)[7]

Vigabatrin (it is a pro-absence drug that may

induce absence status epilepticus)[7]

Tiagabine (it is a pro-absence drug that may induce absence status epilepticus)[7]

Phenytoin

cases and particularly those with persistent myoclonic jerks the best add-on drug is clonazepam which in one small dose (0.5–2 mg) before sleep may have a dramatic effect.[7] Ethosuximide should be added only for uncontrolled absence seizures. Levetiracetam, topiramate and Zonisamide are promising and may be better options than currently available drugs.

> A 28-year-old man with 'IGE and phantom absences' had at least one episode of absence status every month, which often ended with GTCS despite treatment with sodium valproate 1500 mg and lamotrigine 175 mg daily. No more seizures occurred in the next 3 months after adding levetiracetam 500 mg bd.   (Personal case)

DRUG WITHDRAWAL

In childhood absence epilepsy treatment may be slowly withdrawn 1–3 years after controlling all absences.[7] All other syndromes of IGE are probably lifelong and confront the usual textbook advice of withdrawal of medication after 2–3 years from the last seizure. Relapses are probably unavoidable. However, if seizures were mild and infrequent, drug withdrawal may be attempted. This should be in small decrements, probably over years, warning the patient that re-appearance of even minor seizures such as absences or myoclonic jerks mandates continuation of treatment. EEG confirmation of the seizure-free state is needed during the withdrawal period.[7]

TREATMENT OF STATUS EPILEPTICUS IN IDIOPATHIC GENERALISED EPILEPSIES

In IGEs convulsive (generalised tonic-clonic) status epilepticus is relatively rare in comparison to other and mainly symptomatic epilepsies or epileptic encephalopathies. Conversely, non-convulsive status epilepticus has high prevalence, although it is often unrecognised because symptoms may be mild. The treatment of convulsive and non-convulsive status epilepticus is the same irrespective of cause. There are recent major publications and reviews for reference.[444–450]

Convulsive status epilepticus is a medical emergency and should be managed urgently and properly according to established and well-publicised protocols (although these vary).[444–450] The aim of treatment is to prevent neuronal damage caused by systemic and metabolic disturbances and by the direct excitotoxic effect of electrical seizure discharges. Control of overt and electrical seizures is imperative.

Compensatory mechanisms to prevent brain damage are relatively satisfactory during the first 30 minutes but break down subsequently with an increasing speed if the seizures are not stopped. Neuronal damage leads to transient or permanent neurological, epileptic and cognitive sequelae or even death. The risk of brain damage increases progressively if continuous convulsive status persists for more than 30 minutes and particularly after 1–2 hours.

Drug treatment in the first 30 minutes is with intravenous administration of a fast-acting benzodiazepine. Benzodiazepines – mainly diazepam, lorazepam or midazolam – are the most effective agents. Diazepam is the traditional drug; then lorazepam came into prominence as the first choice drug.[448] Recently midazolam infusion has become increasingly popular as an effective and well-tolerated therapeutic agent.[451] Most cases are controlled with this approach, if not, the patient carries an appreciable morbidity and treatment is as for established status epilepticus. First line drug options at this stage include sub-anaesthetic doses of phenobarbitone, phenytoin or fosphenytoin. If seizures are not controlled at this stage the patient enters into the refractory state which requires general anaesthesia.

Because regimens for the treatment of convulsive status epilepticus vary it is important to follow an established protocol; this has been shown to reduce morbidity and mortality.[448]

Non–convulsive status epilepticus[346,347,452] has high incidence in IGE (10–20%) and in some syndromes such as IGE with phantom absences or perioral myoclonia this may be as high as 50%. Additionally, nearly all patients are fully aware of this state and know well that this may inevitably inflict them with a GTCS, although this is avoidable:

> It is the same feeling of: 'slowing down', 'not being in the same world as everyone else', 'uncontrollable rush of thoughts', 'losing control of my mind', 'taking me much longer to formulate my response which occasionally is inappropriate and bumbled'. Then I know that I will have the fit. If I can, I just go in a private place and wait for it.

This stage is unlikely to be considered as a genuine status epilepticus by the physicians of accident and emergency departments. Therefore, advice to the patient regarding therapeutic options for self-administration of drugs is imperative.

Benzodiazepines – mainly diazepam, lorazepam or midazolam – are the most effective agents.

Self–adminstration: Rectal diazepam (10–20 mg for adults and 0.5 mg/kg for children) as soon as the first symptoms appear may stop non-convulsive status but often this is not applicable. Rectal absorption of liquid diazepam is very rapid, reaches the brain within minutes and has a near-intravenous efficacy. Proprietary rectal tubes (Stesolid) of ready-made liquid diazepam are the most widely used formulation. Suppositories of diazepam are not useful because of slow absorption. Diazepam rectal gel is now available in the USA. However, adult patients rarely use this, either because of embarassment or inconvenience. Taking a bolus dose of sodium valproate (usually twice the daily prophylactic dose) from onset of symptoms is often effective in terminating the status and preventing GTCS (most patients prefer this to anything else).

Bucchal[453] or intranasal[318] application of midazolam may be the best practical and effective therapeutic option. The efficacy and rapid action of bucchal administration of midazolam are equal to those of rectal diazepam. This approach is more convenient and less traumatising than rectal tubes of diazepam. Midazolam (10 mg) drawn up from an ampoule (diluted with peppermint, otherwise it smells and tastes terrible) should be swirled in the mouth for 4–5 minutes and then spat out.

Clonazepam orally (1–4 mg) may be used at onset of non-convulsive status epilepticus and this is the preferred option of patients with mainly myoclonic jerks.

> This helps me to go to sleep and when I wake up I am fine

Hospital management: With intravenous administration of any type of the above benzodiazepines non–convulsive status epilepticus usually stops abruptly. The problem is that this condition is not recognised and the patients are not believed when they seek such treatment, even when they produce a relevant letter from their treating physician.

> She started doing the same silly things. I recognised it. The doctor told me that she is ok. No, no I said. She is going to have the fit.

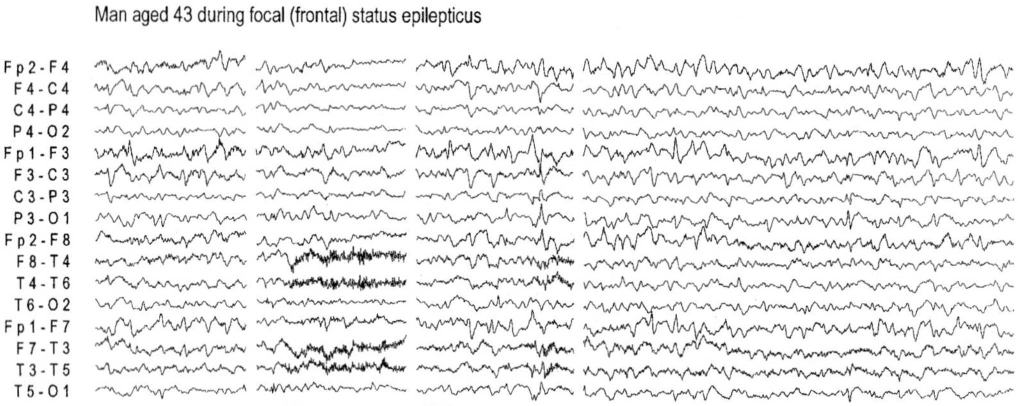

Man aged 43 during focal (frontal) status epilepticus

Moderately confused, unable to recall personal details, talking irrelevantly, behaving strangely and looking happy

Figure 6.15 Compare this EEG of focal (frontal lobe) non-convulsive status epilepticus with the EEG of fig 6.14 of generalised (absence) status epilepticus.

From video-EEG of 43 years old man while in focal status epilepticus. He was confused, disorientated in time and place, with bizarre behaviour, laughing and making inappropriate jokes.

Note a. the frequent but irregular appearance of sharp-slow waves, which are mainly localised in the bifrontal electrodes and mainly on the left, b. the relative preservation of alpha activity, and c. short discontinuation of the ictal pattern.   Actual time of the recording is shown with numbers.

FAMILIAL (AUTOSOMAL DOMINANT) FOCAL EPILEPSIES

7

There have been recent significant advances in identifying the clinical, genetic and molecular basis of certain epilepsies, particularly the familial (autosomal dominant) focal epileptic disorders.[454–457] These came to light through genetic contributions from familial aggregation and twin studies, positional cloning of specific genes that raise risk, and clinical descriptions of families. Familial aggregation studies are consistent in showing an increased risk of epilepsy in the relatives of patients with focal epilepsies that occur in the absence of environmental factors. Susceptibility genes have been localised and in some these have been identified. Nearly all genes discovered to date code for ion channel subunits, either ligand-gated or voltage-gated, which indicates that, at least in part, familial (autosomal dominant) focal epilepsies are a family of channelopathies.[458] Autosomal dominant lateral temporal lobe epilepsy was the first non-ion channel disease of this group to be described. Berkovic and associates have been the main protagonists of these discoveries.

The following syndromes have been recognised in the new diagnostic scheme:[10]

Benign familial neonatal seizures (see page 42)

Benign familial infantile seizures (see page 53)

Autosomal dominant nocturnal frontal lobe epilepsy

Familial temporal lobe epilepsy

Familial focal epilepsy with variable foci (syndrome in development)

AUTOSOMAL DOMINANT NOCTURNAL FRONTAL LOBE EPILEPSY [454,459–468]

Autosomal dominant nocturnal frontal lobe epilepsy (ADNFLE) is the first described distinctive syndrome of focal epilepsy with single gene inheritance.[469]

Demographic data: Onset is mainly in late childhood, 7–12 years (mean 11 years), although it ranges from infancy (2 months) to adulthood (56 years of age). Overall, 90% of the patients have their first seizure before the age of 20. Men and women are equally affected. Prevalence is unknown but the increasing numbers of publications from 1994 indicate that ADNFLE may not be a sparse disease.

Clinical manifestations: ADNFLE manifests with frequent, nearly every night, clusters of brief (20–50 seconds) nocturnal motor seizures, with hyperkinetic/dystonic features or tonic manifestations. Seizures are of sudden, thrashing onset and termination void of post-ictal symptoms. Motor symptoms consist of sudden, hyperkinetic movements and dystonic posturing (shoulder or pelvic thrashing movements, bipedal and fencing postures) or tonic stiffening of the limbs and the body, often with superimposed clonic components. Patients may be thrown out of bed or find themselves prone in a crawling position. Injuries may occur. Paroxysmal arousals or awakening during non-rapid eye movement sleep may also represent mild seizures that may or may not be associated with transient dystonic posturing. Two thirds of patients experience a non-specific aura of somatosensory, sensory, psychic and autonomic symptoms. Consciousness is usually preserved. Sleep is abruptly interrupted but immediately resumes with the end of the seizure. Post-ictal state is entirely normal. See also seizures from the supplementary sensorimotor area (page 181).

Secondary GTCS, occurring in two thirds of patients, are very infrequent also during sleep and mainly happen in untreated patients or after withdrawal of medication.

There is marked intra- and inter-family variability in severity. Affected family members usually have clusters of seizures with a weekly or monthly frequency, but some patients have attacks every night. A few have mild and rare attacks identified only during systematic family study.

Circadian distribution: Seizures are most likely to occur in the hypnagogic state of sleep or shortly before awakening. Diurnal attacks are rare.

Precipitating factors: Stress, fatigue and alcohol increase the frequency of the fits. Seizures in children provoked by movement and sound stimulation are reported.[465]

Aetiology: ADNFLE is an autosomal dominant disease probably with reduced penetrance. ADNFLE has been linked to chromosome 20q and 15q but many other families showing genetic heterogeneity are not linked to these chromosomes. At least three mutations have been described in the M2 domain of the neuronal nicotinic acetylcholine receptor alpha 4 subunit (CHRNA4) gene. CHRNB2 is a second acetylcholine receptor subunit associated with ADNFLE.[470]

Despite this genetic heterogeneity, the clinical phenotypes appear markedly homogeneous in all families and difficult to separate on clinical grounds irrespective of chromosomal linkage and mutations.

Diagnostic procedures: Brain imaging is normal. Interictal and ictal EEG are usually normal and unhelpful.

Prognosis: The occurrence of seizures is lifelong, although in mild cases they may appear only for a brief period. Spontaneous remissions and relapses occur. Some patients have frequent attacks that are refractory to medication. Attacks may become milder in their fifth or sixth decade of life, described as fragments of their previous seizures.

Differential diagnosis: Misdiagnosis of seizures as benign nocturnal parasomnias, night terrors, nightmares, psychiatric and medical disorders is common. 'Nocturnal paroxysmal dystonia'[471] and 'hypnic tonic postural seizures of frontal lobe origin'[472] are certainly frontal lobe seizures and most patients probably have ADNFLE. Some clinical features such as the awakenings with feeling of choking, the abnormal motor activity during sleep and the excessive daytime sleepiness are relatively common both in obstructive sleep apnoea syndrome and in nocturnal frontal lobe epilepsy. An all-night video-polysomnographic monitoring is needed to provide a firm diagnosis.

Management: Carbamazepine monotherapy is frequently effective but one third of the patients are resistant to treatment. Clonazepam or clobazam add-on may be useful. Phenytoin may also be effective. In refractory cases, multiple antiepileptic drugs are often ineffective. Newer drugs licensed for focal epilepsies may be effective (see page 205).

FAMILIAL TEMPORAL LOBE EPILEPSY [454,473–479]

Familial temporal lobe epilepsy is another autosomal dominant epileptic disease.

Demographic data: Onset is typically in teenage or early adult life with a median in the middle of the third decade of life. No children under the age of 10 years have been identified with this disorder. Women (58%) may be more affected than men. Epidemiology is unknown. Berkovic proposes that this may be a common condition.[473,474,477]

Clinical manifestations: Seizures are generally mild, infrequent and well controlled with antiepileptic medication. Simple focal seizures (90%) are far more common than complex focal seizures (66%) and they may be the only seizure type (18%). Main ictal manifestations consist of déjà vu and other mental illusions and hallucinations (nearly all) alone or together with autonomic disturbances. Emotional symptoms of fear and panic, visual and auditory illusions of distortions of light and sound and somatosensory sensations of diffuse (not localised) numbness and tingling are other common ictal symptoms of simple focal seizures. Raising epigastric sensation does not exist.

GTCS occur in only two thirds of patients with familial temporal lobe epilepsy. Half of them occur before initiation of appropriate treatment. GTCS are again infrequent with the worst possible scenario one GTCS per year.

Patients are neurologically and mentally normal and the condition does not appear to affect their otherwise normal life, particularly when on medication.

Aetiology: Autosomal dominant inheritance with reduced 60% penetrance is the most likely mode of inheritance.[474,476]

It appears that familial temporal lobe epilepsy will be a genetically heterogeneous disorder if one considers the original cases,[473,474,477] the focal epilepsy with auditory features[481,482] (page 166) and those with autosomal dominant temporal lobe epilepsy and febrile seizures.[483]

Diagnostic procedures: MRI is normal[473,474] but exceptionally in more severe cases may show hippocampal atrophy, including some rare examples of familial hippocampal sclerosis.[473] Minor and non-specific abnormality of diffuse small high signal areas on T2-weighted images may be seen. Interictal FDG-PET may show ipsilateral temporal hypometabolism in patients with active seizures.

Interictal EEG is usually normal (half the cases), shows mild focal slow waves (28%) or sparse sharp and slow wave complexes localised in the temporal region and usually unilateral (22%).[474,484] Sleep may occasionally activate epileptiform abnormalities.

There are only three recorded seizures.[477] In one, a right temporal ictal discharge appeared during the attack beginning with fear and followed by loss of awareness, staring, swallowing and left hand automatisms. The other two seizures were in the same patient. No definitive epileptiform changes were recorded in one seizure – comprised of an aura of buzzing in the ears and followed by oral automatisms and impaired awareness. There were no lateralised EEG changes in the other seizure that started with an aura and early left-sided dystonia rapidly progressing to secondarily generalised convulsions.

Differential diagnosis: The main difficulty is probably in differentiating patients with very mild and infrequent seizures of predominantly déjà vu from normal phenomena. This may be impossible in individual cases without other overt seizure symptoms or other family members having temporal lobe epilepsy.

Familial temporal lobe epilepsy should be mainly differentiated from hippocampal epilepsy. The main differentiating features in favour of familial temporal lobe epilepsy are:

- onset in teenage or early adult life
- no febrile convulsions or other antecedent factors for epilepsy
- no ictal symptoms of raising epigastric aura
- mild and infrequent seizures that may remit
- usually normal MRI.

Prognosis: Prognosis is commonly excellent. One sixth (16%) of the cases with mild simple partial seizures alone would never know that they have an epileptic disorder if other family members were not affected. Of the cases with more overt seizure manifestations only 66% have complex focal seizures and GTCS that again are rather infrequent and respond well to antiepileptic medication. It is rare for seizures to continue after drug treatment (10–20%). The cross-sectional nature of the study of Berkovic et al.[473,474,477] precluded accurate determination of remission rates, but the histories of affected individuals suggested that long remissions, with or without therapy, were common. Conversely, in the Montreal series, drawn largely from patients considering surgical treatment for epilepsy, a more severe clinical spectrum was observed.[476]

Management: Seizures are usually easily controlled with carbamazepine or phenytoin.

FAMILIAL FOCAL EPILEPSY WITH VARIABLE FOCI [485–488]

Familial focal epilepsy with variable foci is an autosomal epileptic disorder.

Demographic data: Age at onset varies markedly (range 0.75–43 years), although the mean age of seizure onset is 13 years. To date, seven unrelated families have been reported.

Clinical manifestations: The defining feature of this syndrome is that different family members have focal seizures emanating from different cortical locations that include temporal, frontal, centroparietal or occipital regions. Each individual patient has the same electro-clinical pattern of single location focal epilepsy. Seizures are often nocturnal. There is great intrafamilial variability. Severity varies among family members; some may be intractable to medication but usually these are infrequent, easily controlled or even asymptomatic manifesting only with an EEG focus.

Aetiology: This is a rare inherited epilepsy syndrome with an autosomal dominant inheritance with ~60% penetrance. In two families the disease has been mapped to a locus of a 3.8-cM interval on chromosome 22q11-q12, between markers D22S1144 and D22S685.[487] However, the original Australian family was not found to link to chromosome 22, indicating genetic heterogeneity. In this family a genome-wide search failed to demonstrate definitive linkage, but a suggestion of linkage was found on chromosome 2q.[485]

Diagnostic procedures: Neuroimaging is usually normal.

Electroencephalography: Interictal focal epileptiform abnormalities occur in most patients. Their location varies within family members in the temporal, frontal, centroparietal or occipital regions but for each individual a single focus remains constant over time. They are facilitated or brought up in sleep EEG. Clinical seizures are concordant with EEG localisation. EEG severity varies significantly in different individuals and does not correlate with seizure frequency. Normal family members may also have an EEG epileptiform focus, thus indicating that this is likely to be a marker for the familial partial epilepsy with variable foci trait.

Prognosis: Development is usually normal and seizures well controlled with medication, if needed.

Management: The effects of different antiepileptic drugs were not directly evaluated but carbamazepine, phenytoin and valproate appeared to be effective.

SYNDROMES OF AUTOSOMAL DOMINANT INHERITANCE NOT YET RECOGNISED

Of those syndromes not yet recognised by the ILAE Task Force the most important and well documented is:

- **Autosomal dominant lateral temporal lobe epilepsy, which is the same disease as autosomal dominant focal epilepsy with auditory features.**

Others are:

- **Autosomal dominant Rolandic epilepsy and speech dyspraxia.**[489,490]

- **Partial epilepsy with pericentral spikes with evidence for linkage to chromosome 4p15.**[491]

AUTOSOMAL DOMINANT LATERAL TEMPORAL LOBE EPILEPSY

AUTOSOMAL DOMINANT FOCAL EPILEPSY WITH AUDITORY FEATURES [480,481,492–497]

Autosomal dominant lateral temporal lobe epilepsy is the same disease as the autosomal dominant focal epilepsy with auditory features, as they are due to defects in the same gene. It is the first non-ion channel idiopathic epilepsy.[495,497]

It is characterised by:[475]

- Autosomal dominant inheritance with high penetrance. It is due to mutations in the LGI1/Epitempin gene on chromosome 10q24.
- Mild seizures with mainly auditory hallucinations.
- Mainly nocturnal and infrequent.
- GTCS excellent response to treatment.

Demographic data: Onset is typically in teenage or early adult life but this may be earlier, 5–10 years, or later.

Clinical manifestations: Seizures are generally mild, infrequent and well controlled with antiepileptic medication. Simple focal seizures that are the commonest of all mainly consist of simple auditory hallucinations like ringing, humming, clicking or unspecified noises. These may infrequently progress to complex focal seizures and GTCS. Other sensory symptoms such as visual (lights, colours and simple figures), olfactory, vertiginous or cephalic are frequent with simple focal seizures while autonomic, mental and motor symptoms are less common.

Secondary GTCS are rare and predominantly nocturnal.

Aetiology: Autosomal dominant inheritance with high (~80%) penetrance. Genetic analysis showed linkage to chromosome 10q and localised a gene in a common overlapping region of 3-cM at 10q24 (LGI1/Epitempin gene).[495,497] Familial temporal lobe epilepsy with aphasic seizures and linkage to chromosome 10q22-q24 has been described.[480]

Diagnostic procedures: EEG and MRI are often normal or show usually mild and non-specific abnormalities. Interictal EEG epileptiform abnormalities rarely occur.

Prognosis: Prognosis is excellent. Patients are neurologically and mentally normal and the condition does not appear to affect their otherwise normal life particularly when on medication.

Differential diagnosis: Autosomal dominant lateral temporal lobe epilepsy should be mainly differentiated from other structural causes of lateral temporal lobe epilepsy (see Chapter 8) which lack a similar family history. It is markedly different from hippocampal epilepsy.

Autosomal dominant lateral temporal lobe epilepsy versus familial temporal lobe epilepsy

Differentiating patients with this syndrome from those of familial temporal lobe epilepsy may sometimes be difficult for overlapping cases. Auditory hallucinations are the main ictal symptom of autosomal dominant lateral temporal lobe epilepsy but these may not occur in some patients. Conversely, déjà vu and other mental illusions and hallucinations are the predominant seizure manifestations of familial temporal lobe epilepsy.

Management: Response to carbamazepine is excellent.

AUTOSOMAL DOMINANT ROLANDIC EPILEPSY AND SPEECH DYSPRAXIA [489,490]

'Autosomal dominant rolandic epilepsy and speech dyspraxia: a new syndrome with anticipation' appears to be a rare hereditary condition described by the Australian team of Scheffer and associates.[489] They extensively studied a family of nine affected individuals in three generations with nocturnal oro-facio-brachial focal seizures, secondarily generalised focal seizures, and centrotemporal epileptiform discharges, associated with oral and speech dyspraxia and cognitive impairment. The authors assessed that 'The speech disorder was prominent, but differed from that of Landau–Kleffner syndrome and of epilepsy with continuous spike and wave during slow wave sleep'; and that 'The electroclinical features of this new syndrome of autosomal dominant rolandic epilepsy resemble those of benign rolandic epilepsy, a common inherited epilepsy of childhood. This family shows clinical anticipation of the seizure disorder, the oral and speech dyspraxia, and cognitive dysfunction, suggesting that the genetic mechanism could be expansion of an unstable triplet repeat. Molecular studies on this syndrome, where the inheritance pattern is clear, could also be relevant to identifying a gene for benign rolandic epilepsy where anticipation does not occur and the mode of inheritance is uncertain'.

However, the clinical presentation of these patients with permanent neurological deficit, sometimes preceding the seizures can hardly be considered as 'resembling benign Rolandic epilepsy' or 'epitomise the archetypal benign rolandic epileptic attack'.

Patients of previous generations were not so severely affected but they also had neurological deficits, mainly of oral and speech dyspraxia, without evidence of dysarthria.

FOCAL EPILEPSY WITH PERICENTRAL SPIKES [491]

This is based on the study of a family in which affected family members manifested a variety of seizure types, including hemiclonic, hemitonic, GTCS, simple focal (stereotyped episodes of epigastric pain) and complex focal seizures consistent with temporal lobe semiology. The syndrome is benign, either requiring no treatment or responding to a single antiepileptic medication. Seizure onset is in the first or second decades of life, with seizures in individuals up to the age of 71 years and documented EEG changes up to the age of 30 years. A key feature of this syndrome is a characteristic EEG abnormality of spikes or sharp waves in the pericentral region (centroparietal, centrofrontal or centrotemporal). The syndrome may be overlooked because of the variability in penetrance and seizure types among affected family members. There is evidence for linkage to chromosome 4p15.

> Syndromes of autosomal recessive inheritance such as 'autosomal recessive rolandic epilepsy with paroxysmal exercise-induced dystonia and writer's cramp'[498] have not been yet recognised but should be considered in future revisions.

SYMPTOMATIC AND PROBABLY SYMPTOMATIC FOCAL EPILEPSIES

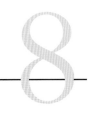

Focal (topographical or localisation-related) epilepsies may be symptomatic, probably symptomatic (cryptogenic) or idiopathic.[9] Ictal symptoms particularly at onset are determined by localisation and not by aetiology.

The new ILAE diagnostic scheme[10] recognises:

LIMBIC EPILEPSIES

Mesial temporal lobe epilepsy with hippocampal sclerosis

Mesial temporal lobe epilepsy defined by specific aetiologies

Other types defined by location and aetiology.

NEOCORTICAL EPILEPSIES

Rasmussen syndrome

Hemiconvulsion-hemiplegia syndrome

Other types defined by location and aetiology

Migrating focal seizures of early childhood.★

I present all of them according to their topographical origin:

- **Temporal lobe epilepsie**s
- **Frontal lobe epilepsies**
- **Parietal lobe epilepsies**
- **Occipital lobe epilepsies.**

★Syndrome in development

Considerations on classification

The new diagnostic scheme of the ILAE Task Force, by recognising 'symptomatic (or probably symptomatic) focal epilepsies' as a separate group, differentiates them from 'idiopathic focal epilepsies'.[10] This is because of the significant progress made in recent years through the investigation of neurosurgical cases, technological advances in brain imaging methodologies and genetics. The practical need for this is that prognosis and treatment of idiopathic focal epilepsies differ significantly from those of symptomatic focal epilepsies. There is now concrete evidence to accept, diagnose and treat certain focal epilepsies on the basis of aetiology rather than simply localisation. Hippocampal epilepsy, amongst the commoner and most distinct epileptic diseases, is a striking example of this. The ILAE Task Force has not yet completed the list, definitions and characterisation of the focal epilepsies. It is for this reason and for didactic purposes that I present the focal epilepsies in an anatomical (topographical) order but detailing the syndromes of the new ILAE diagnostic scheme.[10]

Abbreviations

AED = antiepileptic drugs
GnRH = gonadotropin-releasing hormone
LTLE = lateral temporal lobe epilepsy

MTLE = mesial temporal lobe epilepsy
RTC = randomised clinical trials
SMA = supplementary sensorimotor area

TEMPORAL LOBE EPILEPSIES

Simple and complex focal seizures may account for 60–70% of all epilepsies and nearly half of them originate from temporal lobe structures.[499–501] Thus, temporal lobe epilepsy may have a prevalence of 30–35% of all epilepsies. Two thirds are from the mesial and the other one third from the lateral temporal lobe regions. Temporal lobe epilepsies are categorised as:[10]

LIMBIC EPILEPSY

- **Mesial temporal lobe epilepsy with hippocampal sclerosis**
- **Mesial temporal lobe epilepsy defined by specific aetiologies**

NEOCORTICAL EPILEPSY

- **Lateral temporal lobe epilepsy**

MESIAL TEMPORAL LOBE EPILEPSY WITH HIPPOCAMPAL SCLEROSIS

HIPPOCAMPAL EPILEPSY

The clinical features and prognosis of hippocampal epilepsy derive almost exclusively from neurosurgical series of cases that are medically

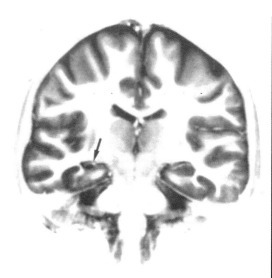
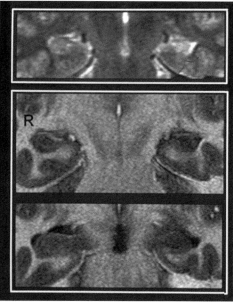

Figure 8.1   MRI findings in hippocampal sclerosis.

Left: Coronal T1-weighted MRI scan showing right hippocampal sclerosis (arrow).

Right: Coronal T2-weighted and magnified T1-weighted MRI showing left hippocampal sclerosis.

Figure courtesy of Professor John S. Duncan and the National Society for Epilepsy MRI Unit.

intractable;[253,502–506] therefore, they may not accurately represent the clinical spectrum of hippocampal epilepsy, particularly in respect of severity and prognosis. The neurosurgical cases may be the iceberg (~20%) with the worst cases on the top. The vast majority (80%) is not seen in these specialised centres and some of them may be very mild and easily controlled with appropriate antiepileptic drugs. A more complete clinical picture is expected to emerge now that MRI enables an in vivo diagnosis of hippocampal sclerosis/atrophy (Figure 8.1).

Demographic data: Onset is in late childhood or adolescence. Hippocampal epilepsy is the commonest form of focal epilepsy, probably around 20% of patients with epilepsies. It accounts for 65% of cases with mesial temporal lobe epilepsy.[507]

Clinical manifestations:[253,502–506] Patients with hippocampal epilepsy usually have a history of complex febrile convulsions before the onset of non-febrile seizures. Complex focal seizures or generalised convulsions are the initial non-febrile seizures that attract medical attention. These by rule are preceded by simple focal seizures that may have been undermined, sometimes for years, as normal phenomena.

Epigastric aura, fear and oro-alimentary automatisms are the most common ictal symptoms.

> It starts with that strange stomach feeling and my panic and then I pass out

Ascending epigastric or visceral aura is by far the commonest symptom in mesial temporal lobe seizures. Irrespective of quality, this sensation often moves upwards in a slow or fast fashion, within seconds, and when it reaches the level of the throat the patient loses consciousness. Downwards movement towards the feet is exceptional. Epigastric aura is often initially described as pain but on further questioning this is rarely pain. It is a strange 'difficult to describe' sensation felt in the upper half of the abdomen for which the most common descriptions are 'if the organs inside are squeezed and twisted'. Other descriptions are of emptiness, rolling, turning, whirling, tenderness, fluttering, butterflies, pressure, burning, nausea and their variations. This is usually short, a few seconds, but becomes longer when other symptoms are added at seizure progress.

Ictal fear is not specific for mesial temporal lobe seizures only. Although it is mainly associated with the amygdaloid, periamygdaloid and hippocampal stimulation, neocortical areas can also be responsible. Typical, for example, is the fear of frontal lobe seizures. However, there is a main difference, I could suggest from experience, between fear of temporal versus frontal lobe epilepsy:

Fear in mesial temporal lobe seizures is predominantly subjective 'I am scared, I am in terrible panic' which does not show to the observer. Conversely, in patients with frontal seizures 'fear' is predominantly expressive 'his face is fearful'. 'Fear' is mainly *emotionally felt* in mesial temporal lobe seizures and is mainly *facially expressed* in frontal seizures.

Oro-alimentary automatisms consist of lip-smacking, chewing, swallowing, licking and tooth-grinding movements. They are often followed by simple gestural automatisms. Oro-alimentary automatisms are characteristic of mesial temporal lobe epilepsy only if preceded by epigastric aura, fear and mental symptoms of the 'dreamy state' of Jackson, alone or in combination.

Gestural automatisms consist of fiddling, fumbling, picking, tapping, patting or plucking, rubbing or scratching the face and other gestural movements.

Dreamy states,[508] **experiential phenomena,**[509] **intellectual aura, mental or psychic symptoms** are the most widely used terms to denote symptoms of mainly temporal lobe seizures that uniquely relate to the patient's personality regarding identity, experience, emotion, thought and memory. These terms are not necessarily synonymous, because they are used in the relevant literature to encompass either limited or much wider ictal manifestations. Currently, the most popular term used is 'experiential phenomena/symptoms'.

Experiential symptoms of mainly temporal lobe seizures are hallucinations, illusions, or both, that may involve any faculty of the human mind: thinking, emotion, memory and recollection, chronological order and speed, sensation, reality and unreality and their interactions with past, present and imaginary experiences. Events and experiences may be reproduced intact or disturbed, present may be misplaced to the past and past to the present, real may be presented as unreal and vice versa, time may be speeded up or slowed down, shape and other morphology may be natural or unnatural, deformed or undistorted. Mental ictal symptoms may be very simple and natural like the 'déjà vu' phenomenon or a sensation of 'fear and panic' or a 'mild sense of depersonalisation – who I am?' that may also be experienced by normal people who do not have seizures. On other occasions, they may be more complicated with a complete distortion of time, space, morphology, direction, experience and normality.

Mental ictal manifestations of temporal lobe seizures typically combine elements of perception, memory and affect that, as in real life, are often encompassed together in a unified subjective symptom.[509] Perceptual, mnemonic or affective aberrations usually cluster in various combinations and various degrees of disturbance. However, one may be more involved than another. Sometimes one of them may be exclusively affected and may occur in isolation. Depending on the predominant mental aberration they are subdivided under various names such as: *ideational* (impairment of thoughts), *dysmnesic* (impairment of memory), *affective* (emotional impairment)[510] or *dyscognitive* (impairment of perception, cognition).

Simple focal seizures of hippocampal epilepsy mainly start with an ascending epigastric aura and less often with fear. Mental hallucinations and illusions of déjà vu and its variations occur but are not as common as in other extra-hippocampal epilepsies. Olfactory and gustatory hallucinations are less common.

Simple focal seizures may be the only seizure type, although they often progress to **complex focal seizures** with impairment of consciousness that typically associates with oro-alimentary automatisms in ~70%. The initial objective symptoms in this stage of impairment of consciousness are staring, motor restlessness or motor arrest, oro-alimentary automatisms and unforced head deviation. The patient has no recollection of this phase but may still be responsive. Gestural automatisms, other forms of automatisms, vocalisations and dystonic posturing may occur soon afterwards. Dystonic posturing, occurring in 20–30% of patients, is contralateral to the side of seizure onset while gestural automatisms occur ipsilaterally. Early head turning is ipsilateral to seizure onset.

Complex focal seizures last for 2–3 minutes, occur on average once or twice per week and usually appear in clusters of two or three. They may also occur during sleep and in some women they are exclusively or predominantly catamenial.

Nausea and marked autonomic signs including borborygmi, belching, pallor, flushing of the face, cardiac abnormalities, arrest of respiration and pupillary dilatation are common.[9]

Post-ictal symptoms of mainly complex focal seizures are very frequent and often severe.

Secondary GTCS are infrequent in properly treated patients.

Complex focal status epilepticus features particularly in untreated patients. It is less common than absence status epilepticus of IGEs but its prevalence may be underestimated.

> A patient with typical right-sided hippocampal sclerosis had frequent seizures starting with an abdominal sensation of discomfort in the stomach 'as though being in a lift that stops abruptly' often ascending upwards and progressing to a feeling of disorientation and 'shivering' and sometimes déjà vu before losing consciousness witnessed as: 'stares and fiddles or drums with his fingers on a table'. He also had clusters of the same 'intense abdominal discomfort and a feeling of shivering' lasting for 2–5 minutes, becoming repetitive at intervals of 1 hour for approximately half a day to 2 days. Within that period he may have longer attacks of half an hour or longer.

Neurological examination is usually normal; facial asymmetry contralateral to the epileptogenic zone may be apparent in some patients. Specific baseline and follow-up memory testing are needed.

Aetiology: A hypocellular and gliotic (hence the word 'sclerotic') hippocampus is the pathological substrate of hippocampal epilepsy (Figure 8.1). Hippocampal sclerosis presents with a unique pattern of cellular loss, not found in other brain diseases.[507]

Its cause is unknown. There are two views supported with equally valid arguments:

1. Hippocampal sclerosis is caused by prolonged febrile convulsions and other cerebral insults in early life.[511–514]

2. Pre-existing hippocampal abnormalities predispose to febrile convulsions which in turn cause further hippocampal damage evolving to hippocampal sclerosis that may manifest with temporal lobe epilepsy.[515,516]

Biological basis: **How does this 'atrophic' and 'sclerotic' organ become one of the most powerful and common epileptogenic agents of human epilepsy?**

This is due to synaptic remodelling and re-organisation of the hippocampal region with GABA increasing the synchrony of firing thresholds and mossy fibres providing convergent excitation.[507]

Diagnostic procedures: MRI is the most important investigational tool. Current MRI scanners are of sufficiently high resolution to allow in vivo visualisation of hippocampal sclerosis in all patients (Figure 8.1).[50,517,518] Two thirds of patients with mesial temporal lobe epilepsy have unilateral or bilateral hippocampal atrophy. In some of them there is also evidence of other 'double pathology' such as cortical malformations.

Straightforward cases of unilateral hippocampal epilepsy confirmed with MRI may not need other tests.

Functional brain imaging and new methodologies such as proton magnetic resonance spectroscopic imaging are of high sensitivity, offer significant insights and practically eliminate the need for invasive techniques (Figure 1.10).[519–524] (See also pages 33-35 regarding the clinical applications of functional brain imaging.)

Electroencephalography: In half or more of patients with hippocampal epilepsy a single, routine, half an hour, EEG may be normal or may show mild and non-specific abnormalities. The classical spike or sharp and slow wave focus in the anterior temporal electrode is seen only in one third of the patients (Figure 8.2).[505,525] Prolonged EEG monitoring also with sleep EEG increases the yield to approximately 70–80%. Regional temporal interictal runs of slow waves

Two patients with hippocampal epilepsy

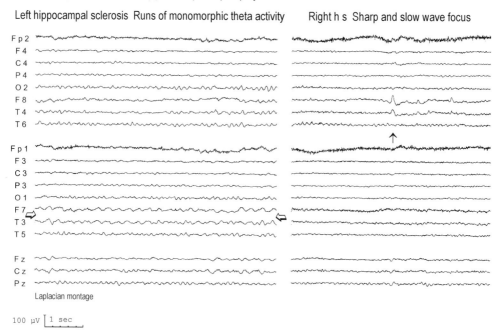

Left hippocampal sclerosis Runs of monomorphic theta activity   Right h s Sharp and slow wave focus

Laplacian montage

100 μV 1 sec

Figure 8.2 EEG samples from two patients with hippocampal epilepsy.

Left: Discrete runs of monomorphic theta activity are localised in the left anterior temporal regions in this patient with left hippocampal sclerosis. There were no spikes or other 'conventional' epileptogenic abnormalities.

Right: The conventional epileptogenic focus of sharp and slow wave complexes is localised in the right anterior temporal electrode. The patient had right hippocampal sclerosis.

which are of lateralising value are recorded in about half of the patients (Figure 8.2).[526]

Ictal EEG usually manifests with rhythmic slow activity, around 4–7 HZ, that appears over the affected temporal lobe, before or simultaneously with clinical events (Figure 8.3).[505] Fast spiking is exceptional.

Differential diagnosis: Hippocampal epilepsy needs differentiation from non-epileptic conditions and from seizures arising from other brain locations.

a. **Non-epileptic conditions:** Simple focal seizures of epigastric aura and 'panic attacks' are unlikely to raise suspicion of epilepsy either by the patient or the general physician (Figure 8.3). These patients are often investigated for gastro-enterological and psychological disorders[527] or hypoglycaemia until more salient seizure features appear with the development of complex focal seizures and secondarily GTCS. Patients are often re-assured with normal relevant tests or told that their symptoms are the result of anxiety. It is rare at this stage that a general physician would request an EEG, but again if this normal (as is the case for two thirds of the patients), a diagnosis of stress-related events would be re-inforced.

The diagnosis of hippocampal seizures should be suspected by their very brief duration, the ascending character of the epigastric sensations, their sometimes nocturnal appearance and often an associated feeling of depersonalisation.

Pseudo-seizures may be difficult to differentiate. An increase of prolactin post-ictally may be helpful in the differentiation between epileptic seizures and 'pseudo-seizures'.[528]

b. **Mesial temporal epilepsy with other than hippocampal sclerosis aetiologies:** The differential diagnosis of hippocampal from other mesial temporal lobe epilepsy is impossible without MRI (see page 177).

c. **Mesial versus other temporal lobe seizures:** The epigastric aura and early oro-alimentary automatisms predominate in mesial temporal epilepsy compared with other neocortical temporal lesions. Conversely, hippocampal epilepsy is unlikely when seizures manifest with early focal motor, somatosensory, visual or auditory ictal symptoms or frequent secondary GTCS, or occur in patients with neurological or cognitive deficits other than memory impairment.

d. **Mesial versus familial temporal lobe epilepsy:** The clinical manifestations of familial temporal lobe epilepsy with mild, easily controlled seizures where ictal mental illusions and hallucinations predominate are also significantly different from hippocampal epilepsy (page 163).

e. **Typical absence seizures:** Typical absence seizures are more likely to be misdiagnosed as complex focal seizures than vice versa (Table 6.1). Although often not appreciated, rarely patients with absence seizures may also have hallucinations and illusions of any sort thus imitating complex focal seizures.[336]

Prognosis: Despite high prevalence and known pathology, prognosis and many other important aspects of hippocampal epilepsy are largely unknown. The

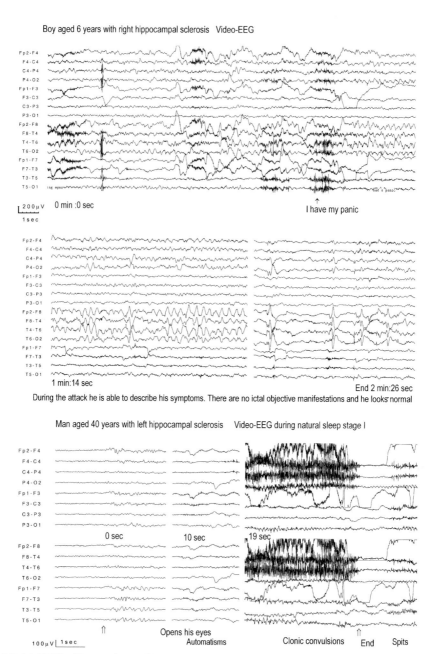

Boy aged 6 years with right hippocampal sclerosis   Video-EEG

0 min :0 sec

I have my panic

1 min:14 sec

End 2 min:26 sec

During the attack he is able to describe his symptoms. There are no ictal objective manifestations and he looks normal

Man aged 40 years with left hippocampal sclerosis   Video-EEG during natural sleep stage I

0 sec

10 sec

19 sec

Opens his eyes
Automatisms

Clonic convulsions   End   Spits

Figure 8.3 Ictal EEG of two patients with hippocampal epilepsy.

Top and middle: This was the first EEG of a boy aged 6 referred for episodes of panic attacks and a recent GTCS. The resting EEG was entirely normal but one of his seizures was recorded from onset (0 minutes: 0 seconds) and lasted for 2 minutes and 26 seconds. The child looked disturbed, complaining, 'I have my panic'. He was able to communicate well during the whole seizure. Speech and cognition were normal. Brain MRI documented right hippocampal sclerosis.

Bottom: Sample of video-EEG during a brief seizure of a man aged 40 years with increasing numbers of complex focal seizures typical of hippocampal epilepsy. MRI documented left hippocampal sclerosis. Note that towards the end of the attack the patient had mild clonic convulsions although he never had GTCS. Also note that he immediately spits after the cessation of the seizure.

neurosurgical cases show a specific clinical pattern. Initially, patients have a rather mild or uneventful course of hippocampal seizures that may be controlled with medication. Later, within years from onset, seizures become worse, intractable to any medication and may be associated with memory and other psychological abnormalities.[253,502–506]

Management: Medical treatment of hippocampal epilepsy may be relatively effective in 80% of patients; for the other 20% and probably many more with intractable seizures neurosurgical resection of the offending epileptogenic region is usually successful.

Drug treatment: Drug treatment is similar to that for any other type of focal seizures (pages 205-213).

If treatment with one or two of the main drugs fails, the chances of achieving medical control in hippocampal epilepsy are negligible. Polypharmacy will add more misery, memory problems and drowsiness rather than any benefit.[529,530] These patients, even in childhood,[531] need urgent evaluation for neurosurgical treatment for which they are the best candidates and the most likely to have excellent and sustained benefit.

Neurosurgical treatment: With early surgical intervention, patients with hippocampal epilepsy have an excellent chance of cure and a subsequent normal life.[504,505,532,533] Around 60% become seizure-free even after stopping all antiepileptic medication, 20% have reduced numbers of seizures but need to continue with antiepileptic drugs, 10% have no benefit, 10% get worse. Significant neurosurgical complications rarely occur.

MESIAL TEMPORAL LOBE EPILEPSY DEFINED BY SPECIFIC AETIOLOGIES OTHER THAN HIPPOCAMPAL SCLEROSIS

This encompasses mesial temporal lobe epilepsy with aetiologies other than hippocampal sclerosis.[253,502–506]

> Seizure symptomatology is the same irrespective of cause and location within the mesial temporal lobe structures. MRI commonly determines structural causes.

Clinical manifestations: The overall view is that seizure symptomatology is the same irrespective of cause and location within the mesial temporal lobe structures. Thus, seizures of hippocampal sclerosis are considered indistinguishable from those caused by other lesions in the mesial temporal lobe. Their differentiation is also practically impossible with surface EEG. High-resolution MRI provides anatomical evidence of localisation in nearly all symptomatic cases. The sensitivity of MRI in the diagnosis of tumours and other lesions of the temporal lobe is estimated to be around 90%[517] but soon this will be exceeded.

Aetiology: Structural causes are malignant and benign tumours (astrocytomas, gangliogliomas, dysembryoplastic neuroepithelial tumours), vascular (cavernous and venous angiomas, arteriovenous malformations), developmental (malformations of cortical development), traumatic and other injuries, viral and other infective agents, cerebrovascular disease.[534] Of 63 children with new-onset temporal lobe epilepsy, 18 had hippocampal epilepsy, 34 were either cryptogenic or idiopathic with normal neuroimaging and no significant past history and 10 had long-standing, non-progressive temporal lobe tumours and malformations.[535]

Drug treatment: Drug treatment is similar to any other type of focal seizures (page 205).

Neurosurgical treatment: Surgical intervention is possible, often with an excellent chance of cure and a subsequent normal life in certain pathological conditions of mesial temporal lobe epilepsy.

LATERAL TEMPORAL LOBE EPILEPSY [9,503,504,536]

Lateral temporal lobe epilepsy (LTLE) is neocortical as opposed to mesial temporal lobe epilepsy, which is limbic.

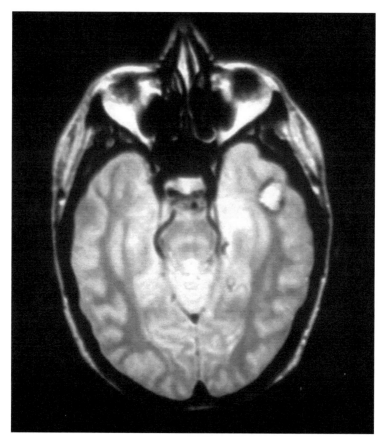

Figure 8.4 Axial PD MRI scan showing left temporal lobe cavernoma.

Figure courtesy of Professor John S. Duncan and the National Society for Epilepsy MRI Unit.

Clinical manifestations: Simple seizures of LTLE are characterised by auditory hallucinations or illusions, vestibular phenomena, mental illusions and hallucinations of the dreamy states and visual misperceptions. Language disturbances occur in dominant hemispheric focus.

Motor ictal symptoms include clonic movements of facial muscles, grimacing, finger and hand automatisms, dystonic posturing of an upper extremity, leg automatisms, restlessness, and unformed vocalisations. Rotation of the whole body is frequent and of value in differentiation from mesial temporal lobe epilepsy.

These symptoms may progress to complex focal seizures through spreading to mesial temporal or extratemporal structures. Impairment of consciousness is not as pronounced as with mesial temporal lobe epilepsy.[504]

Aetiology: Structural causes are similar to those of mesial temporal lobe epilepsy other than hippocampal sclerosis.

Diagnostic procedures: MRI often determines the structural causes of LTLE (Figure 8.4). Scalp interictal EEG shows unilateral or bilateral midtemporal or posterior temporal spikes (Figure 8.5).[9,504]

Differential diagnosis: Lateral temporal lobe seizures usually lack features commonly exhibited in mesial TLE such as:

- Ascending epigastric aura or fear are rare and variable (15%).[504]
- Eye blinking and aggressive behaviour.
- Contralateral dystonia, searching head movements, body shifting, hyperventilation and post-ictal cough or sigh.[536]

Drug treatment: Drug treatment is similar to that for any other type of focal seizures (page 205).

Neurosurgical treatment: Surgical intervention is possible, often with excellent chance of cure and a subsequent normal life in certain pathological conditions of LTLE.

Woman aged 24 with lateral temporal lobe epilepsy

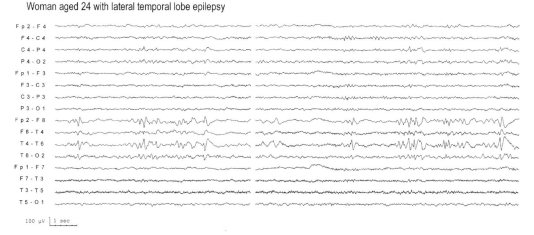

100 µV | 1 sec

Figure 8.5 EEG of a woman with lateral temporal lobe epilepsy. Note the marked focal abnormalities of slow waves and sharp slow wave complexes around the right anterior-midtemporal regions.

FRONTAL LOBE EPILEPSIES

Frontal lobe seizures have greatly variable clinical and EEG manifestations depending on the origin and spread of the epileptogenic focus.[537–546] The frontal lobe is as big as the other three brain lobes. On the basis of cytoarchitectural and functional studies, the frontal lobe can be subdivided into the primary motor cortex, premotor cortex, prefrontal cortex, and the limbic and paralimbic cortices,[543] with distinct cortico-subcortical organisations and immense connections with the temporal and parietal cortices.[540,547] Thus, there is a great variability in the clinical and EEG manifestations of frontal lobe seizures due to the complex and varied patterns of spread of seizure discharges.[539,548] Anatomical origins of some epilepsies are difficult to assign to specific lobes. Such epilepsies include those with pre- and post-central symptomatology (perirolandic seizures). Such overlap to adjacent anatomic regions also occurs in opercular epilepsy.[9]

Seizures arising from the primary motor cortex and the supplementary motor area have been relatively well defined, but seizures generated in other regions of the frontal lobe are less well specified.

Demographic data: Frontal lobe epilepsies may start at any age and equally affect both sexes. They are probably rare, ~1–2% of all epilepsies although they are second, after temporal lobe epilepsies, in neurosurgical series. Also, in a prospective community-based study[549] the prevalence of frontal seizures (22.5%) among focal epilepsies was comparable to that of temporal lobe (27%) and central sensorimotor cortex (32.5%). The others had frontotemporal (5.6%), parietal (6.3%) and other posterior cortex (6.3%) localisations.[549]

Clinical manifestations: According to their origin within the frontal lobe various seizure patterns have been recognised, although multiple frontal areas may be involved rapidly and specific seizure types may not be discernible.[9] Motor manifestations are the commonest and most characteristic ictal symptom, occurring in 90% of the seizures.

In general, frontal seizures:[9]

- Manifest with prominent motor manifestations (tonic, clonic or postural) and complex gestural automatisms, which are frequent at onset. Frequent 'falls' occur when the discharge is bilateral.

- Are short, usually from seconds to hardly a minute.

- Progress to rapid secondary generalisation (more common than in temporal lobe epilepsy).

- Show no or minimal post-ictal confusion.

- Often occur several times a day and mainly during sleep.

Considerations on classification:
Frontal lobe epilepsies other than Kozhevnikov-Rasmussen syndrome have not yet been detailed in the new ILAE diagnostic scheme.[10] The syndromes of frontal lobe epilepsy have been well described in the 1989 Classification of ILAE and these are presented in this section modified in accordance with new evidence.[9]

The following are the most common of frontal lobe seizures.

SEIZURES FROM THE MOTOR CORTEX [9]

Seizures originating from the motor cortex are mainly simple focal seizures. Symptoms depend on the side and topography of the area involved. Focal motor seizures (with or without march) originate from the contralateral Rolandic area (precentral gyrus). In the lower prerolandic area there may be speech arrest, vocalisation or dysphasia, tonic-clonic movements of the face on the contralateral side, or swallowing. Generalisation of the seizure frequently occurs. In the paracentral lobule, tonic movements of the ipsilateral foot may occur as well as the expected contralateral leg movements. Post-ictal or Todd's paralysis is frequent.[9]

Simple focal motor clonic or tonic-clonic seizures with or without Jacksonian march. They manifest with localised clonic movements, rhythmic or arrhythmic, that may affect thumb only, thumb and ipsilateral side of lips, hand, the whole arm or any other contralateral to the focus body part. Distal segments are more frequently affected than proximal segments. Hand and mainly thumb, face and mainly lips are preferentially affected because of their larger cortical representation (homunculus of Penfield). These ictal motor manifestations may remain highly localised for the whole of the seizure or march in an ordinary anatomical fashion to neighbouring motor regions, which constitute the classical Jacksonian (or Bravais-Jackson) seizure.

Myoclonic seizures that may be unilateral or bilateral are predominantly distal or facial. Epilepsia partialis continua of Kozhevnikov is one type of this (page 186).

Tonic postural motor seizures associated with clonic movements are unilateral or bilateral and asymmetric.

SEIZURES FROM THE SUPPLEMENTARY SENSORIMOTOR AREA

Seizures from the supplementary sensorimotor area (SMA) have distinct and characteristic clustering of symptoms and they are usually stereotyped (Figure 8.6).[550–555]

Hypermotor seizures[556] of bizarre bilateral, asymmetric tonic posturing and movements. The characteristic hypermotor seizure of SMA consists of sudden and explosive, bilateral and asymmetric tonic posturing of limb girdles at shoulder and pelvis often with contraversion of the eyes and head, vocalisation or speech arrest.

'Fencing posturing'[557] is the most well-known descriptive term for these SMA seizures although this may not be frequent.[555] In fencing posturing one arm raises semi-extended above the head while the other remains by the body semi-flexed at the elbow. Bilateral asymmetrical posturing is the most common.

M²E posture is another term used to describe flexion of the elbow of one arm, abduction of the shoulder to 90°, with associated external rotation. The head may look at the postured hand, and the opposite arm may show slight flexion. The leg ipsilateral to the involved arm extends, while the opposite leg flexes at the hip and knee.

In reality, posturing in SMA is extremely variable amongst patients with SMA seizures but it is stereotypical for each individual patient. This reflects well in other descriptive terms of SMA seizures such as complex gestural automatisms, extreme motor restlessness, complex motor automatisms and agitation, frenetic complex motor automatisms of both arms and legs, intensely affective vocal and facial expression associated with powerful bimanual-bipedal and axial activity, repetitive rhythmical and postural movements accompanied by bizarre vocalisation, complex motor automatisms with kicking and thrashing, complex and global gesticulations.

> *Hypermotor seizures* consist of 'complex, organised movements which affect mainly the proximal portions of the limbs and lead to a marked increase in motor activity. Consciousness may be preserved. They are most frequently associated with frontal lobe epilepsy'.[295,556]

Somatosensory or other ill–defined auras (not epigastric), vocalisations and speech arrest are common ictal manifestations of seizures of the SMA.

Somatosensory auras are described by more than half, probably ~80%,[558] of the patients, mainly at onset. Unilateral somatosensory sensations usually accurately predict contralateral lateralisation.[559] Cephalic sensations are probably the most frequent.[558] Auras are described as 'pressure on the chest', 'difficult to breathe', 'floating away', 'paraesthesia of a hand', 'dizziness and light-headedness', 'cephalalgia' or 'electrical sensation in the head', 'discharge in the whole body', 'sensation of body heat', 'feeling of coldness or heat in the back and the head', 'vertebral column shivering', 'moving outside oneself', 'crawling sensation in both, one leg or somewhere in the body'.[556,558,560,561]

Epigastric auras are not described.

Vocalisations: One third of the patients manifest with vocalisations that may vary from a brief deep breath or air expiration, pallilalic vocalisations to the most bizarre, loud and scaring noises.

Speech arrest is a well-documented and frequent ictal manifestation. Pure paroxysmal speech arrest without other motor activity is exceptional.

Consciousness is usually well preserved; by rule these are simple focal seizures.

Other characteristics of seizures from the supplementary sensorimotor area are:

- Abrupt onset and abrupt termination

- Nocturnal circadian distribution, rarely occur in awake states

- High frequency, sometimes many per night

- Lack of post-ictal confusion.

Negative motor seizures (ictal loss of localised muscle power or inability to produce a voluntary movement) and absences are other types of epileptic events associated with the frontal lobe.

SEIZURES FROM OTHER FRONTAL LOBE REGIONS

Seizures from other frontal lobe regions are less common and these topographically are:[9]

Cingulate are complex focal seizures of complex motor gestural automatisms at onset. Autonomic signs are common, as are changes in mood and affect.

Anterior frontopolar seizure patterns include forced thinking or initial loss of contact and adversive movements of head and eyes, with possible evolution including contraversive movements and axial clonic jerks and falls and autonomic signs.

Orbitofrontal are complex focal seizures with initial motor and gestural automatisms, olfactory hallucinations and illusions, and autonomic signs.

Dorsolateral seizure patterns may be tonic or, less commonly, clonic with versive eye and head movements and speech arrest.

Opercular seizure characteristics include mastication, salivation, swallowing, laryngeal symptoms, speech arrest, epigastric aura, fear and autonomic phenomena. Simple focal seizures, particularly focal clonic facial seizures, are common and may be ipsilateral. If secondary sensory changes occur,

Man aged 23 years with seizures from the supplementary sensorimotor area from age 4 years

Sample of a hypermotor seizure during all night video-EEG recording

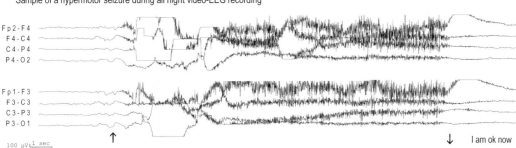

Abrupt and explosive right hand and leg posturing, body turning 180 degress to the left side from supine to prone position

Figure 8.6 Hypermotor seizure of the sensorimotor supplementary area.

Sample from one of 10 stereotypical hypermotor seizures recorded during an all-night video-EEG. Note the abrupt and explosive character of the seizure, which lasted for14 seconds only. There are no discernible ictal EEG abnormalities although occasionally some bilateral slow waves preceded the onset of the seizures. Frequent EEGs, ictal and interictal, over a 20-year period, failed to reveal any conventional epileptogenic abnormalities.

The patient is an intelligent man with numerous nocturnal hypermotor seizures from age 4 years. He is fully aware of the attacks but he cannot speak during them although he hears and understands. He has a sensory aura of 'a tight sensation in my chest and a feeling that I cannot breathe as all holes of my body are closed'. All possible drug treatments failed. High-resolution brain MRI and PET scans were normal.

numbness may be a symptom, particularly in the hands. Gustatory hallucinations are particularly common in this area.

The following frontal seizures are of particular clinical interest:[539,545,562,563]

a. 'Frontal absences' which are similar, often indistinguishable, from generalised absence seizures in clinical and EEG manifestations (Figure 8.7).[562,564]

b. Seizures characterised by unusual symptoms of 'forced thinking' that is an obsessive thought associated with a fairly well-adapted attempt to act on this thought (forced acts),[565,566] 'eye directed automatisms' and 'pseudo-compulsive behaviour'. Tonic deviation of the eyes preceding head deviation (frontal eye field involvement) may occur independently or associated with these strange symptoms.[539,545,563]

> The patient is compulsively 'forced to fix something with the eyes', 'the brain commands to do something that he should not do', 'a sensation of being forced to open the eyes'. This is often associated with forced motor bizarre actions of hypermotor seizures.

Aetiology: Frontal lobe epilepsies may be symptomatic, cryptogenic and idiopathic. In neurosurgical series, two thirds are symptomatic[563] from cortical dysplasia (57.4%), tumours (16.4%), traumatic and other lesions (26.2%).[567] Of the idiopathic forms, autosomal dominant nocturnal frontal lobe epilepsy is detailed on page 161.

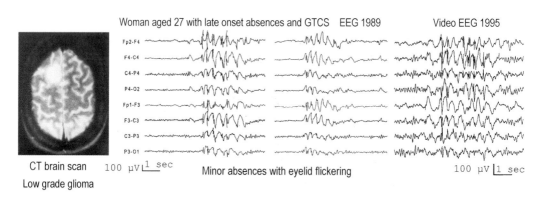

Woman aged 27 with late onset absences and GTCS EEG 1989   Video EEG 1995

CT brain scan   100 μV⌊1 sec   Minor absences with eyelid flickering   100 μV⌊1 sec
Low grade glioma

Figure 8.7 Typical absence seizures of late onset due to frontal lobe glioma.

Left: Brain CT scan showing a left-sided frontal glioma of a woman who started having absences at age 28 years (1989).
Middle right and left: Initially, the EEG discharges of spikes/multiple spikes and slow waves were entirely symmetrical; there was nothing to suggest that these were symptomatic absences. Clinically during the discharges there were minor and occasional errors on breath counting with consistent eyelid flickering. In her daily life, these were manifested as 'losing control of thoughts, repeating simple phrases and occasional mild jerking of the head to the right'. This could last for seconds to a minute and once she had non-convulsive status epilepticus with mild confusion and expressive dysphasia.
Right: Video-EEG 6 years later continued having similar generalised discharges which were asymmetrical.

Diagnostic procedures: High–resolution brain MRI shows abnormalities in around 60% of the patients. Functional neuroimaging is important for localisation.

EEG, interictal and ictal, is usually normal in seizures originating from the mesial frontal regions and this is a contributing factor to misdiagnosis.

If abnormal, interictal EEGs may show background asymmetry, frontal spikes or sharp waves (either unilateral or frequently bilateral or unilateral multilobar).[9]

If abnormal, ictal EEG patterns consist of (a) frontal or multilobar, often bilateral, low-amplitude fast activity, mixed spikes, rhythmic spikes, rhythmic spike waves, or rhythmic slow waves; or (b) bilateral high amplitude single sharp waves followed by diffuse flattening. Uncommonly, the EEG abnormality precedes the seizure onset, providing important localising information.[9,568]

Differential diagnosis: The typical motor seizure with or without Jacksonian march is unlikely to impose any diagnostic difficulties.

However, hypermotor seizures with the bizarre movements, posturing and vocalisations are frequently misdiagnosed as pseudo-seizures[569] or other episodic movement disorders.[555] Usually normal interictal and often ictal EEG reinforces this error. Nowadays, this should be an unlikely misdiagnosis because the constellation of hypermotor seizures is probably unique:

- sudden onset and termination within seconds to a minute,
- usually stereotypic appearance and
- typically nocturnal occurrence in clusters.

Frontal lobe hypermotor seizures should be differentiated from non-epileptic paroxysmal movement disorders[570–572] such as:
   psychogenic movement disorders[573]
   familial paroxysmal dystonic choreoathetosis[574]
   paroxysmal kinesigenic choreoathetosis [575–577]
   episodic ataxia type 1[571,578–581]

Familial paroxysmal dystonic choreoathetosis[574] is a non–epileptic hyperkinetic movement disorder characterised by attacks of involuntary chorea, dystonia and ballism with onset in childhood. Attacks typically last half to several hours (with no signs of abnormality between attacks) and may occur several times each week. There is no impairment of consciousness and EEG is normal during the episodes. Attacks are precipitated by a variety of factors, including caffeine, alcohol and emotion. Contrary to frontal lobe seizures, attacks in familial paroxysmal dystonic choreoathetosis can be relieved by short periods of sleep in most subjects.

Non-epileptic paroxysmal kinesigenic choreoathetosis is characterised by recurrent, brief attacks of involuntary movements induced by sudden voluntary movements.[575,576,582,583] The involuntary movements combine tonic, dystonic and choreoathetoid features on one or both sides. They often associate with dysarthria, upward gaze and sensory aura. Consciousness is entirely intact. Duration is usually 10–30 seconds and no more than 3 minutes. EEG during the attacks is normal. There may be tens per day for more than half of the patients. Onset is in mid-teens with a range from 5 to 16 years. For nearly all patients spontaneous remissions occur between 20 and 30 years of age. Most patients respond well to antiepileptic medication such as carbamazepine, phenytoin or phenobarbitone.[584]

Paroxysmal kinesigenic choreoathetosis is distinct from reflex epilepsy. However, patients may have a previous history of benign infantile seizures between the ages of 3 and 8 months.[585] There are no differences in the clinical presentation of cases with and without infantile seizures.[585] In addition there is an 8% prevalence of family history of epileptic seizures.

Episodic ataxia type 1: Of the various types of episodic ataxias[578–581] only type 1 may impose differential problems. In episodic ataxia type 1 patients suffer from brief (seconds to minutes) attacks of ataxia and dysarthria often associated with continuous inter-attack myokymia. Attacks are diurnal and may occur several times per day. EEG is frequently abnormal and patients may also have seizures. Episodic ataxia type 1 is a rare, autosomal dominant potassium channelopathy caused by at least 10 different point mutations in the KCNA1 gene on chromosome 12p13.

Symptomatic frontal lobe absences may have similar clinical and EEG features of some typical absence seizures (Figure 8.7).

Management: The focal seizures of frontal lobe epilepsies are usually resistant to any antiepileptic drug and their use is usually to protect the patients against secondary GTCS. Drug treatment is similar to that for any other type of focal seizures (page 205). Neurosurgery has had limited success.[553]

SPECIFIC FORMS OF NEOCORTICAL FRONTAL LOBE SEIZURES AND SYNDROMES

The ILAE Task Force diagnostic scheme recognises:[10]

1. **A seizure type:** *Epilepsia partialis continua of Kozhevnikov* (previously known as Kozhevnikov syndrome type 1)[9] of many aetiologies including Kozhevnikov-Rasmussen syndrome and

2. **A syndrome:** *Rasmussen syndrome*[10] (Kozhevnikov syndrome type 2 is the name used in the syndromic classification of ILEA[9,23]).[587]

EPILEPSIA PARTIALIS CONTINUA OF KOZHEVNIKOV

Epilepsia partialis continua of Kozhevnikov is rightly considered to be a seizure/status epilepticus type (and not a syndrome) caused by various heterogeneous conditions in children and adults.[588–595]

Demographic data: Onset is at any age from the very young to the very old but probably one third start in children under 16 years. Both sexes are equally affected. Prevalence is extremely small.

Clinical manifestations: The cardinal and defining symptom of epilepsia partialis continua is 'spontaneous regular or irregular clonic muscle twitching of cerebral cortical origin, sometimes aggravated by action or sensory stimuli, confined to one part of the body, and continuing for a period of hours, days, or weeks'.[588]

Epilepsia partialis continua is a prolonged segmental myoclonic seizure of a few milliseconds each repeated nearly every second for hours, days or months. The twitching is limited to a muscle or a small group of contiguous or unrelated muscles in one side of the body. Agonists and antagonists are simultaneously contracted. Facial and hand muscles are preferentially affected.

Nearly all patients with epilepsia partialis continua also have other seizures such as motor focal seizures in the same side and secondarily GTCS. These may start before or after the onset and more often intersperse with epilepsia partialis continua.

Aetiology: There are multiple and diverse causes of epilepsia partialis continua such as focal or multifocal brain lesions, systemic diseases affecting the brain and metabolic or other derangement. Kozhevnikov-Rasmussen syndrome and malformations of cortical development are the main causes in children. Cerebrovascular disease and brain space-occupying lesions are the main causes in adults. Non-ketotic hyperglycaemia is the commonest of the reversible causes. Other metabolic, mitochondrial or hereditary disorders are well described. Dereux (1955)[596] in a thesis of 102 cases found that more than 50% were caused by an 'encephalitic process'.

Russian spring-summer tick-borne encephalitis is another cause of epilepsia partialis continua. There is an assumption[586] that the cases described from Kozhevnikov were due to this disease, which is not correct.[587]

Pathophysiology: The generators of the epilepsia partialis continua are mainly in the primary motor cortex.

Diagnostic procedures: The yield of investigative procedures is cause-dependent. Around two thirds have abnormal brain MRI and EEG which are getting worse in progressive disorders such as Kozhevnikov-Rasmussen syndrome. Ictal EEG may or may not show epileptiform abnormalities concomitant with the jerks (Figure 8.8). Typically jerk locked back-averaged cortical potentials appear in the contralateral primary motor area preceding the jerks by a few milliseconds, sensory evoked potentials are of high amplitude (Figure 8.9) and there is a rostro-caudal pattern of muscle recruitment with co-contraction of agonists and antagonist muscles. PET and SPECT scans often localise the abnormal region but they are not specific. Screening for metabolic and mitochondrial disorders may be needed and a few cases are of unknown origin.

Prognosis: Prognosis is cause-dependent and it is usually poor, often associated with residual or progressive neuromental deficits.

Management: Epilepsia partialis continua is resistant to antiepileptic drug treatment, with clonazepam, sodium valproate and carbamazepine probably the most effective.

Normal girl aged 12 years with frequent episodes of epilepsia partialis continua from age 4 years   Video-EEG

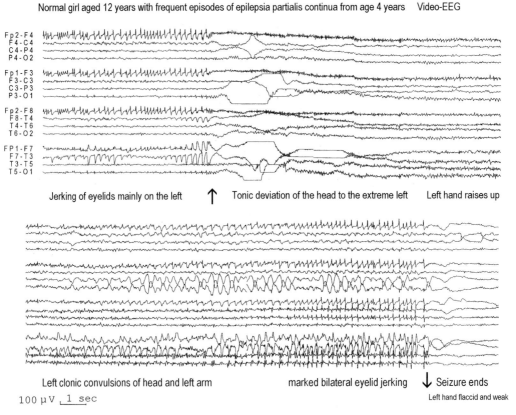

Jerking of eyelids mainly on the left   ↑   Tonic deviation of the head to the extreme left   Left hand raises up

Left clonic convulsions of head and left arm   marked bilateral eyelid jerking   ↓ Seizure ends

100 µV ⌐1 sec   Left hand flaccid and weak

Figure 8.8   Epilepsia partialis continua of 3 days duration ending with hemiconvulsions.

This is sample from a video-EEG of a girl aged 12 years. She has epilepsia partialis continua, which started at the age of 4 years and continues to date at increasing frequency and duration. This is fast (3–10 Hz) twitching of the left eyelids simultaneously with the left rectus abdominis (she points close to the midline by the umbilicus) and a muscle in the arm-pit (probably the latissimus dorsi). This lasts for hours to 2–3 days and is continuous day and night. This is interspersed with left-sided focal tonic-clonic motor seizures affecting face and upper limb mainly. Additionally, there is post-ictal and probably ictal left hemiparesis of mainly the upper limb. She does not lose consciousness during these attacks and communicates well. Also during the focal motor seizures, she is able to understand but cannot speak. She never had a full-blown GTCS.

Initially, the seizures were once or twice per year but now they occur every 2 weeks. Neurological and mental status are normal. High-resolution brain MRI was normal. All appropriate tests for metabolic or other diseases associated with epilepsia partialis continua were normal. Drug treatments failed; only rectal diazepam during the attacks offers temporary relief.

Differential diagnosis of the case: Epilepsia partialis continua is a non-specific seizure type that may occur in a number of diverse conditions and causes. In a child the first syndrome that comes to mind is Kozhevnikov-Rasmussen chronic encephalitis. However, her good clinical state throughout the years as well as the normal MRI and the lack of background EEG abnormalities is rather against this diagnosis although there are on the record some unusual cases where deterioration appeared 10 years after onset of epilepsia partialis continua.

Dermatomal Somatosensory Evoked Potentials – DSSEP

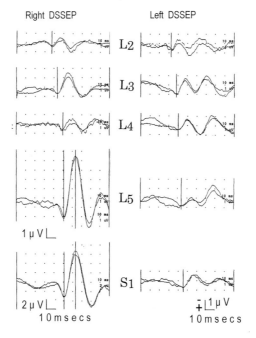

Somatosensory Evoked Potentials from the Tibial Nerve

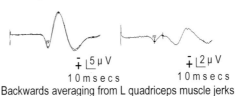

Backwards averaging from L quadriceps muscle jerks

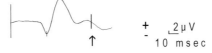

Figure 8.9

Neurophysiological investigations of a man aged 26 years who started having epilepsia partialis continua from age 25. This consisted of continuous and arrhythmic twitching of various muscles of the left leg and particularly the toes. There was great variation in intensity, spread and severity. It was exaggerated on dorsiflexion of the foot and improved when resting. On five occasions this progressed in a Jacksonian manner to GTCS. The clonic movements of the toes spread to the foot and then to the knee for 5 minutes prior to GTCS. On neurological examination there were mild pyramidal signs of the left leg. All possible tests to discover the cause of this were negative including high-resolution MRI, PET scan, CSF with appropriate metabolic screening. Mitochondrial disease was also excluded. After a short course of steroids and drug treatment with mainly clonazepam the situation improved dramatically. Ten years later he is well although he infrequently has some clusters of irregular twitching of the toes of the left leg and he is still on clonazepam.

Top and middle: Dermatomal and somatosensory potentials are gigantic on the right side (from stimulation of the left). Note that the maximum amplitude of the dermatomal potentials is obtained when the S1 dermatome is stimulated.

Bottom: Jerk locked back-averaged cortical potentials appear in the contralateral primary motor area preceding the jerks by 25 milliseconds (positive peak).

KOZHEVNIKOV-RASMUSSEN SYNDROME

Kozhevnikov[597]-Rasmussen[598] syndrome★ is a severe, probably acquired, neurological neocortical disorder characterised by intractable mainly motor focal seizures, epilepsia partialis continua and progressive neuropsychiatric deterioration with hemiparesis and mental deficits.[586,593,599–602]

Demographic data: Onset is in childhood from age 1 to 10 years with a peak at 5–6 years. Late onset, in adolescence or adulthood, is rare. Both sexes are equally affected. This is a very rare disease.[593] Highly specialised tertiary centres may see one case per year.

Clinical manifestations: Kozhevnikov-Rasmussen syndrome typically affects otherwise normal children that start having motor focal seizures, localised clonic muscle twitching of epilepsia partialis continua, complex focal seizures without automatisms or secondary GTCS. Epilepsia partialis continua occurs in 60% and may last for days, often interspersed with hemi-tonic–clonic convulsions that may also become generalised. Hemiplegia is initially transient associated with seizures but gradually becomes permanent.

The clinical course follows three stages:

The first stage is characterised mainly by simple motor or somatosensory seizures. Less frequently onset may be with epilepsia partialis continua, complex focal seizures without automatisms or secondary GTCS. A combination of these types of seizures may occur. Gradually, over weeks or months, seizures become more frequent. Hemiparesis is initially post-ictal and transient but slowly becomes permanent.

In the second stage, seizures become more frequent, more widespread and of longer duration. It is at this stage, varying from 3 months to 10 years from seizure onset, that permanent neurological and mental deficits appear with a progressive intensity. These consist of moderate to severe hemiparesis, hemi-hypoaesthesia, visual field defects and intellectual/language impairment (including dysphasia and dysarthria).

In the third stage, the disease appears to burn out regarding seizure frequency and severity as well as progression of neurological deficits.

Progressive deterioration of the neurological and psychological state, either with or without seizure deterioration, is a typical feature of Kozhevnikov-Rasmussen syndrome. This may appear within 3 months to 10 years from seizure onset.

Diagnostic procedures: There is no specific diagnostic procedure or abnormality in Kozhevnikov-Rasmussen syndrome. At onset, all functional and structural modalities may be normal. It is the progression and their localisation that may be consistent with this diagnosis.

Cerebrospinal fluid shows non-specific abnormalities in half of the patients. Oligoclonal or monoclonal bands may be found.

Brain imaging: Serial CT brain scan and preferably MRI show progressive hemi-atrophy. This usually starts in the temporo-insular region with enlargement of the temporal horn and Sylvian fissure.

---

*The reason for this eponymic nomenclature has been detailed elsewhere.[587]

Magnetic resonance spectroscopy (MRS) demonstrates decreased relative N-acetylaspartate signal intensity over the cortex and white matter of the entire affected hemisphere, which is more prominent in the anterior periventricular region and progresses in time.

Functional brain imaging with single photon emission computed tomography (SPECT) and 5-fluoro-D-glucose positron emission tomography (PET) demonstrates interictal hypoperfusion and hypometabolism in the affected side that is widely distributed, more intense in the Rolandic and temporo-insular regions, worsens with progression of the disease and may be abnormal at a stage where MRI is normal. Ictally, there is regional hyperperfusion corresponding to the epileptogenic locus.

Electroencephalography: may be initially normal but soon after focal slow, usually polymorphic high amplitude delta waves appear that gradually dominate in one hemisphere and often become bilateral with lateralised predominance. Gradual disappearance and poverty of physiological rhythms in the affected side is the rule. Focal slow waves may appear before MRI abnormalities. Nearly all EEG show interictal spikes or sharp and slow waves. A single focus is rare.

Onset of ictal EEG patterns is variable and exceptionally remains localised. More commonly, seizures have multifocal onset either confined in one hemisphere or less frequently from one or the other side. Focal motor seizures may occur without concomitant EEG changes. Conversely, ictal EEG paroxysms may frequently occur without discernible clinical manifestations.

Epilepsia partialis continua is notorious regarding the lack of clinico-EEG correlations. The myoclonic jerks do not have a chronological relation with the interictal spikes. It is exceptional to have jerks associated with EEG discharges.

With progress of the disease abnormalities tend to become bilateral. Thus background slow and poverty of physiological rhythms affects both hemispheres, epileptiform abnormalities become more widespread and multifocal also affecting the contralateral hemisphere.

Aetiology: This is unknown. Chronic encephalitis, as the main aetiological factor, is the main issue. Pathology reveals an inflammatory process, initially relatively localised but progressing in a confluent rather than a multifocal manner to more extensive unilateral or bilateral mainly cortical involvement. The pathological abnormalities vary from those of active to those of remote disease. Converging lines of evidence suggest that an autoimmune process may be important in the pathogenesis of this syndrome. Direct analysis of resected brain tissue for virus by polymerase chain reaction or in situ hybridisation has yielded inconsistent results, perhaps as a consequence of the variable presence of non-disease-related viral genomes, either in neural cells or in inflammatory cells in the lesions.

Proposed causes of the pathological changes are:

1. chronic viral infection – but so far no virus has been isolated

2. acute viral infection leading to a local immune response

3. independent autoimmune process, not linked to infection, but results are either in favour or against this hypothesis.

Differential diagnosis: The diagnosis of Kozhevnikov-Rasmussen syndrome at the initial stages is impossible, particularly before the appearance of epilepsia partialis continua. At this stage high-resolution brain imaging is mandatory to exclude other more likely and common causes such as malformation of cortical development, brain tumours, tuberous sclerosis, vascular anomalies, parasitic (such as cysticercosis) or other infectious disorders. An EEG is also mandatory as this may reveal functional spikes of Rolandic seizures or other ictal and interictal abnormalities that may suggest a possible diagnostic seizure category. Also, these tests are important as a baseline for follow-up comparisons.

Other more serious diseases such as MELAS (mitochondrial myopathy, encephalopathy, lactic acidosis and stroke) are less likely to cause diagnostic difficulties despite high prevalence of epilepsia partialis continua. Acute encephalitis of any cause producing hemiplegia and seizures should also be apparent from onset. Russian spring-summer and other tick-borne encephalitides should also be considered in patients with acute onset symptoms in endemic areas.

Prognosis: This is a progressive disorder of increasing seizure frequency and severity with the development of fixed neurological deficits, mainly hemiplegia and intellectual and language deficits, ranging from mild to severe.

Management: Seizures are usually refractory, with little response to antiepileptic drugs. There is no effective treatment other than the dramatic functional hemispherectomy.

PARIETAL LOBE EPILEPSIES [9,603–611]

The syndromes of parietal lobe epilepsy manifest with seizures originating from a primary epileptic focus anywhere in the parietal lobe. The clinical seizure characteristics, electroencephalographic findings and results of neuroimaging studies in patients with carefully documented parietal lobe origin of seizure have been detailed recently.[603–608,611,612]

Demographic data: Parietal lobe epilepsies may start at any age and equally affect both sexes. Age at onset is much later in tumoral than in non-tumoral

---

Considerations on classification:

Parietal lobe epilepsies have not yet been classified in the new ILAE diagnostic scheme.[10] Also, the 1989 Classification of ILAE described seizure characteristics rather than parietal lobe syndromes.[9]

groups of patients. Parietal lobe epilepsy is relatively rare, probably 6% in neurosurgical series.

Clinical manifestations: Seizures mainly manifest with:

- subjective somatosensory symptoms
- subjective disturbances of body image (somatic illusions)
- vertiginous complaints
- visual illusions or complex formed visual hallucinations and
- receptive or conductive linguistic disturbances.

Somatosensory seizures are by far the commonest type (around two thirds) and consist of various types of paraesthetic, dysaesthetic and painful sensations described as tingling, numbness, thermal, burning, tickling, pricking, creeping, tight, crawling, electric and their variations. Pain, sometimes exacerbating, is experienced by one quarter of patients with somatosensory seizures. Somatosensory seizures are of lateralising significance occurring contralateral to the side of seizure origin. Face (mainly lips and tongue), hand (mainly thumb) and arm that have the largest cortical representation (homunculus of Penfield) are more likely to get involved. Symptoms may be static or may march in a Jacksonian manner.

Somatic illusions are the second most common ictal symptom of parietal lobe seizures. These include illusions of distorted posture, limb position or of movement, and a feeling that an extremity or a body part is alien or absent. They mainly emanate from the non-language-dominant cerebral hemisphere. Inability to move one extremity or a feeling of weakness in the hand contralateral to the epileptogenic zone is also reported.

Vertigo and other vertiginous sensations of an illusion of movement are well reported, probably ~10% as ictal manifestations of parietal lobe seizures. They are elicited predominantly from the temporoparietal border.

Visual illusions and complex formed visual hallucinations occur in ~12% of patients with parietal lobe epilepsy. Images may be larger or smaller, close or far away or moving although static. Ictal visual illusions such as micropsia, metamorphopsia and palinopsia most likely emanate from the non-dominant parietal regions.

Linguistic disturbances: Language-dominant temporal-parietal lobe seizures are associated with a variety of linguistic disturbances, alexia with agraphia and significant calculation defects. Non-dominant parietal-occipital-temporal seizure activity usually results in significant spatial disturbances.

Genital sensations, sometimes well lateralised, may occur with paracentral involvement. Orgasm is well documented.[613]

Simple focal seizures often spread to extra-parietal regions producing unilateral focal motor clonic manifestations (57% of patients), head and eyes deviation (41%), tonic posturing of usually one extremity (28%) and automatisms (21%).

Most of the patients also suffer from secondary GTCS.

Of *post-ictal symptoms,* Todd's paralysis (22%) and dysphasia (7%) are common.

Seizures may be provoked by movements of the affected part of the body, tapping or other somatosensory stimuli.

Duration of seizures varies from a few seconds to 1–2 minutes.[606] Prolonged isolated sensory auras analogous to epilepsia partialis continua but without any spread to motor regions have been reported[565,607,608] and this condition may be misdiagnosed as functional psychogenic seizures.[614]

Aetiology: This is diverse, from symptomatic, possible symptomatic and idiopathic causes. Of 82 non–tumoral patients with parietal lobe epilepsy, 43% had a history of head trauma, 16% a history of birth trauma and the cause was unknown in 20% of patients.[607] The remaining 21% had a history of encephalitis, febrile convulsions, gunshot wounds to the head, forme fruste of tuberous sclerosis, hamartoma, vascular malformations, tuberculoma, arachnoid or porencephalic cysts, microgyria and post-traumatic thrombosis of the middle cerebral artery.[607] In reports with MRI,[603,604] lesions were small, indolent or non-progressive and could have been found only on pathological examination. Focal cortical dysplasia is frequent.[612]

Of tumours, astrocytomas (62%) were more common than meningiomas (14%), haemangiomas (9%), oligodendrogliomas (9%) and ependymoblastomas (3%).[608] However, patients with more aggressive tumours, like glioblastomas, are unlikely to feature in these series of neurosurgical epilepsy evaluation.

Diagnostic procedures: Brain high–resolution MRI shows abnormalities in around 60% of the patients. Functional neuroimaging is important for localisation.

Electroencephalography: EEG, interictal and ictal, may be of lateralising but not of localising value. Normal interictal and ictal EEG is usually the case, contributing to diagnostic errors.

Ictal EEG may be normal in 80% of simple focal sensory seizures.[612]

Differential diagnosis: Somatosensory seizures, if reported, are likely to be misdiagnosed as psychogenic, imaginatory, transient ischaemic attacks or migraine with aura, in that order.

Patients with simple sensory seizures alone, brief or prolonged, are a challenging proposition. Commonly, it is only when these progress to motor symptoms or alteration of consciousness that seizures are suspected and appropriate investigations are instituted. When patients with pure sensory seizures also have psychiatric complaints, the chances of misdiagnosis or delay of diagnosis are high. The diagnosis is also particularly difficult for patients with somatosensory symptoms at seizure onset that progress to loss of consciousness and amnesia for the aura. These patients often have more intense seizures, and EEG changes are usually bilateral. Further, patients may not volunteer information on sensory symptoms until thoroughly interrogated about an aura.

Differentiating pure sensory seizures from psychogenic seizures or psychiatric disturbances may be extremely difficult, as emphasised by Lesser et al.[614] and indicated by the fact that simple focal seizures are only associated with ictal EEG changes in 21% of patients.[612]

Parietal lobe seizures of ictal pain, sensory epilepsia partialis continua, genital and orgasmic manifestations are more likely to be diagnosed as psychogenic phenomena.

Sensory Jacksonian seizures may imitate migraine with sensory aura.[615] In older patients, transient ischaemic attack is the most likely diagnostic error.

Management: Drug treatment, similar to that for any other type of focal seizures (page 205), is usually effective.

Neurosurgery is performed for severe symptomatic cases. Sixty-five percent of patients with non-tumoral parietal lobe epilepsy became seizure-free or had rare seizures. Completeness of resection of the epileptogenic zone correlated with better outcome. More favourable outcome in a few patients with lesional parietal lobe epilepsy has recently been reported in the MRI era.[603,604]

OCCIPITAL LOBE EPILEPSIES [25,605,616–621]

Occipital seizures originate from an epileptic occipital focus that is triggered spontaneously or by external visual stimuli. These may be idiopathic, symptomatic or probably symptomatic.

Demographic data: Symptomatic occipital seizures may start at any age and at any stage after or during the course of the primary disorder. Idiopathic occipital epilepsy usually starts in late childhood (page 103). Prevalence of occipital epilepsies is around 5–10% of epilepsies.[25] In neurosurgical series prevalence is around 5%,[619] which is comparable to that (6%) of demographic studies.[622]

Clinical manifestations: Ictal clinical symptoms of occipital lobe epilepsy are subjective, objective and both. The cardinal symptoms are mainly visual and occulo-motor.

Visual symptoms include:

- elementary and less often complex visual hallucinations,
- blindness,
- visual illusions and
- pallinopsia.

Other visual or ocular symptoms include:

- sensory hallucinations of ocular movements and
- ocular pain.

Ictal oculo-motor symptoms include:

- tonic deviation of the eyes (pursuit-like rather than oculotonic),
- oculoclonic or nystagmus and
- repetitive eyelid closures or eyelid fluttering.

Considerations on classification:

Occipital lobe epilepsies have not yet been detailed in the new ILAE diagnostic scheme.[10] Also, the 1989

Classification of ILAE describes occipital seizures rather than occipital lobe syndromes.[9]

Elementary visual hallucinations are the commonest and most characteristic, most likely the first and often the only seizure clinical manifestation. Ictal elementary visual hallucinations mainly consist of small multi-coloured circular patterns that often appear in the periphery of a temporal visual field, becoming larger and multiplying in the course of the seizure, frequently moving horizontally towards the other side (Figures 5.7 and 8.10). Flashing or flickering achromatic lights or non-circular patterns are rare. They develop fast in seconds and they are usually brief, for seconds to 1–3 minutes, rarely longer. Patients do not have the over 4 minutes linear, zigzag, achromatic or black and white patterns characteristic of migraine visual aura. Elementary visual hallucinations may progress and co-exist with other occipital seizure symptoms such as illusions of ocular movements and ocular pain, pursuit-like tonic deviation of the eyes, eyelid fluttering or repetitive eye closures and oculoclonic-epileptic nystagmus.

Complex visual hallucinations, visual illusions and other symptoms from more anterior ictal spreading occur in the seizure progress that may terminate with hemiconvulsions or generalised convulsions. Complex visual hallucinations do not have the emotional and complicated character of temporal lobe seizures. They may be the first ictal symptom but more often follow elementary visual hallucinations.

Ictal blindness, appearing ab initio or less commonly after other occipital seizure manifestations, usually lasts for 3–5 minutes, although status amauroticus may occasionally occur. Blurring of vision as an initial seizure manifestation before visual hallucinations may be common if investigated.

Seizures may spread from the occipital to other more anterior regions of the brain generating symptoms from the temporal, parietal and frontal lobes and secondary hemiconvulsions or generalised convulsions. Progress to

Imagine that these visual fields below are as you see them in front of you

1. Where are they and how they look at the beginning of the event

2, Where are they and how they look at the very peak (maximum) of the visual effect

Left visual field   Midline (nose)   Right visual field   Left visual field   Midline (nose)   Right visual field

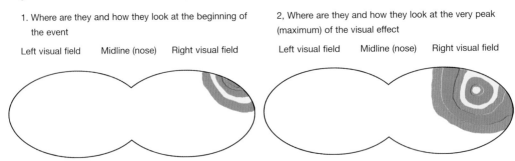

Figure 8.10 Visual seizures as perceived and drawn by a patient with symptomatic occipital epilepsy.

From Panayiotopoulos (1999)[621] with the permission of the Editor of *Epileptic Disorders.*

temporal lobe seizure symptomatology is rather exceptional in idiopathic cases.

Consciousness is not impaired during the elementary and complex visual hallucinations, blindness and other occipital seizure symptoms, but may be disturbed or lost in the course of the seizure, usually prior to convulsions.

Ictal or post-ictal headache frequently associate with occipital seizures. Post-ictal headache, often indistinguishable from migraine, is far more common in occipital (more than half) than other focal seizures and may occur even after brief visual seizures.

Visual seizures occur, often in multiple clusters, daily or weekly. Commonly there may be several per day. They are usually diurnal but some patients may often wake up with elementary visual hallucinations.

Some patients suffer from occipital status epilepticus.[623]

Aetiology: Aetiology may be idiopathic, structural or metabolic. In symptomatic occipital epilepsy lesions may be congenital, residual or progressive, resulting from vascular, neoplastic, metabolic, hereditary, congenital, inflammatory, parasitic and systemic diseases and infections. Malformation of cortical development is a common cause increasingly recognised with MRI.[619] Metabolic or other derangement such as eclampsia may have a particular predilection for the occipital lobes and may cause either occipital 'seizures that do not require a diagnosis of epilepsy' or permanent occipital lesions leading to symptomatic occipital epilepsy.[624] There is an interesting association between coeliac disease and occipital lobe epilepsy.[307] Occipital seizures may be the first manifestation of a devastating course such as in Lafora disease[625–627] or mitochondrial disorders.[628]

Pathophysiology: Elementary visual hallucinations generate from the visual cortex, complex visual hallucinations from occipito-parietal-temporal junction areas, visual illusions from the non-dominant parietal regions.[25]

Diagnostic procedures: The discovery of the underlying cause in symptomatic occipital epilepsies may need haematology, biochemistry, screening for metabolic disorders, molecular DNA analysis or even skin or other tissue biopsy.[25] All patients with occipital lobe epilepsy require a high-resolution MRI (Figure 8.11).[25] Unsuspected residual or progressive lesions, tumours, vascular malformations and malformations of cortical development are all shown with MRI. CT is much inferior to MRI and insensitive to focal cortical dysplasia. Conversely, calcifications of coeliac disease may be missed with MRI but this is rare. Functional brain imaging for localisation is of practical value.[629]

Electroencephalography: EEG is essential.

Interictal EEG: In symptomatic cases background EEG is usually abnormal with posterior lateralised slow waves. Unilateral occipital spikes and occasionally occipital paroxysms occur and there may be photosensitivity but there are also fast multiple spikes either posterior or generalised and these are often facilitated by sleep.[25] Worsening of the background EEG is also significant for diagnosis.

In idiopathic cases (classified differently) background inter-ictal EEG is normal (page 103).[25] Occipital spikes and occipital paroxysms – spontaneous, evoked, or both – are often abundant but disappear with age, frequently long after cessation of occipital seizures (page 104).

Ictal EEG: Surface ictal EEG in occipital seizures, irrespective of cause, usually manifests with paroxysmal fast activity, fast spiking or both, localised in the occipital regions with occasional gradual anterior spreading and generalisation with irregular spike wave discharges or monomorphic spike and wave activity (Figure 8.12). Brief occipital flattening may be seen before the fast rhythmic pattern. Often, in patients with symptomatic occipital lobe epilepsy, the ictal discharge is more widespread (regional) rather than of a precise occipital localisation. Usually, there is no post–ictal localised slow activity unless the seizure is prolonged or progressed to secondary GTCS. One third (30%) of ictal surface EEG do not show any appreciable changes.[25]

Differential diagnosis: Occipital seizures should not be difficult to diagnose and these should be first differentiated from migraine (Table 8.1), normal phenomena and psychogenic or other causes unrelated to seizures.[25] The main differentiation is between symptomatic and idiopathic cases. Normal neurological state (including visual fields) is not exceptional in symptomatic occipital epilepsy.[25,619]

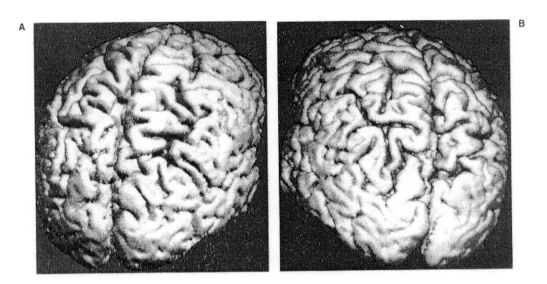

Figure 8.11 Patient with visual seizures and focal status epilepticus of occipital lobe epilepsy.[623] Three-dimensional reconstruction of the brain demonstrating abnormal gyral patterns on the right.

(A) Surface rendering of cortex viewed from right posterosuperior occipital aspect, demonstrating abnormally enlarged gyral pattern.

(B) Surface rendering of cortex viewed from left posterosuperior occipital aspect, with normal gyral pattern shown for comparison.

From Walker et al. (1995)[623] with the permission of the authors and the Editor of *Epilepsia*.

Occipital seizures manifesting with elementary visual hallucinations, blindness, vomiting and headache alone or in combination may imitate migraine, which is the reason that they are often mistaken for migraine with aura, acephalgic or basilar migraine (Table 8.1).[25,306,621] The main reason that visual seizures are misdiagnosed for migraine is two-fold. Firstly, visual seizures are not examined in a synthetic manner. Secondly, their differential diagnostic criteria have not been adequately addressed. The quality and the chronological sequence of ictal elementary visual hallucinations are markedly different from the visual aura of migraine. As a rule, brief (less than a minute), elementary visual hallucinations that may cluster in a daily frequency with coloured and circular patterns are probably pathognomonic of visual seizures and may be followed by severe headache and vomiting. EEG may be normal, show non-specific abnormalities or reveal slow focal or occipital spikes. A high-resolution MRI is mandatory as this may detect a structural lesion requiring early attention and management.

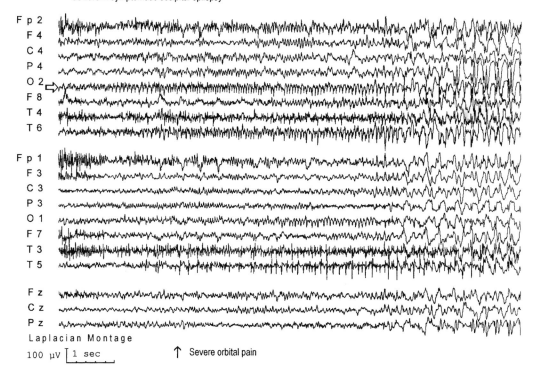

Seizure in symptomatic occipital epilepsy

Laplacian Montage

100 µV ⌐ 1 sec

↑ Severe orbital pain

Figure 8.12

Ictal EEG of an occipital seizure starting with fast spikes in the right occipital electrode (horizontal arrow) with rapid spread anteriorly and contralaterally.

The patient complained of severe pain behind both eyes (vertical arrow) just after the onset of the ictal discharge.

Prognosis: Frequency, severity and response to treatment vary considerably from good to intractable and progressive, mainly depending on the underlying cause and extent of the lesions.[25]

Management: Drug treatment, similar to that for any other type of focal seizure (page 205), is usually effective and this should be initiated as soon as possible.[25] Carbamazepine is the drug of choice.

Neurosurgery is reserved for severe symptomatic cases and this may be selectively effective.[610,630–632]

Table 8.1 Differential diagnosis of occipital seizures from basilar migraine or migraine with aura

	Occipital epilepsy	Migraine with aura	Basilar migraine
Visual hallucinations			
Duration for seconds to a minute	Exclusive	None	None
Duration for 1–3 minutes	Frequent	Rare	Rare
Duration for 4–30 minutes	Rare	As a rule	As a rule
Daily in frequency	As a rule	Rare	None
Mainly coloured circular patterns	As a rule	Rare	Exceptional
Mainly achromatic or black and white linear patterns	Exceptional	As a rule	Rare
Moving to the opposite side of the visual field	Exclusive	None	None
Expanding from the centre to the periphery of a visual hemifield	Rare	As a rule	Frequent
Evolving to blindness	Rare	Rare	As a rule
Evolving to tonic deviation of eyes	Exclusive	None	None
Evolving to impairment of consciousness without convulsions	Frequent	Rare	Frequent
Evolving to impairment of consciousness with convulsions	Frequent	Exceptional	Rare
Associated with post-ictal/post-critical headache	Frequent	As a rule	Frequent
Blindness and hemianopia			
Without other preceding or following symptoms	Frequent	None	Frequent
Other neurological symptoms			
Brain stem symptoms	None	None	Exclusive
Post-ictal/post-critical vomiting	Rare	Frequent	Frequent
Post-ictal/post-critical headache			
Post-ictal or post-critical severe headache	Frequent	As a rule	Frequent

Modified from Panayiotopoulos (1999)[621] with the permission of the editor of *Epileptic Disorders.*

HYPOTHALAMIC (GELASTIC) EPILEPSY [633–635]

Hypothalamic (gelastic epilepsy) is a rare epileptic disease of hypothalamic hamartomas manifesting with gelastic seizures. :

Demographic data: Onset of habitual seizures typically begins in the neonatal period or early childhood with a peak at 2–3 years. Boys are affected twice as often as girls. Hypothalamic gelastic epilepsy appears to be extremely rare, probably 0.1%. In my experience of 1500 patients only 2 had hypothalamic gelastic epilepsy.

Clinical manifestations: Laughter is the defining, inaugural and starting clinical ictal manifestation of hypothalamic gelastic epilepsy. Gelastic seizures may manifest only with laughter particularly at onset and may not even be recognised as pathological. The laughter may be silent, a facial expression of a smile, or loud, with the natural vocalisations at various intensities and combinations. There is no emotional element of pleasure or amusement associated with this; it is a mirthless laughter. The laughter is unmotivated; the attacks come out of the blue, out of place and they are inappropriate. Dacrystic (crying) attacks alone or together with laughter may occur in 13% of the patients.[634]

The attacks are usually brief (10–30 seconds), of sudden onset and termination, occurring on a daily basis.[634] Subjectively, patients may be conscious of laughing but they cannot prevent it or stop it.[634] They feel embarrassed about this, often inventing various excuses to justify it if this occurs at school, church or social meetings. A few patients report a warning that they cannot describe. Other subjective symptoms include disorientation, localised tingling, and auditory sensations. The attacks are usually diurnal but exceptionally they may also occur during sleep.[634,636]

Gelastic seizures may be associated with impairment of consciousness in half of the patients.[634] The commoner pattern is that of simple focal gelastic seizures becoming longer with impairment of consciousness and, other than laughter, clinical ictal manifestations such as automatisms.

Autonomic symptoms associated with the attacks of laughter are common, occurring in one third of patients.[634,637] These include changes of the respiratory or cardiac rhythm, blood pressure, facial flush or pallor, moaning, pupillary dilation, sniffing and urinary incontinence. Gelastic seizures are accompanied by an abrupt sympathetic system activation, probably due to the

---

Considerations on classification:
Hypothalamic gelastic epilepsy has not been recognised as a separate syndrome.[10] The new diagnostic scheme correctly recognises gelastic seizures as a seizure type of various aetiologies[10] but ignores the fact that some of them are aetiologically linked to the hypothalamus. The association between hypothalamic hamartoma and gelastic seizures, often with precocious puberty, is now well established thus constituting an epileptic entity (disease).

direct paroxysmal activation of limbic and paralimbic structures or other autonomic centres of the hypothalamus and medulla.[638]

More than half of the patients (66%) also suffer from other types of seizures in addition to gelastic attacks.[634,639,640] These are usually generalised seizures such as tonic, atonic, generalised tonic-clonic and absences, alone or in combination. Complex focal seizures without laughter are less common. These additional types of seizures may start at the same time with laughter attacks or usually later within one to a few years.[634]

There are no objective or subjective post-ictal symptoms in non-convulsive seizures of hypothalamic gelastic epilepsy. Pre-ictal activity continues as if nothing had happened.

Although by rule unmotivated, some of the attacks may be triggered by a pleasant situation.

Aetiology: By definition the aetiology of hypothalamic gelastic epilepsy is due to hypothalamic hamartomas that usually originate in the region of the tuber cinereum and the mamillary bodies.[641] Hamartoma is a non-neoplastic, developmental tumour-like nodule that results from aberrant differentiation. Typically, it is a mass composed of disorganised but mature cells, all of which are indigenous to the site of origin (the hypothalamus in these cases of hypothalamic gelastic epilepsy). Hypothalamic hamartomas are directly involved in the pathogenesis of gelastic and dacrystic seizures and they have intrinsic epileptogenicity. There is direct evidence with intracranial recordings that the gelastic seizures of hypothalamic gelastic epilepsy arise from the hamartoma itself.[642] The fact that seizures may also respond to long-acting gonadotropin-releasing hormone (GnRH) analogue prescribed for precocious puberty may indicate that the epileptogenic generators reside in the same cells that autonomously produce GnRH.[643]

Diagnostic procedures: A clinical diagnosis of hypothalamic gelastic epilepsy would demand confirmation with high-resolution MRI.

Electroencephalography: Interictal EEG is not informative. It may be normal or more commonly show non-specific and non-lateralising episodic abnormalities. Low voltage episodic fast rhythms with simultaneous suppression of background activity is the typical ictal pattern in surface EEG (Figure 8.13).

Differential diagnosis: Hypothalamic seizures need differentiation from non-epileptic conditions and from seizures arising from other brain locations. Gelastic seizures may be initially so mild and appear so natural that they are understandably unrecognised as pathologic. It is only after the appearance of other more conventional seizure manifestations and impairment of consciousness that medical advice is sought.

The fact that gelastic seizures may arise from brain locations other than the hypothalamus and particularly the temporal and frontal lobes is well documented.[633,645,646] It is difficult to establish exact differential criteria between gelastic seizures of different origins in the brain. My understanding is that gelastic seizures of hypothalamic epilepsy are unique regarding:

- seizure onset of laughter as the first and often the only ictal manifestation
- daily seizure frequency
- lack of mirth
- awareness of ictal laughter.

This clustering of events does not occur in either temporal or frontal gelastic seizures. For example, laughter in the middle of other ictal manifestations,

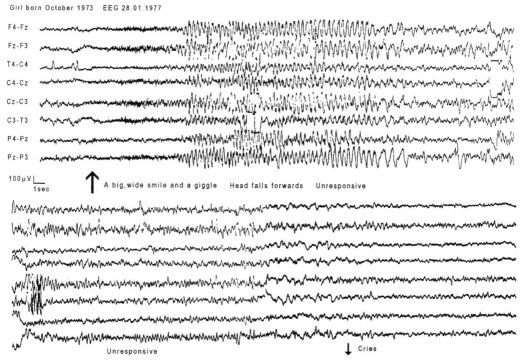

Figure 8.13

Surface ictal EEG of a girl aged 3 years and 3 months with normal neuropsychological development and frequent daily gelastic seizures.[644] First noticed at age 2 years when her parents observed that when told 'how beautiful' she is or 'come and get these candies' she reacted with a 'facial grimace', something like a 'frozen smile', 'a smile that freezes', 'right-sided deviated lips with a smile'. This initially lasted for only a few seconds, occurred every fortnight and was always provoked as above. Subsequently, within months, this occurred daily, nearly every morning, without precipitating factors, became longer and it was also associated with small giggles. At the first arrow, her mother says, 'here it is her big smile'. The girl suddenly has a big and wide smile and this is associated with a mild giggle. This lasts for only a few seconds followed by head falling forwards and complete unresponsiveness until the end of the seizure when recovering is notified by a cry (second arrow). Interictal EEG was normal with well-organised and symmetrical alpha rhythm. The seizure starts (first arrow) with fast episodic activity at around 22 Hz, which is widely spread with some left-sided emphasis. This is concordant with the gelastic manifestations of the seizure. The rest of the EEG ictal events are self-evident.

laughter associated with emotions, infrequent complex seizures of laughter or gelastic seizures starting in adolescence are not features of hypothalamic gelastic epilepsy.

Gelastic seizures of temporal lobe origin are well documented.[633] Age at onset is variable but several cases starting in childhood were described. Gelastic seizures have been produced by stimulation of the temporobasal cortex in two candidates for surgery for non-gelastic seizures and explored with subdural electrodes.[647]

In the large majority of cases, the laughter is devoid of any sensation and is accompanied by a break of contact. In half of the cases other types of seizure also occur concomitantly with the gelastic seizures or precede them.[633]

Drug treatment, mainly with carbamazepine, may control the seizures; others become seizure-free after neurosurgical removal of the epileptogenic brain region.

Gelastic seizures of frontal lobe origin:[633,646] There are around 15 well-documented cases of gelastic seizures originating from the frontal lobe. Onset of seizures is usually before the age of 6 years but one third may start in adulthood. Most common lesions involve the cingulate gyrus. Laughter is described as unnatural and not associated with feelings of mirth. Laughter usually lasts less than 30 seconds, seizures generally less than 2 minutes. Other types of seizures may pre-date or follow the gelastic attacks.

Prognosis: Hypothalamic gelastic epilepsy is often a progressive seizure disorder. Typically, neonates or children are normal before the onset of seizures. Brief attacks of laughter with time become more and more frequent and longer with associated impairment of consciousness. Later generalised seizures of any type appear as of symptomatic generalised epilepsies. Additionally, progressive cognitive and behavioural impairment develops for most patients. More than half (59%) of them suffer from precocious puberty.[634]

The acquired cognitive and behavioural symptoms probably result from a direct effect of the seizures.[648] Children with hypothalamic hamartomas and precocious puberty, but without seizures, do not develop cognitive and behavioural problems.

Management: Medical treatment of hypothalamic gelastic epilepsy is often ineffective and polytherapy may do more harm than good.[634] A new and possibly exciting development was reported recently.[643] While treating precocious puberty in two such patients with long-acting gonadotropin-releasing hormone (GnRH) analogue, gelastic seizures stopped. The matter demands further trials in patients with and without precocious puberty.

Surgical removal of the hamartoma is technically difficult but it is highly effective if successful. Complete lesionectomy results in freedom from seizures and prevents neurobehavioural deterioration. In incomplete removal, improvement may occur. Stereotactic radiofrequency lesioning of the hamartoma resulting in seizure remission without complications after surgery was reported recently.[649,650]

DRUG TREATMENT OF FOCAL EPILEPSIES

The treatment of focal epilepsies is with antiepileptic drugs. If this fails, neurosurgical options are now becoming more widely available and often life-saving for symptomatic cases.

Existing evidence indicates that 15–30%[651,652] of those with newly diagnosed focal epilepsy (of any cause) fail to achieve reasonably sustained remission with optimal antiepileptic medication. The figure is probably significantly higher (35%) for those with symptomatic focal epilepsy.[651] Of those failing to respond, 25–50% develop intractable disease that is a continuation of seizures beyond 2–3 years despite optimal drug treatment.

This is only a brief guide on antiepileptic drugs in the treatment of focal epilepsies derived from an extensive review of the literature, inquiries I have made regarding the clinical experience of leading epileptologists and my personal experience of treating over 10,000 patients in the last 35 years. Recent books[445,653–656] and reviews[657–671] exhaustively detail the treatment of focal epilepsies and these are recommended for study. Readers are also advised to consult the prescribing information provided by the drug manufacturers. This is widely publicised and frequently updated regarding indications, drug doses, titration, drug interactions, recommendations and adverse reactions of antiepileptic drugs.

New antiepileptic drugs, if appropriately used,[669] make the treatment of epilepsies more promising, more challenging and more rewarding.

Antiepileptic drugs effective for focal seizures

According to evidence-based medicine all antiepileptic drugs (AEDs) entered into randomised clinical trials (RCTs) have approximately equal efficacy in controlling focal seizures with the old ones, but the new drugs are better tolerated than the older AEDs.[657,658,672] The reality in clinical practice often contradicts these conclusions for many reasons.[657,673,674] It is extremely difficult to find the balance. There is a significant and rapidly changing swing with the increasing experience obtained from the clinical application of licensed new drugs and the introduction of new antiepileptic agents. The following may be applicable at the *present time*.

Evidence-based medicine

Overall, randomised control trials usually in comparison with old AEDs showed that:

- New drugs such as vigabatrin, lamotrigine, gabapentin, ox-carbazepine, zonisamide, tiagabine, topiramate and levetiracetam (in chronological order) are of nearly equal efficacy to sodium valproate, carbamazepine and phenytoin (phenobarbitone and clobazam rarely enter these studies).[657,658,672]

- According to a meta-analysis of available clinical trials in terms of efficacy for focal seizures, there is no statistical difference in the responder rates between new antiepileptic drugs,[675] although there are no direct comparisons between them.

● No new drug was superior in efficacy to carbamazepine or phenytoin but new AEDs were better tolerated.[657,658,672]

Clinical practice

In developed countries:

1. **Old AEDs:** Carbamazepine is the superior drug, controlling focal seizures in more than 70% of patients (10% of the patients develop idiosyncratic reactions). Sodium valproate, a superior drug in generalised epilepsies, is inferior in focal epilepsies with significant concerns in the treatment of women. Phenytoin, as effective as carbamazepine, is dramatically falling out of use, mainly because of chronic toxicity. Phenobarbitone and primidone, less efficacious, have been practically eliminated, mainly because of their adverse effects on cognition. Clobazam (although often highly beneficial in selective cases) is rarely used as continuous AED treatment.

2. **New AEDs:** Ox-carbazepine, probably of equal efficacy with carbamazepine and possibly producing less idiosyncratic reactions, is gaining ground.[676] Topiramate is the most efficacious of the new drugs (but with concerns regarding cognitive and other adverse reactions). Gabapentin rarely controls seizures and is now used mainly for neurogenic pain. Vigabatrin has been practically discarded for the treatment of focal epilepsies because of common and often irreversible visual field defects. Tiagabine is cautiously used because of fears of adverse reactions similar to those of vigabatrin. Levetiracetam is becoming increasingly popular because of combined high efficacy, comparative poverty of adverse reactions and rapid titration.

In developing countries:

Carbamazepine, phenytoin and phenobarbitone are by far the most used main agents for treating focal epilepsies.

MONOTHERAPY AND RATIONAL POLYTHERAPY FOR FOCAL EPILEPSIES

Monotherapy for focal epilepsies is the primary aim – nearly all of the old AEDs and lamotrigine of the new AEDs are currently licensed for this purpose. Carbamazepine remains the first choice of most physicians but 10% of patients develop acute idiosyncratic reactions (mainly rash). In numerous comparative studies, no other drug has shown better efficacy than carbamazepine in focal seizures although some new drugs were better tolerated. If this fails at maximal tolerated doses, all other licensed drugs are alternative options for monotherapy. Topiramate, levetiracetam and zonisamide are increasingly used by modern epileptologists. Personally, I also use clobazam in selective cases. Thus, this section provides more information regarding the most successful of the new drugs (lamotrigine, levetiracetam, topiramate) and also comments on the use of sodium valproate and clobazam in focal epilepsies.

Rational polytherapy is often needed. All new drugs are licensed for this purpose. Initially, a second drug is added to the agent that showed better efficacy and tolerability in monotherapy. The choice of the second or sometimes a third drug depends on many factors such as efficacy, modes of action, adverse effects and interactions. Polytherapy with more than three drugs is discouraged because adverse reactions become more prominent with little if any seizure improvement.

Drugs licensed in monotherapy for focal seizures with or without secondary GTCS (in order of usefulness)

Carbamazepine (10% of patients may not be able to tolerate it because of idiosyncratic reactions)

Lamotrigine (It is one of the best drugs regarding cognitive adverse effects, but idiosyncratic reactions – which exceptionally may be fatal – are a realistic threat)[677,678]

Phenytoin (10–20% of patients may not be able to tolerate it because of idiosyncratic reactions which exceptionally may be fatal. Also long-term use is associated with unacceptable adverse reactions including dysmorphic features)

Sodium valproate (RCTs found it of nearly equal efficacy to carbamazepine[679] but this is rarely the case in clinical practice. Sodium valproate is likely to remain the first choice drug in generalised but of limited use in focal epilepsies)

Phenobarbitone and primidone (Still very valid antiepileptic drugs although their use is often barred by cognitive adverse reactions)

Drugs licensed as adjunctive medication for focal seizures with or without secondary GTCS (listed alphabetically)

Clobazam (It is a very useful drug that should be tried in all intractable patients or those with adverse reactions to other drugs. Tolerance to this drug has been overemphasised; the truth is in between and many patients may remain seizure-free despite continuing use)[680,681]

Gabapentin (Rather poor efficacy even at very high doses although with fewer adverse reactions. It is now mainly used for neurogenic pain)[682]

Levetiracetam (It may soon become a first line drug; see details below)

Ox-carbazepine (May be an alternative for those sensitive to carbamazepine but this is not certain)

Tiagabine (Visual field defects, although not yet confirmed, may be a reality because of its mechanism of action which is similar to vigabatrin)

Topiramate (Probably the most effective of all but handicapped by adverse reactions and particularly cognitive effects, sometimes relentless weight loss and others such as acute angle-closure glaucoma. See details below)

Vigabatrin (The high risk of visual field defects probably prohibits its use in focal epilepsies)[683]

Zonisamide (It is one of the most popular drugs in Japan. Nephrolithiasis occurred in 4% of patients in a USA study particularly in patients with a family history of kidney stones.[439] Drowsiness occurs in one quarter of patients)

ON THREE MOST COMMONLY USED NEW ANTIEPILEPTIC DRUGS

LAMOTRIGINE

Lamotrigine, first licensed for clinical practice in 1993, is now established as one of the best antiepileptic drugs of its generation. It is a highly effective, broad-spectrum antiepileptic drug for all types of focal and generalised seizures except myoclonic jerks.[678,684–690] Its efficacy has been documented in children[684,685] and adults[678,687,688] for all epileptic syndromes with the exception of predominantly myoclonic epilepsies such as Dravet syndrome. Lamotrigine appears to be the drug of first choice for women in relation to sodium valproate. The other major advantage of lamotrigine is that is non-sedating with improved global functioning, which includes increased attention and alertness reported in both paediatric and adult trials.[686] Lamotrigine use has already reached 3 million patient exposures worldwide. Idiosyncratic reactions, mainly rashes that can become very serious and sometimes fatal, are a significant disadvantage.[691,692]

Current main applications are: All focal or generalised, idiopathic or symptomatic epileptic syndromes of all age groups including neonates[80] and children.[684,685] There are only a few exceptions as noted above.

In polytherapy, lamotrigine is at its best when combined with sodium valproate, because of very efficacious pharmacodynamic interactions.[693] This combination may be ideal for drug-resistant generalised epilepsies including those with myoclonic seizures.[694] Usually, small doses of lamotrigine added to sodium valproate render previously uncontrolled patients seizure-free.[7,693,695,696]

Important interactions with other antiepileptic drugs

Sodium valproate inhibits lamotrigine metabolism, doubling or tripling its half-life.[691]

Enzyme inducers, such as carbamazepine, phenytoin and phenobarbital, accelerate its elimination, but lamotrigine itself has no effect on hepatic metabolic processes.[697]

With lamotrigine added to carbamazepine, symptoms of carbamazepine neurotoxicity (headache, diplopia, ataxia) may occur (probably because of pharmacodynamic interaction rather than elevated carbamazepine epoxide levels); this necessitates reduced carbamazepine dosage when lamotrigine is introduced.

Dose (monotherapy): Children 2–8 mg/kg/day in two divided doses; adults 200–400 mg daily in two divided doses.

Dose (polytherapy): Because of the effect of other drugs on lamotrigine metabolism and elimination (see above) polytherapy requires adjustment of monotherapy dosage upwards with enzyme-inducing antiepileptic drugs (300–500 mg daily in adults) and downwards with sodium valproate (100–300 mg daily in adults).

Cautions on titration: Probably, slower dosage titration reduces the risk for skin rash and possibly of the generalised hypersensitive reaction.[692] Therefore, it is mandatory to follow the manufacturer's recommendations regarding initial dose and subsequent slow dose escalation of lamotrigine. For monotherapy in children this is approximately 0.3 mg/kg/day in the first 2 weeks to 0.6 mg/kg/day in the next 2 weeks. For monotherapy in adults this is in weekly steps of 25–50 mg. Polytherapy should follow the same principles as above depending on concurrent medication with sodium valproate or enzyme-inducing antiepileptic drugs.

Therapeutic range: Lamotrigine can be efficacious even at very small dosage although occasionally higher than recommended doses may be needed. There is no need for serum level monitoring.

Main adverse reactions: An allergic skin rash is the commonest and probably the most dangerous adverse effect prompting withdrawal of lamotrigine.[692] Children are at higher risk that also increases with over-rapid titration when starting therapy and when lamotrigine is prescribed in combination with valproate. Skin rash occurs in approximately 10% of patients, usually in the first 4–8 weeks. Serious rashes leading to hospitalisation, including Stevens-Johnson syndrome and hypersensitivity syndrome, occur in approximately 1 in 300 adults and 1 in 100 children (<16 years of age) treated with lamotrigine.[692] The incidence of skin rash can be reduced by starting treatment with a low dose spread over longer intervals, particularly in patients receiving concomitant sodium valproate, which inhibits lamotrigine metabolism. Other common side-effects with lamotrigine include headache, nausea, diplopia, dizziness, ataxia and tremor.

Teratogenicity: Lamotrigine is probably relatively safe but it may be a long time before this is firmly documented. It is categorised as a pregnancy C drug.

Comments:

Lamotrigine is an excellent drug for nearly all forms of seizures and epilepsies (with the exception of myoclonic seizures).

Lamotrigine's efficacious therapeutic pharmacodynamic interaction with other drugs and more notably with sodium valproate makes it an ideal drug for adjunctive medication for all epilepsies including those with myoclonic seizures (its weak point).

Lack of cognitive and behavioural adverse reactions with lamotrigine an d its friendly profile in relation to women make lamotrigine even more advantageous and attractive. Conversely, idiosyncratic reactions are a realistic threat and should be seriously considered. The physician's responsibility is to follow the manufacturer's recommendations regarding titration and to address a proper warning to the patient or guardians of immediate withdrawal of this drug if suspicious rashes appear, unless the rash is clearly not drug-related.

LEVETIRACETAM

Levetiracetam, licensed in 1999, is the newest of the antiepileptic drugs and the most promising of all.[666,698–705] It appears to be a broad-spectrum new class antiepileptic drug with a unique mechanism of action. Its effectiveness in focal seizures is well established through well-controlled studies.[441,706] Its effectiveness in generalised seizures of any type is promising as regards its profile in experimental[707] and uncontrolled studies. This includes myoclonus[442,708] and photosensitivity.[437] The fact that levetiracetam is considered one of the most adverse reaction–free drugs[709] makes it extremely valuable. Other significant advantages of levetiracetam are:

- the starting dose of 1000 mg/day is often therapeutic and

- levetiracetam does not influence other antiepileptic drugs in a clinically meaningful way and conversely other antiepileptic drugs do not interfere with the pharmacokinetics of levetiracetam.

> A 25-year-old woman had surgery at age 21 for drug-resistant focal epilepsy due to left temporal lobe cavernoma. There was no improvement; she continued having four complex focal seizures per week and one GTCS per month despite the fact that appropriate combinations of all available drugs were tried. A breakthrough in her life came when levetiracetam was added. She is now seizure-free and obtained her driving licence on levetiracetam 1500 mg daily and carbamazepine at reducing doses of 200 mg bd. (Case courtesy of Professor JWAS Sander.)

Current and future main applications are: All focal or generalised, idiopathic or symptomatic epileptic syndromes of all age groups. There may be no exceptions to this but probably it is too early to speculate.

In polytherapy, levetiracetam has a significant proven efficacy for intractable focal seizures with or without secondary generalisation[441,706] and probably all other idiopathic or symptomatic generalised seizures. Addition of levetiracetam to standard medication seems to have a positive impact on health-related quality of life.[709] There are no known drug interactions.[699]

Main adverse reactions: Few major adverse effects were reported in the clinical trials and overall their incidence in the levetiracetam groups was little higher than reports from the placebo groups.[710] The most common adverse effects are headache, asthenia, somnolence, infection (common cold, upper respiratory infections which were not preceded by low neutrophil counts that might suggest impaired immunological status), anorexia, pharyngitis, dizziness and pain. No withdrawal-related adverse events were reported during the cross-titration period.[700,701] Caution should be exercised when administering levetiracetam to individuals who may be prone to psychotic or psychiatric reactions.[702]

Teratogenicity: It is categorised as a pregnancy C drug.

Dose: Adults. Initial dose of 1000 mg/day (twice-daily dosing), which itself may be sufficient for seizure control. If needed, levetiracetam can be titrated at steps of 500 mg/week to a maximum of 3000 mg/day (twice-daily dosing).

Children. Preliminary recommendations are that maintenance doses for children should be 30–40% higher on a weight basis than for adults. The reason for this is that levetiracetam clearance in children is 30–40% higher than in adults.[711]

Dose adjustment is required for patients with renal dysfunction but not for patients with liver disease.

Therapeutic range: Levetiracetam can be efficacious from the starting dose. There is no need for serum level monitoring.

Comments: Levetiracetam has had only 3 years exposure in clinical practice. Therefore, it may be too early to say but levetiracetam appears to fulfil significant expectations for a near-perfect antiepileptic drug (providing that there are no unwanted future disasters with increasing experience during the clinical use of this drug).

- It is efficacious for all forms of seizures and epilepsies (including the difficult to treat myoclonic seizures).

- Adverse reactions appear minimal and reversible. No idiosyncratic reactions have been reported (a great relief for most epileptologists and patients who usually show cross-sensitivity).

- It respects cognitive functions (a major problem with most of the old and new antiepileptic drugs).

- The starting dose is often therapeutic (thus avoiding slow titration schemes which are undesirable for patients' safety and medical economics).

- There are no practical unwanted interactions with other drugs either way (thus making its use easy for polytherapy).

- It does not interfere with liver function (a major problem with some other antiepileptic drugs).

TOPIRAMATE

Topiramate, first licensed in 1995, is one of the most effective broad-spectrum antiepileptic drugs for adults and children.[712–720] It is highly efficacious in all types of seizures, focal or generalised, idiopathic or symptomatic. Adverse effects are the main problem with topiramate that may hamper its clinical use.

Current clinical use: all focal or generalised, idiopathic or symptomatic epileptic syndromes of all age groups. There may be no exceptions to this but probably it is too early to speculate.

Adverse reactions are significant:[721,722] Somnolence, anorexia, fatigue, nervousness are also common with other antiepileptic drugs. However, difficulty with concentration/attention, memory impairment, psychomotor slowing, speech disorders and related problems are often very severe with Topiramate even when starting with small doses and when titration is slow. Behavioural and cognitive problems are a limiting factor in some children. Weight loss (10% of the patients) may be considered as beneficial for some women but this is sometimes relentless and problematic.[712] Nephrolithiasis (0.6% in paediatric patients and 1.5% in adults) is an additional handicap. Recent case reports of acute angle-closure glaucoma and other ocular abnormalities are also alarming.[723] Withdrawal rates were low in the controlled trials (4.8%), but appear to be more frequent in non-comparative and post-marketing studies.[712,724]

Topiramate lacks significant idiosyncratic reactions.

Teratogenicity: It is categorised as a pregnancy C drug.

Dose: Adults. Topiramate should be initiated slowly starting with 25 mg/day and gradually titrating the doses every 1–2 weeks until an effective dose is reached or adverse reactions appear. Maximum recommended dose is 200–400 mg/day (twice-daily dosing).

Children. Maximum dose for children older than 2 years is 5–9 mg/kg/day with the same recommendations regarding titration as for adults.

Comments: Topiramate is one of the most effective drugs in epilepsies but with a significant number of adverse reactions and the need for slow titration.

- It is efficacious for all forms of seizures and epilepsies (including the difficult to treat myoclonic seizures and Lennox-Gastaut syndrome).
- Adverse reactions mainly affect cognitive function but others are also of clinical concern. No idiosyncratic reactions have been reported.
- The starting dose should be small and titration slow (in weeks).
- It does not interfere with liver function (a major problem with some other antiepileptic drugs).

NOTE ON THE APPLICATION OF TWO OLD ANTIEPILEPTIC DRUGS IN THE TREATMENT OF FOCAL EPILEPSIES

CLOBAZAM [680,681,725–733]

Based on recent evidence clobazam is a very useful antiepileptic drug both in polytherapy and monotherapy. It is neglected in current clinical practice mainly because it is erroneously considered of high tolerance, of similar effectiveness regarding seizure type to that of clonazepam and because it is a diazepine.

Current main applications are:

A. Adjunctive medication in all forms of drug-resistant epilepsy in adults and children.[681,725–732] It is particularly effective in focal rather than generalised seizures. Clobazam was found to have equivalent efficacy to carbamazepine and phenytoin as monotherapy for childhood epilepsy.[680,733]

B. Intermittent clobazam administration 5 days before and during the menses in catamenial epilepsy[734] is the most popular textbook recommendation.

Dose: Children older than 3 years, 5–15 mg; adults, 10–40 mg daily (divided into a smaller dose in the daytime and a larger dose before going to sleep). Small doses (10 mg nocte) are sometimes highly effective as adjunctive therapy in focal seizures.

Main adverse reactions: As for all benzodiazepines but much milder than most of them.[681,732] Somnolence may be partly prevented by administering the drug in small doses 1 hour before going to sleep. The cognitive and behavioural effects of clobazam appear to be similar to those of standard monotherapy with carbamazepine or phenytoin.[680]

Tolerance may develop, but this aspect has been largely over-emphasised, as documented in many recent studies.[681,733] More than a third of patients do not develop tolerance.[728] When clobazam is effective, patients continue to benefit for years without drug dependence or unwanted side-effects.[728]

Comments: Clobazam should be tried in all drug-resistant epilepsies as adjunctive medication at 10–30 mg nocte (half this dose in children older than 3 years old). It is more effective in focal than generalised epilepsies and can also be used as monotherapy. Probably only 1 out of 10 patients will have a clinically significant improvement but this may be very dramatic and render the patient seizure-free.

Avoid over-medication. Small doses (10–20 mg) 1 hour before going to sleep may be effective and well tolerated.

SODIUM VALPROATE

Sodium valproate is the superior AED for generalised epilepsies (see page 156); however, its use as monotherapy in focal epilepsies may be in doubt.

A recent meta-analysis of randomised controlled trials found that sodium valproate was only of minor inferiority to carbamazepine in controlling focal seizures.[679] However, two points should be noted as regards these studies. First, 'Misclassification of patients may have confounded the results … The age distribution of adults classified as having generalised seizures indicated that significant numbers of patients may have had their seizures misclassified …'[679] Second, 'systematic reviews cannot up-grade poor primary research. Also, a major hurdle is that of publication bias, as trials with a positive result are more likely to be published than those with a negative result.[735] It is not surprising that a review of trials with positive results will come up with a positive answer.'[736] Personally, after consistent failures to introduce sodium valproate as monotherapy in focal seizures, I use sodium valproate only adjunctively in patients with focal and secondary GTCS because:

- Effective required doses of sodium valproate are much higher for focal than generalised epilepsies,
- Side-effects, particularly in some women, make its use undesirable.
- There are now other more effective and safer drugs for focal seizures.

The treatment of focal and indeed of all epilepsies requires thorough knowledge of the AEDs regarding mechanisms, pharmacokinetics, doses, indications, drug interactions, acute and chronic adverse effects. These could not be provided in this brief guide in detail but are widely available through books, journal reviews and manufacturer's prescribing information sheets.

It is also important to remember that special groups of patients with epileptic disorders require particular attention and management.[737] Children,[656,738–741] the elderly,[742] women (particularly of childbearing age)[743–745] and disabled people are more vulnerable and their treatment is more demanding.

REFLEX SEIZURES AND REFLEX EPILEPSIES

Epileptic seizures can arise in a 'spontaneous' unpredictable fashion without detectable precipitant factors, or they can be provoked by certain recognisable stimuli.

Factors and stimuli that contribute towards the initiation of a seizure are provided by the internal and external environment of the subject. Hormones, electrolytes, state of consciousness and body temperature are examples of internal factors that alter the epileptogenic threshold. External stimuli may be sensory, electrical and biochemical. A complex interaction between external and internal factors may explain why the effectiveness of a well-defined seizure-precipitating stimulus may vary and why a patient may experience both 'spontaneous' and 'reflex' seizures.

Reflex or stimulus-sensitive or triggered or sensory-evoked epileptic seizures are synonyms denoting epileptic seizures that are consistently elicited by a specific stimulus. 'Reflex' is the preferred name in the new ILAE diagnostic scheme.[10] Reflex seizures have 4–7% prevalence among patients with epilepsies.[435,746,747] Aetiology may be idiopathic, symptomatic or probably symptomatic.

Definitions

Reflex seizures are 'Objectively and consistently demonstrated to be evoked by a specific afferent stimulus or by activity of the patient. Afferent stimuli can be: elementary, i.e. unstructured (light flashes, startle, a monotone) or elaborate, i.e. structured. Activity may be elementary, e.g. motor (a movement); or elaborate, e.g. cognitive function (reading, chess playing), or both (reading aloud)'.[11]
Reflex epilepsy syndrome: is 'A syndrome in which all epileptic seizures are precipitated by sensory stimuli. Reflex seizures that occur in focal and generalised epilepsy syndromes that are also associated with spontaneous seizures are listed as seizure types. Isolated reflex seizures can also occur in situations that do not necessarily require a diagnosis of epilepsy. Seizures precipitated by other special circumstances, such as fever or alcohol withdrawal, are not reflex seizures'.[10]

Author's note:
In the definition of reflex epilepsy syndromes '**all** seizures are precipitated by sensory stimuli' may be too restrictive. Most patients also suffer from spontaneous seizures. Should '**all**' be replaced by '**all or nearly all**'?

The term 'precipitating stimulus' should be differentiated from 'facilitating stimulus'. In certain patients with IGE for example, EEG discharges or seizures may increase during IPS (**facilitating** stimulus) but these are not consistently evoked by IPS (as would be expected with **precipitating** stimuli).

Abbreviations:

COE = childhood occipital epilepsy
FOS = fixation-off sensitivity
GTCS = generalised tonic-clonic seizures
ILAE = International League Against Epilepsy
IPOE = idiopathic photosensitive occipital lobe epilepsy
IPS = intermittent photic stimulation
OPS = occipital seizures precipitated by photic stimuli
PPR = photoparoxysmal responses
VGS = video game-induced seizures

Reflex epilepsies are determined by the specific precipitant stimulus and the clinical–EEG response.[435,746,747]

The precipitating stimulus

The stimulus evoking an epileptic seizure is specific for a given patient and may be extrinsic, intrinsic or both.

I. Extrinsic stimuli are:

- *simple* such as flashes of light, elimination of visual fixation, tactile
- *complex* such as reading or eating.

The latency from the stimulus onset to the clinical or EEG response is typically short (1–3 seconds) with simple stimuli and long (usually many minutes) with complex stimuli.

II. Intrinsic stimuli are:

- *elementary* such as movements or
- *elaborate* such as those involving higher brain function, emotions and cognition (thinking, calculating, music, or decision-making).

The response to the stimulus

The response consists of clinical and EEG manifestations, alone or in combination. EEG activation may be subclinical only. Conversely, ictal clinical manifestations may be triggered without conspicuous surface EEG changes.

Reflex seizures may be:

- **generalised** (absences, myoclonic jerks, GTCS) or
- **focal** (visual, motor or sensory).

Myoclonic jerks are by far the most common, manifested in the limbs and trunk or regionally, such as in the jaw muscles (reading epilepsy) or the eyelids (as in eyelid myoclonia with absences).

GTCS may constitute the first clinical response, may follow a cluster of absences or myoclonic jerks, or may be secondary to a focal, simple or complex seizure.

The electroclinical events may reflect activation of the stimulus-related (receptive) brain region only (such as photically induced EEG occipital spikes), or become much wider (as in photosensitive focal seizures that propagate in extra-occipital areas), and even generalised (as in photoparoxysmal response, associated with generalised seizures). Inter-individual responses to the same stimulus vary widely. For example, photic stimuli or reading may trigger both focal and generalised seizures.

The role of the EEG is fundamental in establishing the precipitating stimulus in reflex epilepsies because it allows subclinical EEG or minor clinical ictal events to be reproduced on demand with application of the appropriate stimulus. However, there are cases in which the stimulus–seizure relationship is difficult to document, as exemplified with video games-induced seizures.

IPS elicits photoparoxysmal responses in 70% of these patients, documenting photosensitivity (Figure 9.1). The provocative factors in the other 30% remain unknown and speculative; sleep deprivation, mental concentration, fatigue, excitement, borderline threshold to photosensitivity, fixation-off sensitivity, proprioceptive stimuli (praxis) or more complex visual or auditory stimuli, alone or in combination, are all possibilities.[25,748,749] There are also epileptic syndromes in which EEG 'epileptogenic activity' is consistently elicited by a specific stimulus but its provocative relevance to the clinical situation is difficult to prove. This is exemplified by certain cases of benign focal childhood seizures where somatosensory (tapping) or visual (elimination of fixation and central vision) stimuli consistently elicit spike activity, although these children appear to have 'unprovoked' seizures which mainly occur during sleep (Chapter 5).[25]

Table 9.1 Precipitating stimuli and reflex seizures/syndromes listed in the new ILAE Classification Scheme[10]

Precipitating stimuli for reflex seizures
    Visual stimuli
        Flickering light – colour to be specified when possible
        Patterns
        Other visual stimuli
    Thinking
    Music
    Eating
    Praxis
    Somatosensory
    Proprioceptive
    Reading
    Hot water
    Startle

Reflex seizures
    Reflex seizures in generalised epilepsy syndromes
    Reflex seizures in focal epilepsy syndromes

Reflex epilepsies
    Idiopathic photosensitive occipital lobe epilepsy
    Other visual sensitive epilepsies
    Primary reading epilepsy
    Startle epilepsy

Conditions with epileptic seizures that do not require a diagnosis of epilepsy
    Reflex seizures

From Engel (2001)[10] with the permission of the author and the Journal of *Epilepsia*.

Table 9.1 lists the types of precipitating stimuli, reflex seizures and epileptic syndromes according to the new ILAE diagnostic scheme.[10] Table 9.2 is an analytical list of reflex seizures, related reflex epileptic syndromes and their precipitating stimuli. Some of these are well known and common such as photosensitivity while others are extremely rare in humans but may be common in animals, such as audiogenic seizures.

Table 9.2   Reflex seizures, related reflex epilepsies and the precipitating stimuli (for details see refs[746,747])

I. Somatosensory stimuli

1. *Exteroceptive somatosensory stimuli*
   a. Tapping epilepsy and benign childhood epilepsy with somatosensory evoked spikes[312,750,751]
   b. Sensory (tactile) evoked idiopathic myoclonic seizures in infancy[752]
   c. Tooth-brushing epilepsy[753]

2. *Complex exteroceptive somatosensory stimuli*
   a. Hot water epilepsy[754,755]

3. *Proprioceptive somatosensory stimuli*
   a. Seizures induced by movements[756]
   b. Seizures induced by eye closure and/or eye movements[757]
   c. Epileptic paroxysmal kinesiogenic choreoathetosis[758]

4. *Complex proprioceptive stimuli*
   a. Eating epilepsy[759,760]

II. Visual stimuli

1. *Simple visual stimuli*
   a. Photosensitive epilepsies[434] (including self-induced photosensitive epilepsy)[434,761,762]
   b. Pattern-sensitive epilepsies[434,763] (including self-induced pattern-sensitive epilepsy)[761,764]
   c. Fixation-off sensitive epilepsies[765]
   d. Scotogenic epilepsy[765]

2. *Complex visual stimuli and language processing*
   a. Reading epilepsy[766–770]
   b. Graphogenic epilepsy[771]

III. Auditory, vestibular and olfactory stimuli[756,772]
   a. Seizures induced by pure sounds or words[756]
   b. Musicogenic epilepsy (and singing epilepsy)[773,774]
   c. Olfactorhinencephalic epilepsy[746]
   d. Eating epilepsy triggered by tastes[760]
   e Seizures triggered by vestibular and auditory stimuli[756]

IV. High-level processes such as cognitive, emotional, decision-making tasks and other complex stimuli[772]
   a. Thinking (noogenic) epilepsy[775,776]
   b. Reflex decision-making epilepsy[777,778]
   c. Epilepsia arithmetica (mathematica)[779]
   d. Emotional epilepsies[780,781]
   e. Startle epilepsy[782,783]

Modified from Panayiotopoulos (1996)[435] with the permission of the Editor S. Wallace and the publishers Chapman & Hall.

In this chapter common and principal forms of simple and complex reflex seizures and epilepsies are reviewed with particular emphasis on the syndromes listed in the new ILAE diagnostic scheme.[10] Classical references or reviews are cited for the remainder (Table 9.2).

VISUAL-INDUCED SEIZURES AND EPILEPSIES [434,435,746,747,784]

Seizures triggered by visual stimuli are the commonest type of reflex seizures. Visual seizures are triggered by the physical characteristics of the visual stimuli and not by their cognitive effects. Photosensitivity and pattern sensitivity are the two main categories (with frequent overlap) of simple reflex epilepsies with short (typically within seconds) time between stimulus and response. Photosensitivity and pattern sensitivity are genetically determined.

PHOTOSENSITIVITY, EPILEPTIC SEIZURES AND EPILEPTIC SYNDROMES

Photosensitivity, the propensity to seizures induced by light, is a genetically determined trait that may be asymptomatic throughout life or may manifest with epileptic seizures.[785,786]

'Photosensitive epilepsy' is a broad term comprising all forms of heterogeneous epilepsies in which seizures are triggered by photic stimulation. It is not an epilepsy syndrome.

Demographic data: Photosensitive seizures and epilepsies affect 1 in 4000 of the population (5% of patients with epileptic seizures); two thirds are women, and the peak age at onset is 12–13 years.[434] The overall annual incidence of cases with a newly presenting seizure and unequivocal photosensitivity in the UK was 1.1 per 100,000 and 5.7 per 100,000 in the age group from 7 to 19 years.[787,788] Clinical photosensitivity was found in 2% of patients of all ages presenting with seizures and 10% of patients presenting with seizures in the age range 7–19 years.[787,788]

In healthy males aged 17–25 years EEG photosensitivity is very low (0.35%).[789]

Clinical manifestations: These vary considerably depending on the underlying syndrome and severity of photosensitivity. Of seizure patients with photoparoxysmal responses (PPR), 42% have only photically induced without spontaneous seizures (pure photosensitive epilepsy), 40% have spontaneous and photosensitive seizures and the remaining 18% have spontaneous seizures only.[25,434,790–792]

> Generalised seizures are far more common than occipital; any other focal seizures from other than occipital brain regions are exceptional ab initio.

Generalised seizures: Myoclonic jerks, absences and GTCS in this order by prevalence, can occur in photosensitive patients. Some subjects may have only one type, but most suffer from any combination, particularly myoclonic jerks and GTCS. The fact that myoclonic jerks are by far the commonest may appear contradictory to the commonly stated view that GTCS prevail.[434] Thus, GTCS are reported far more commonly (55–84%) than absences (6–20%), focal seizures (2.5%) and myoclonic jerks (2–8%). This prevalence is based on clinical historical evidence, which is likely to over-exaggerate GTCS in relation to minor seizure events although these predominate. Seventy-five percent of patients with PPR experience impaired consciousness during IPS or show motor phenomena such as involuntary opening of the eyes or jerking on one or both sides of the body; in one third these were not reported in clinical history.[791,793] In my personal experience with video-EEG of over 300 patients, PPR commonly associate with eyelid manifestations (a blink, fluttering, flickering, myoclonia) and less often with myoclonic jerks of the head, eyes, body or limbs (Figure 9.2). Absences followed in prevalence and only one patient had an accidental GTCS. Patients are often unaware of the minor seizures although some of these are marked. These facts have been illustrated on many occasions in this book (see for example Figures 1.3 and 6.8).

Photically induced occipital seizures are much more frequent than originally appreciated after the use of IPS in EEG testing (see page 226). These may occur alone or progress to symptoms from other brain locations and GTCS.

Extra-occipital focal seizures from onset are exceptional.[794]

Subjective symptoms during PPR are of doubtful significance; some are ictal phenomena but most others are not.[784] Many patients cannot tolerate the light at all.[784]

Aetiology: Photosensitivity is genetically determined.[785,786]

Diagnostic procedures: Photosensitivity is best demonstrated in EEG with appropriate intermittent photic stimulation (IPS) eliciting abnormal photoparoxysmal responses (PPR).[434,435,791,795,796] IPS has not yet been standardised and the IPS techniques used vary significantly in various publications and departments. I follow the recommendations of Jeavons.[434] Adding a quadrille pattern of small squares (2 mm x 2 mm) of fine black lines (1/3 mm) in the front of the glass of the stroboscope increases the possibility of obtaining PPR.[797]

Photoparoxysmal responses are broadly categorised as:[434,792]

a. ***Generalised spike/polyspike waves.*** They are of higher amplitude in the anterior regions, but onset – particularly if patterned IPS is employed – is often with occipital spikes. They are highly associated (90%) with clinical photosensitivity particularly if they outlast the stimulus train (Figure 9.1). Generalised PPR often (60%) associate with clinical events such as jerks, impairment of cognition or subjective sensations but their detection may require video-EEG.[792]

b. ***Posterior (temporo-parieto-occipital with occipital emphasis) spike/polyspike waves.*** This is the mildest form of PPR and does not spread to the anterior regions. It consists of occipital spikes, polyspikes or slow

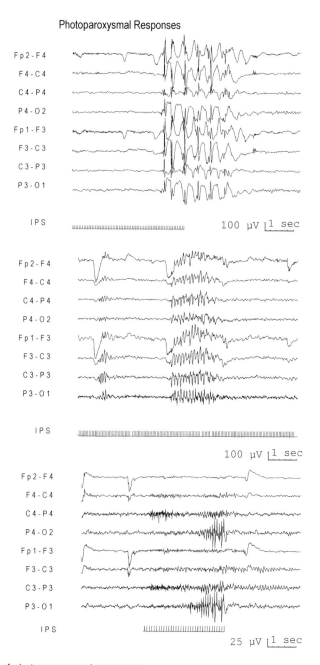

Figure 9.1 Examples of photoparoxysmal responses.

Top: Generalised 3–4 Hz spike/polyspike waves associated with an absence. The discharge outlasts the duration of the stimulus.

Middle: Generalised polyspike discharge of a patient with symptomatic spontaneous and photically induced mainly GTCS which are resistant to appropriate antiepileptic medication. These types of discharges usually associate with myoclonic jerks but these did not feature in this case. Note that the discharge occurs only after eye blinks or eye closure and does not outlast the stimulus train.

Bottom: Typical occipital spikes time-locked to each flash of IPS. The patient is a woman with idiopathic occipital epilepsy (probably a variant of Gastaut-type COE who never had attacks precipitated by lights) (case report of ref [798]).

waves intermixed with small, larval spikes (Figures 9.1 and 9.2). Occipital spikes are often time-locked to the flash with a latency of approximately 100 milliseconds, coinciding with the positive P100 of the visual evoked response (Figure 9.1).[799] Half of the subjects with posterior PPR have epileptic seizures (spontaneous, photically elicited or both).[434]

Note on the duration of the PPR and their relation to the IPS train: Emphasis is often placed on whether PPR outlast the stimulus train or they are self-limited, i.e. they stop before or with the end of the IPS.[795,796] The rationale is that photoparoxysmal discharges that outlast the stimulus train may strengthen their association with epilepsy. This may be artificial because the duration of the discharge as a rule depends on the duration and strength of the IPS and the time that this was stopped after the appearance of the photoparoxysmal discharges.

Ictal clinical manifestations during the discharges may be one of the most important factors regarding risk of seizures but this aspect has not been studied and not emphasised in the consensus report of experts.[795,796]

The resting EEG of patients with idiopathic photosensitive seizures is usually normal or frequently (20–30%) shows eye closure-related paroxysms occurring within 1–3 seconds after closing of the eyes. These are usually brief EEG paroxysms lasting for 1–4 seconds and have similar features to those elicited by IPS for each individual patient. They disappear if eye closure occurs in total darkness.

Precipitating factors: By definition all patients are sensitive to flickering lights. Many artificial or natural light sources can provoke epileptic seizures. Video games, television, visual display units of computers, discotheques and natural flickering light are common triggers in that order.

Video game-induced seizures (VGS) can occur not only with games using an interlaced video monitor (TV) and computers but also with small hand-held liquid crystal displays and non-interlaced 70 Hz arcade games.[748,787,803–805] Most patients (87%) are aged 7–19 years. There is a preponderance of boys, probably because more boys than girls play video games. Two thirds of patients are photosensitive. For the other third there are other triggers such as sleep deprivation, fatigue, decision-making, excitement or frustration and praxis that may operate alone or in combination. One third of VGS are occipital seizures and these occur in patients with or without photosensitivity.

Television (TV) epilepsy denotes seizures triggered by TV and it is not a syndrome. TV-induced seizures mainly affect children aged 10–12 years. There is a two-fold preponderance of girls. Seizures are more likely to occur

Clarifications on eyes open, eyes closed and eye closure during IPS

The state of the eyes during IPS is probably the most significant internal factor that modifies the response to IPS.[800] Eye closure (closing of the eyes while IPS continues) is by far the most potent.[434,800] Of the other two states, eyes open is more susceptible than eyes closed to patterned flickering lights. Conversely, eyes closed appeared to be more susceptible than eyes open to direct unpatterned light, probably because of a diffusion effect of light by the eyelids. When light with a diffuser is applied, eyes open is again more effective than eyes closed because of an intensity loss by the closed eyelids.

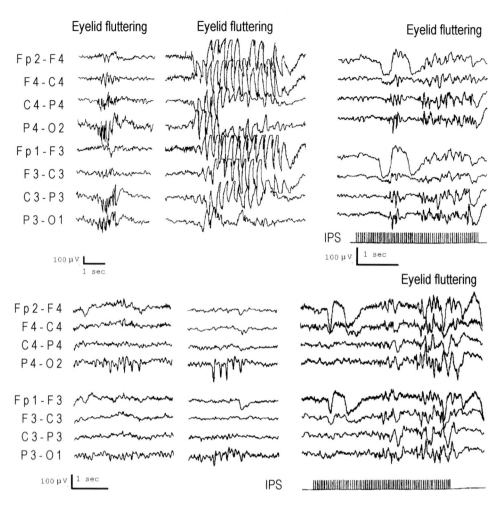

Figure 9.2 Samples from video-EEG of spontaneous EEG paroxysms and photically induced posterior or maximum posterior PPR in two children with photically induced occipital seizures. These 2 patients probably have IPOE as detailed (cases 12.1 and 12.2 in ref 25).

Top left and middle: Spontaneous occipital spikes and polyspikes and generalised discharges are associated with eyelid fluttering which is conspicuous on video-EEG viewing. Neither the patient nor her relatives were aware of these.

Top right: IPS consistently elicited posterior spikes that were also associated with ictal eyelid fluttering. This patient had typical multi-coloured visual seizures from age 5 years (case 12.1 in ref[25]). They were elicited by environmental lights and occasionally progressed to GTCS. She improved over the years but at age 20 and while on medication with sodium valproate she had a visual seizure with GTCS while watching TV from near touch distance. High-resolution MRI was normal.

Bottom left and middle: Spontaneous occipital paroxysms without discernible clinical manifestations. *Bottom right:* IPS consistently elicited PPR with maximum posterior emphasis. These were often associated with conspicuous eyelid fluttering. This patient illustrates the links of IPOE with the benign childhood seizure susceptibility syndrome (case 12.2 in ref [25]). She initially had typical Rolandic seizures, she then developed frequent visual seizures often with secondary GTCS. These were sometimes photically induced but more often occurred during sleep. High-resolution MRI was normal.

From Panayiotopoulos (1999)[25] with permission of the publisher John Libbey.

when the patient is watching a faulty (i.e. flickering) TV set, or is very near to the TV screen. Myoclonic jerks often precede the GTCS and history-taking reveals that these may have occurred in the past without GTCS.

> First she jerked a few times, head and hands, and then she had the convulsions. I thought she was electrocuted by an electric fault of the TV.

A substantial number of these patients also have spontaneous attacks. In pure television epilepsy, one or a few overt TV-induced seizures occur without evidence of any other type of spontaneous attacks or seizures induced by other means of precipitation.

Ten percent of patients are 'being drawn like a magnet' and when they reach a certain proximity to the screen they have GTCS. This is called 'compulsive attraction'.

> He was watching TV and then suddenly, off he goes towards the set, eyes fixed in the picture, and he had the fit a few inches away from the screen

> I do not know what happens. My eyes suddenly fixed to the picture, I could not move them away …

Self-induced seizures[761,762,806,807] Self-induction is a mode of seizure precipitation employed by mentally handicapped or normal photosensitive individuals. Its prevalence is debated. Techniques include waving the outspread fingers in front of a bright light, viewing geometric patterns, or slow eye closure. Absences and myoclonic jerks are the commonest seizures in self-induction. Whether eyelid blinking or compulsive attraction to television or bright sun is mainly an attempt for self-induction or part of the seizure is disputed although both may be true.

Diagnostic procedures: Properly applied IPS during EEG is the most important test.

In order to be provocative the IPS has to imply all potent physical characteristics of the stimulus (intensity, frequency, contrast), combine flash with patterns (a linear 2 mm × 2 mm grid, not a chequer-board, in front of the stroboscope may be sufficient), central vision is mandatory (the patient should look at the centre of the stroboscope). IPS on eye closure should be tested.[434,795,796] Monocular stimulation is usually ineffective.

The practical objective of IPS is to determine whether:

1. Seizures (of any type) are aetiologically linked with environmental photic stimuli (TV, video games and others). If PPR occurs this confirms photosensitivity.

2. PPR are associated with ictal events. This can only be achieved with video-EEG recording; otherwise minor events such as eyelid or limb jerks are likely to escape notice.

Prolonged photic stimulation that may cause the patient to have a major seizure should be totally discouraged. There is nothing to learn and no benefit to the patient from this practice. There are plenty of examples of subjects having an IPS-induced seizure during an EEG that was performed for reasons other than epilepsy. To continue a train of photic stimulation after the appearance of EEG ictal discharges or ictal clinical manifestations is unacceptable.

Management:[434] In pure photosensitive seizures, avoidance of the provocative stimulus may be adequate. For example, patients with TV-induced seizures should be advised to view TV in a well-lit room, maintain a maximum comfortable viewing distance (typically, >2.5 m for a 19″ screen),

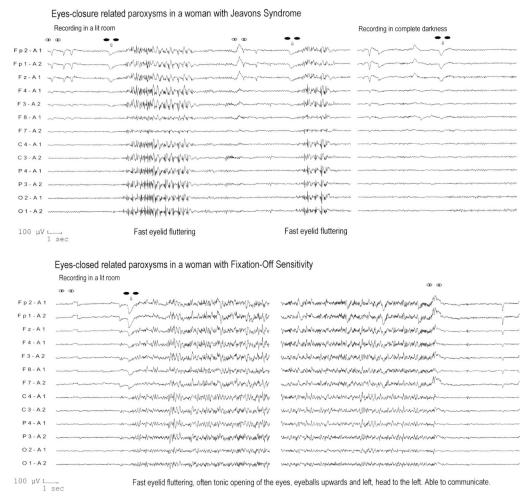

Figure 9.3 Samples from video-EEG to illustrate the differentiation between eye closure (top) and eyes closed (bottom) abnormalities.

Top: Eye closure-related abnormalities in a patient with Jeavons syndrome.[801] High amplitude generalised discharges occur within 1–3 seconds after closing the eyes in a lit room. These are of brief duration, do not continue in the resting period that the eyes are closed and are totally inhibited in complete darkness.

Bottom: Eyes closed-related abnormalities in a woman with possibly symptomatic epilepsy and seizures related to fixation-off sensitivity.[765,802] The EEG paroxysms last as long as the eyes are closed. They are abruptly inhibited when the eyes are opened. The response to fixation off and on by any means (eyes closed, darkness, plus 10 spherical lenses, Ganzfeld stimulation) was similar. The best practical means for testing FOS is underwater goggles covered with opaque tape.

use the remote control and – if it is necessary to approach the screen – cover one eye with their palm, and avoid prolonged watching particularly if sleep-deprived and tired. Occlusion of one eye is also advised when photosensitive subjects are suddenly exposed to flickering lights such as in discotheques.

Patients with VGS can do without video games or significantly restrict the time of playing. They should not play when they are sleep-deprived.

Conditioning treatment or wearing appropriate tinted glasses[808] have been recommended. Small doses of sodium valproate may be needed in patients with possible spontaneous seizures or co-existent spontaneous EEG discharges.

Patients with distinct IGE and photosensitivity are treated accordingly. Sodium valproate controls all seizure types in more than 80% of the patients, clonazepam mainly controls jerks, lamotrigine may be effective, levetiracetam abolishes photosensitivity under experimental conditions.[437]

EPILEPTIC SYNDROMES OF PHOTOSENSITIVITY

Photosensitivity epilepsy was classified among the generalised epilepsies by the ILAE Commission.[9] This is because:

(a) Photoparoxysmal responses were considered primarily generalised;[434,746,809,810] although the initial occipital onset of the discharge was well reported,[799,811] as recently appreciated.[434,812] The evidence is that photosensitivity in humans is mainly generated in the occipital lobes and therefore it is regional (occipital lobar) epilepsy.[434,435,784,792,797,799,811,812]

(b) A quarter of patients with spontaneous seizures and EEG photosensitivity belong to a variety of epileptic syndromes of IGE, such as juvenile myoclonic epilepsy.[435,813] A high prevalence of photosensitivity is also found in certain forms of symptomatic generalised epilepsies like Dravet syndrome (70%),[197] Baltic-Mediterranean myoclonus (90%)[626] and progressive myoclonic epilepsies.[626]

Occipital photosensitivity only recently came into prominence, although it was well known from the time of Gowers (1881).[814] Earlier studies were over-shadowed by the prevailing view that photosensitive epilepsies are mainly generalised. Indeed, with the application of IPS as a provocation method in EEG, it was discovered that the majority of photosensitivity

---

Differentiation between eye closure and eyes closed state (Figure 9.3)

Eye closure is the transient state, which immediately follows closing of the eyes, lasts less than 3 seconds and does not persist in the remaining period of eyes closed. Eye closure is much more potent than eyes open or eyes closed for induction of abnormalities during IPS. Jeavons syndrome is a typical example of eye closure-related seizures and EEG abnormalities. In some photosensitive patients, PPR occur only after eye closure.

Eyes closed is the state which lasts as long as the eyes remain closed. Fixation-off sensitivity is a typical example of eyes closed-related seizures and EEG abnormalities.

patients had generalised discharges and suffered mainly from idiopathic generalised epilepsies.[815,816] The fact that occipital spikes often preceded generalised discharges[799,811,817] was ignored. Reports of photically induced occipital seizures with or without secondary generalisation were scarce. The traditional view that occipital seizures precipitated by photic stimuli (OPS) are rare contrasts with recent findings.[818–820] In one report alone,[821] 45 of 95 patients had occipital seizures precipitated by visual stimuli. There are two recent extensive reviews on OPS.[25,309]

IDIOPATHIC PHOTOSENSITIVE OCCIPITAL LOBE EPILEPSY [10,25,308,309]

The new ILAE diagnostic scheme[10] recognises 'Idiopathic photosensitive occipital lobe epilepsy (IPOE)' as a new syndrome of reflex epilepsy with age-related onset.

Depending on severity, there may be three significant groups of IPOE:[25]

1. **Patients with low occipital epileptogenic threshold to IPS that manifests with seizures only under extreme exposure to the offending stimulation.** These are seizures that do not require a diagnosis of epilepsy.[10] Accidental single isolated occipital seizures in normal young persons[824] or patients with migraine[824] during IPS are most likely due to a low threshold to such events and may not happen again.

2. **Patients with idiopathic occipital epileptogenicity that may be the majority of IPOE.** Patients, usually children, have clinical occipital seizures elicited by various environmental light stimuli (video games are involved far more frequently than television).

3. **Patients, usually children, with idiopathic focal or generalised epilepsies** who also have OPS. These are often demanding cases as regards diagnosis and management.

Considering all these points, the following data may not accurately represent a single syndrome of IPOE.

Demographic data: Of 39 patients with occipital photosensitivity that I reviewed[25] age at onset of the first provoked seizure ranged from 15 months to 19 years with a mean at around 12 years of age. Eighteen were boys and 21 girls. Prevalence is small, ~0.4% of all epilepsies.

Considerations on classification

The boundaries of this syndrome of IPOE are genuinely uncertain. Photosensitive occipital seizures may start in adulthood,[822] be part of Gastaut-type COE,[25,303] develop later in children with Rolandic seizures[25,293] or occur accidentally during IPS of normal or migraine subjects.[25] Gastaut[303] included photosensitivity and IPOE in his syndrome: (a) seven of 63 patients had IPS-evoked occipital spikes, 'not seen in the resting EEG' and 'unrelated to eye opening and closing'; and (b) seven other patients with typical occipital paroxysms had generalised PPR, sometimes associated myoclonus (see also his case no. 11).[303] Also, one third of the patients reported by Terasaki et al. (1987)[823] had photosensitivity. Contrary to this is the view that 'reflex triggering of seizures has not been reported' in Gastaut-type COE.[309]

Clinical manifestations: Occipital seizures are induced by video games and less often by television or other photic stimuli. Seizures consist of multi-coloured circular visual hallucinations often associated with blindness that may also occur alone. Visual symptoms may be the only ictal manifestations,[820] usually lasting for seconds, frequently 1–3 minutes and rarely longer (5–15 minutes) in which case other symptoms also occur.[820,825] Consciousness is not impaired during the phase of visual symptoms.

Progression of visual seizures to other ictal symptoms: Autonomic symptoms and mainly retching and ictal vomiting, like those occurring in Panayiotopoulos syndrome, often follow the occipital symptoms and may end with secondary GTCS.[25,820]

Occipital seizures with bizarre ictal symptomatology mimicking hysterical attacks or migraine are well reported.[25,820] The fact that these symptoms, even the very prolonged and unusual ones, are ictal has been documented with ictal EEG.[820]

Other type of seizures: Patients with IPOE may have exclusively occipital seizures that are only photically induced. Others may also have spontaneous visual or other types of seizures. These may vary from eyelid flickering, myoclonic jerks, absences and GTCS that occur independently of the occipital seizures. In some cases spontaneous secondary GTCS occur only during sleep.[25] There are also patients with Rolandic seizures that may later develop OPS (Figure 9.2).[25,826]

Precipitating factors: By definition, all patients with IPOE are sensitive to flickering lights. Depending on the severity of photosensitivity in some patients seizures may be elicited by minimal photic provocation, in others combined pattern and photic or prolonged exposure may be responsible, while in others (probably the majority of IPOE) photic stimuli are effective only if combined with other precipitating factors such as excitement or frustration, fatigue and sleep deprivation.[25,749]

Diagnostic procedures: All except EEG are normal.

Electroencephalography: By definition, all these patients are photosensitive and IPS elicits abnormal EEG paroxysms of spikes or polyspikes that may be entirely confined to the occipital regions or generalised photoparoxysmal responses of spikes or polyspikes and slow waves that predominate in the posterior regions (Figures 9.2 and 9.4). Spontaneous, mainly posterior spikes often appear in the resting EEG. Centrotemporal spikes may co-exist.[25,749]

Occipital spikes and other posterior abnormalities induced by IPS are considered of much lower epileptogenic capacity than generalised PPR. They may occur in 50% of patients who do not have seizures.[434] Occipital spikes precede generalised PPR in 90% of photosensitive patients when light and pattern are combined during IPS.[25,434,827,828]

Ictal EEGs document the occipital origin and the spreading of the discharges to the temporal regions.[309]

In my experience with video-EEG recordings, most patients with IPOE also have other types of seizures induced by IPS; eyelid flickering and eyelid tremors are the most prominent clinical manifestations during IPS-induced occipital PPR (Figure 9.2).[25]

Visual evoked potentials: These are always of abnormally high amplitude[309] but this is not a specific IPOE-related finding and is of no diagnostic significance.

Aetiology: IPOE by definition is idiopathic and some patients have a family history of similar seizures elicited by photic stimuli. Symptomatic occipital photosensitivity was already known to Holmes in 1927[829] for patients with gunshot wounds.

Differential diagnosis: The differential diagnosis of IPOE includes migraine (rarely an actual problem if symptoms are appropriately analysed), Gastaut-type COE (of no practical significance other than avoidance of precipitating stimuli and classification), idiopathic generalised epilepsies (probably of management importance) and pseudo-seizures (differentiation is sometimes very difficult).

The differential diagnosis of visual seizures from all types of migraine with visual aura (page 200) is not different for IPOE. Some seizures of IPOE may be prolonged, progressing from visual symptoms to nausea and vomiting with altered consciousness.[820,830] The spread of the discharge from the occipital cortex can be slow, and responsiveness may be maintained while the patient is vomiting.[820,830] These seizures may be erroneously diagnosed as migraine proper.[831]

In children and adolescents, the differentiation of IPOE from the Gastaut-type COE is not of any significance other than avoidance of precipitating factors.

Differentiation of IPOE from generalised photosensitive epilepsies should rely on clinical criteria. Occipital spikes often precede generalised discharges in photosensitive epilepsies.

Adult-onset IPOE: In adults, occipital photosensitivity has been documented recently (Figure 9.4).[822] These were patients aged ~30 years presenting with a late onset first GTCS (often preceded by visual symptoms).[822] Of 1550 patients with seizures, 3 women and 2 men (0.3%) had EEG occipital photosensitivity and onset of solitary (3 patients) or infrequent seizures in adulthood (median 31; range 26–35 years). All five patients had generalised convulsions, which were preceded by blurring of vision or elementary visual hallucinations in four. Precipitation by lights, alone or in combination with other factors, was apparent in only two patients. Seizures were diurnal in all but one patient. By inclusion criteria all had EEG occipital spikes elicited by IPS (Figure 9.4). Neurological and intellectual state as well as brain imaging were normal.

Prognosis: Frequency of seizures and overall prognosis vary significantly among affected individuals. This depends on the severity of photosensitivity and exposure to the offending visual stimuli.[25,309,820]

There are rare case reports of normal young people[824] or patients with migraine[824,832] having an occipital seizure during IPS.

Some patients may have only one or two occipital seizures in their life despite exposure to precipitating factors and no drug treatment.[25,309,820] Others, particularly those also having spontaneous seizures, may need medication for 1–3 years together with strict avoidance or cautious exposure to insulting stimuli. However, other patients may have frequent spontaneous and elicited occipital fits alone or in combination with other types of seizures that may be myoclonic jerks, often of the eyelids, infrequent absences and GTCS.[25]

Management: Advice regarding avoidance of precipitating factors is essential. This is similar to that given to patients with any type of photosensitivity. Particular emphasis is needed regarding video games and television.

Drug treatment: Although sodium valproate is the drug of choice in generalised photosensitive epilepsies, it is not certain that this is also the case for IPOE. Cases of IPOE resistant to sodium valproate became seizure-free with add-on carbamazepine.[25] Clobazam may be an alternative. Newer drugs such as lamotrigine and levetiracetam are promising.

Occipital photosensitivity in adults with late onset seizures

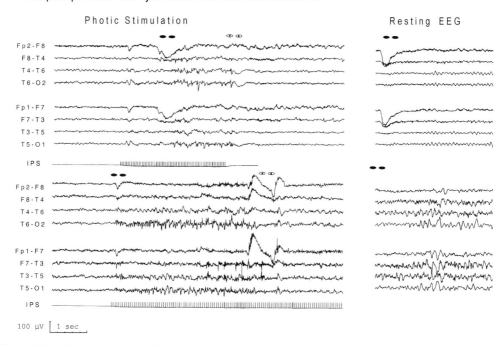

Figure 9.4 4 Adult onset idiopathic photosensitive occipital lobe epilepsy.

Top: Sample from an EEG of a man who had his first seizure at age 35 years while in a lift cradle at work. His vision became blurred, he felt dizzy and within 2 minutes had a GTCS. No further seizures occurred in the next 6 months of follow-up. MRI was normal.

Bottom: Sample from an EEG of a woman who had her first seizure at age 31 years. There was a cluster of precipitating factors. She was dancing exposed to flickering disco lights at 4 a.m. She had consumed a few alcoholic drinks, was sleep-deprived and was 4 months pregnant. She first experienced whirling lights in front of her eyes, visual perception became disturbed and within a minute she had a GTCS. She was well in the next 4 months of follow-up. MRI was normal.

JEAVONS SYNDROME [801,833,834]

EYELID MYOCLONIA WITH ABSENCES

Eyelid myoclonia with absences (Jeavons syndrome) is one of the most distinctive genetic reflex IGE syndromes with well-defined clinico-EEG manifestations. It is characterised by the triad:

1. Eyelid myoclonia with and without absences
2. Eye closure-induced seizures, EEG paroxysms, or both
3. Photosensitivity.

This is a syndrome not recognised by the ILAE Commission[9] and not listed in the new ILAE diagnostic scheme[10] although vividly described by Jeavons and documented in a multi-authored book.[833]

Demographic data: Onset is typically in childhood with a peak at 6–8 years (range 2–14). There is a two-fold preponderance of girls. In our studies in adults all were women except one man who from age 3 to 32 had daily seizures of eyelid myoclonia without any other ictal symptoms or GTCS. Prevalence of Jeavons syndrome is around 3% among adult patients with epileptic disorders and 13% among IGE with absences.[801]

Clinical manifestations: Eyelid myoclonia, not the absences, is the hallmark of Jeavons syndrome (Figure 9.5).[801,834]

Eyelid myoclonia consists of marked jerking of the eyelids, often associated with jerky upward deviation of the eyeballs and retropulsion of the head **(eyelid myoclonia without absences)**. This may be associated with or followed by mild impairment of consciousness **(eyelid myoclonia with absences)**. The seizures are brief (3–6 seconds), happen mainly after eye closure and consistently occur many times per day.

All patients are photosensitive.

GTCS, either induced by lights or spontaneous, are probably inevitable in the long term, particularly provoked by precipitating factors (sleep deprivation, alcohol) and inappropriate antiepileptic drug modifications. Typically GTCS are sparse and avoidable.

Myoclonic jerks of the limbs may occur but are infrequent and random.

Eyelid myoclonic status epilepticus either spontaneously, mainly on awakening, or photically induced occurs in one fifth of the patients. This consists of repetitive and discontinuous episodes of eyelid myoclonia with mild absence rather than continuous non-convulsive absence status (Figure 9.5).

Aetiology: Jeavons syndrome is a genetically determined homogeneous syndrome.[378,836]

Considerations on classification

The new ILAE diagnostic scheme[10] has not recognised 'eyelid myoclonia with absences (Jeavons syndrome)'. Instead, a new seizure type 'eyelid myoclonia with and without absences' has been accepted.[10,834] These seizures occur in many epileptic conditions of idiopathic, symptomatic or possibly symptomatic causes.[834,835] They are the defining seizure symptom in Jeavons syndrome, which has a unique clinical, EEG and often genetic clustering.[378,801,834,836]

Diagnostic procedures: All tests except EEG are normal.

Electroencephalography: Video-EEG is the single most important procedure for the diagnosis of eyelid myoclonia with or without absences. This shows frequent high amplitude generalised dicharges of 3–6 Hz spike/usually polyspike and slow waves (Figure 9.5). These typically are:

- eye closure-related, i.e. they occur immediately (within 0.5–2 seconds) after closing the eyes in an illuminated recording room and

- brief (1–6 seconds; commonly 2–3 seconds).

They are eliminated in total darkness.

Eyelid myoclonia of varying severity often occurs with these discharges.

In addition, photoparoxysmal responses are recorded in all untreated young patients but may be absent in older patients or those on medication. Photosensitivity and fixation-off sensitivity may co-exist.[765]

EEG discharges are also enhanced by hyperventilation.

Sleep EEG patterns are normal. Generalised discharges of polyspikes and slow waves are more likely to increase during sleep, but a reduction may also be observed. The discharges are shorter and devoid of discernible clinical manifestations of any type, even in those patients who have numerous seizures during the alert state.

EEG and clinical manifestations deteriorate consistently after awakening.

A normal EEG is rare, even in well-controlled patients.

Differential diagnosis: The diagnosis of Jeavons syndrome is simple because the characteristic eyelid myoclonia, if seen once, will never be forgotten or confused with other conditions.[335] Furthermore, the EEG with the characteristic eye closure-related discharges and photosensitivity leaves no room for diagnostic errors.

> As a simple rule of thumb, eyelid myoclonia is highly suggestive of Jeavons syndrome. This becomes more likely when eyelid myoclonia is combined with photosensitivity, and it is pathognomonic of the syndrome when it also occurs after eye closure.[373]

Despite all these, eyelid myoclonia is often misdiagnosed as facial tics, sometimes for many years. Also, eyelid myoclonia should not be confused with

a. the rhythmic or random closing of the eyes, often seen in other forms of IGE with absences; and

b. eyelid jerking that may occur at the opening or the initial stage of the discharges in typical absence seizures of childhood or juvenile myoclonic epilepsy.

The main diagnostic problem, probably iatrogenic, is self-induction as debated by Binnie (in favour)[806] and Panayiotopoulos (against).[762] Eyelid myoclonia is

---

Differential diagnosis of Jeavons syndrome

- Non-epileptic conditions – tics and exaggerated normal eye movements
- Symptomatic generalised epilepsy
- Cryptogenic generalised epilepsy
- Self-induced photosensitive epilepsy
- Symptomatic occipital epilepsy
- Idiopathic generalised epilepsy with absences
- Idiopathic occipital epilepsy

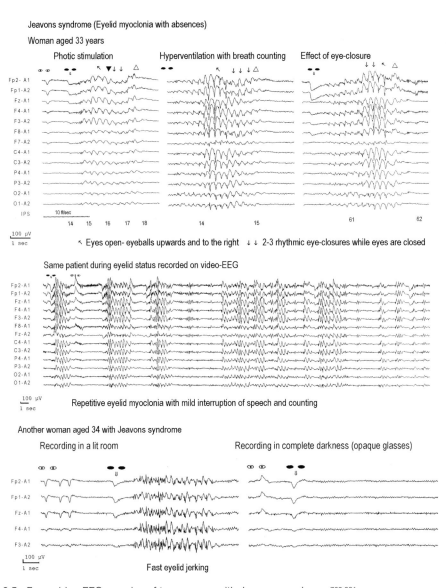

Figure 9.5 From video-EEG samples of two women with Jeavons syndrome.[762,801]

Top: Brief generalised discharges of spikes/multiple spikes and slow waves of similar characteristics are induced by IPS (left) or eye closure (right). They occasionally occur spontaneously (middle). In all illustrated occasions these were associated with marked eyelid myoclonia (denoted with various symbols). Also note that there is no impairment of cognition counting (numbers)

Middle: Repetitive discontinuous seizures of eyelid myoclonia occurred upon awakening when she was erroneously treated with carbamazepine. These lasted for more than half an hour. There was only mild interruption of speech and counting during the discharges. The patient was fully aware of her condition.

Bottom: Long video-EEG of a woman with Jeavons syndrome while on sodium valproate. There were frequent eye closure-related generalised discharges of mainly polyspikes often associated with fast eyelid jerking, mild or violent. The discharges occurred only in the presence of light. They were totally inhibited in complete darkness (complete darkness implies that any means of lights were eliminated).

Symbols of eyes indicate when the eyes were open or closed.

often erroneously considered as a deliberate manoeuvre for self-induction. Self-induced seizures in Jeavons syndrome are rare. Conversely, self-induced photosensitive epilepsy may imitate and should be differentiated from Jeavons syndrome.

The symptom/seizure of eyelid myoclonia alone is not sufficient to characterise Jeavons syndrome because this may also occur in other epileptic conditions, mainly cryptogenic and symptomatic,[370,834,835] that are betrayed by developmental delay, learning difficulties, neurological deficits, abnormal MRI and abnormal background EEG.[370,834,835]

Prognosis: Jeavons syndrome is a lifelong disorder even when well controlled with antiepileptic medication. There is a tendency for photosensitivity to disappear in middle age but eyelid myoclonia persists and may occur on a daily basis.

Eyelid myoclonia is highly resistant to treatment, occurring many times per day, often without apparent absences, and even without demonstrable photosensitivity.[801]

Management: Based on anecdotal evidence, the drugs of choice are those used for other IGEs (page 156).[7] Sodium valproate alone, or most likely combined with clonazepam or ethosuximide, appears to be the most effective regimen. The choice of the second drug depends on the main seizure type. Clonazepam is highly efficacious in eyelid myoclonia and myoclonic jerks; some patients achieve relatively good control with clonazepam monotherapy.

Of the new drugs, levetiracetam and topiramate may prove effective. Lamotrigine may exaggerate myoclonic jerks.

Carbamazepine, vigabatrin and tiagabine are contraindicated, and the same may be true for phenytoin.

Lifestyle and avoidance of seizure precipitants are important.

Non-pharmacological treatments in photosensitive patients often have a beneficial effect and should also be employed in Jeavons syndrome when photosensitivity persists.[837]

PATTERN-SENSITIVE EPILEPSY [434,763,784,816,838–841]

Pattern-sensitive epilepsy refers to epileptic seizures induced by patterns; it is not a particular epileptic syndrome. Pattern seizure sensitivity is closely related to photosensitivity. Nearly all patients with clinical pattern-sensitive epilepsy show PPR (Figure 9.6). Conversely, of clinical photosensitive patients, 30% are also sensitive to stationary and 70% to appropriately vibrating patterns of stripes. Patterns enhance the effect of photic stimulation whether under test conditions or in real life. 'Whether pattern sensitivity ever occurs in subjects who are consistently insensitive to IPS is uncertain.'[763] Pattern-sensitivity without photosensitivity, patients sensitive to non-geometric patterns and self-induced pattern-sensitive epilepsy are rare.

Environmental stimuli: Stimuli that induce seizures in pattern-sensitive patients are those that best match the properties of provocative patterns used in relevant EEG testing and best suit and create the conditions of their spatial and directional presentation to the eyes. These are striped clothes (such as shirts, jackets or ties), escalators, wallpaper and furnishing decorations, Venetian blinds, air-conditioning grills and radiators. Any activity visually involved with these patterns, such as ironing, is likely to induce seizures. Less direct but often very significant is the role of patterns in more complex stimuli such as television viewing and video games.[434,763,784]

Pattern is recognised as a seizure precipitant less often by patients, caregivers and physicians than are environmental flicker and specific agents such as television, discotheque lighting, or video games. Direct questioning implicates pattern as a seizure trigger in 6–30% of photosensitive subjects.[791,840]

Demographic data: Purely pattern-sensitive epilepsy with clinical attacks induced by patterns is exceptional.[816] This is despite the relatively high incidence of patients, mainly photosensitive, who show pattern-induced paroxysmal activity on appropriate EEG testing.[434,763,784,816,838–841]

Clinical manifestations: Clinical manifestations have not been well studied in purely pattern-sensitive epilepsy. All types of generalised seizures have been described. My impression is that absences are more common than GTCS and myoclonic jerks (in that order). I am not aware of patterns inducing occipital seizures, although they should exist considering that the visual cortex is the primary target of pattern stimulus.

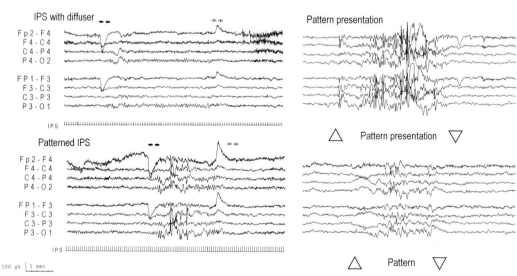

Boy aged 14 with pattern sensitive epilepsy from age 7

Figure 9.6 Samples from video-EEG of a child with pure pattern-sensitive epilepsy from age 8.

Left (top and bottom): Only patterned IPS elicits PPR. Patterned IPS is achieved by adding a quadrille pattern of small squares (2 mm x 2 mm) of fine black lines (1/3 mm) in the front of the stroboscope.[797]

Right (top and bottom): Paroxysmal discharges (generalised or maximum posterior) are consistently elicited by various linear patterns.

Pathophysiology: Pattern seizure sensitivity has been extensively studied with elaborate and intelligent methodology mainly in patients with photically induced seizures. This has revealed many aspects of pattern seizure susceptibility and its pathophysiology:[434,763,784,816,838–841]

1. The seizures are triggered in the visual cortex.

2. The seizures are triggered by normal neural activity.

3. The trigger involves one cerebral hemisphere or both hemispheres independently.

4. The trigger requires the physiological activation of a critical area of cortical tissue.

5. Synchronisation of neural activity is necessary.

Diagnostic procedures: EEG with appropriate pattern presentations is the key test. Pattern sensitivity depends on the spatial frequency, orientation, brightness, contrast and size of the pattern. An optimally epileptogenic pattern should be used for testing.[763,784]

1. An optimally epileptogenic pattern consists of black and white stripes of equal width and sharp contour (a square-wave luminance profile).

2. The image must be well focused, and if the subject has a refractive error, an appropriate correction must be worn.

3. Spatial frequency is critical; this is the number of cycles of the pattern (pairs of dark and light stripes) per degree of visual angle. For most subjects without refractive error, a spatial frequency of 2-4 cycles per degree is the most epileptogenic. Thus, each stripe should subtend 7.5–15 minutes of arc at the eye.

4. The orientation of the lines rarely affects epileptogenicity, except in astigmatic patients.

5. EEG activation in a susceptible subject is not usually seen at a luminance below 10 cd/rn^2, although exceptions exist. For purposes of testing, the space-averaged luminance should be at least 200 cd/rn^2. The Michelson contrast (difference in luminances of light and dark stripes expressed as a proportion of their sum) should be >0.4.

6. Binocular stimulation should be used.

7. Pattern sensitivity, like visual acuity, depends mainly on central vision. Between a lower threshold and an upper saturation level is an approximately log linear relationship between pattern radius and discharge probability for circular patterns of up to 500 visual angle. To determine whether a subject is pattern-sensitive, it is therefore worthwhile using stimuli of at least this size.

Prognosis and management: These have not been systematically studied. Management may be similar to that of photosensitive epilepsy. My impression is that prognosis is worse than for photosensitive epilepsy and it is much more difficult to treat.

FIXATION-OFF SENSITIVITY

'Fixation-off sensitivity (FOS)' is a term that I coined to denote the form/forms of epilepsy and/or EEG abnormalities that are elicited by elimination of central vision and fixation.[765,802] Elimination of central vision and fixation is a specific precipitating stimulus but the response varies. This may be only an EEG response without clinical manifestations and is often limited to the occipital regions; generalised FOS paroxysms may occur.

Of epileptic syndromes, Panayiotopoulos syndrome and Gastaut-type childhood occipital epilepsy are the model examples of FOS (Figure 5.5). However, FOS has been also described in generalised epilepsies (Figure 9.3). FOS may be due to idiopathic, symptomatic or cryptogenic causes.[765,842,843]

The term *scotosensitive* implies seizures and EEG abnormalities induced by the complete elimination of retinal light stimulation; most cases described as scotosensitive are probably FOS.[765]

STARTLE EPILEPSY [782,783,844–848]

Startle epilepsy is recognised as a syndrome although most realistically this consists of a heterogeneous group of patients with startle-induced seizures. Aetiologies, EEG correlates and brain structural abnormalities are variable.

Startle seizures are induced by sudden and unexpected stimuli. Sudden noise is the main triggering stimulus but somatosensory and less often visual stimuli are also effective in some patients. The startle (unexpected and sudden presentation of the stimulus) is the provoking factor although rarely patients may be specifically sensitive to one sensory modality. Habituation to repetitive stimulation occurs.

Demographic data: Onset is in childhood or early adolescence (1–16 years), both sexes are affected, prevalence is very low.

Clinical manifestations: The majority of the patients suffer from static neurological and intellectual handicaps. Infantile hemiplegia predominates.

The startle response is brief (up to 30 seconds) and consists of axial tonic posturing – frequently causing falls, which are often traumatic. The seizures are asymmetric in one quarter of the patients. In hemiparetic patients, the seizure starts with flexion and abduction of the paretic arm and extension of the ipsilateral leg, which rapidly involves the contralateral side. Concurrent symptoms such as marked autonomic manifestations, automatisms, laughter and jerks may occur. Less commonly, startle-induced seizures may be atonic or myoclonic, particularly in patients with cerebral anoxia. Seizures are frequent, occurring many times a day and sometimes progress to status epilepticus.

Spontaneous seizures are common (probably all patients). These are infrequent and may precede or follow the startle-induced seizures.

Aetiology: Startle-induced seizures usually occur in patients with a variety of localised or diffuse static brain pathology (symptomatic startle seizures). Typically, the insults are pre- or peri-natal or occur within the first 2 years of life. Startle-induced seizures appear to be common in Down syndrome.[849]

Diagnostic procedures: Appropriate brain imaging reveals a variety of focal and diffuse usually atrophic and often large cerebral abnormalities. Brain MRI is needed even for those patients with normal neurology.[846] The structural abnormalities predominate in the lateral sensorimotor cortex.

Electroencephalography: Interictal EEG shows a variety of diffuse or focal abnormalities reflecting the underlying brain structural lesions. Ictal EEG consists of an initial vertex discharge followed by diffuse relative flattening or low voltage rhythmic ~10 Hz activity which begins in lesioned motor or premotor cortex and spreads to mesial frontal, parietal and contralateral frontal regions.[783,844,846] On surface EEG, this is often obscured by muscle artefacts.

Differential diagnosis: The main diagnostic confusion is with hyperekplexia (also called startle disease), which is a non-epileptic disorder (see page 49).

Seizures induced by touch, tap or sudden dousing with hot water may have a startle component but this is not a prerequisite for their provocation. In addition, seizures are mainly myoclonic, ictal EEG shows generalised discharges, patients are otherwise normal and there are no structural brain abnormalities.

Prognosis: This is commonly poor, particularly for those with severe pre-existing encephalopathies. There is increased mortality compared with the general population. Total control of the seizures is nearly impossible.

Management: There is no established drug of choice, and therapy is often unsatisfactory. Clonazepam, clobazam and carbamazepine are often used. In a study of four patients, adjunctive lamotrigine therapy had dramatic beneficial effect.[689]

COMPLEX REFLEX EPILEPSIES [746,747]

SEIZURES INDUCED BY THINKING, PROCESSING OF SPATIAL INFORMATION AND SEQUENTIAL DECISION-MAKING

Thinking-induced seizures occur in response to high cognitive functions; effective triggers include mathematical calculations, drawing, playing cards, chess and other board games, and Rubik's cube.[775,776,850,851] Decision-making and spatial tasks are essential elements in seizure provocation. Thinking-induced seizures usually occur in the context of IGE. They usually start during adolescence and are myoclonic, absences and GTCS; focal seizures are rare. Neuropsychological analysis of the stimuli points to right parietal cortical dysfunction.

READING EPILEPSY [767–770]

Reading is a well-documented provocative seizure-inducing stimulus in idiopathic (primary reading epilepsy) and less often cryptogenic/symptomatic epilepsies (Figure 9.7). Myoclonic jerks of the masticatory muscles constitute the commonest and uniform pattern. Some patients have prolonged, focal seizures manifested with alexia and possibly dysphasia,[767] while absences are exceptional. Primary reading epilepsy is a distinctive form of idiopathic reflex epilepsy.

Demographic data: Age at onset is usually between 12 and 19 years with a peak in late teens, i.e. long after reading skills have been acquired. There is a male preponderance of 1.8/1. Prevalence may be very low.

Clinical manifestations: In primary reading epilepsy seizures are elicited by reading (silently or aloud) and consist of brief myoclonic jerks mainly restricted to the masticatory, oral and perioral muscles. They are described as clicking sensations and occur a few minutes to hours after reading, particularly loud reading of texts that are difficult or unusual. Jaw myoclonus is by far the commonest manifestation of reading epilepsy. If the patient continues reading despite jaw jerks, these may become more violent, spread to trunk and limb muscles or generate other seizure manifestations before a generalised tonic-clonic seizure develops. The majority of the patients have one GTCS which is usually self-inflicted because of their curiosity to see what will happen if they continue reading despite jaw jerks or other manifestations. This is usually the first and last GTCS in their life because their condition is effectively treated and the patient learns to stop reading or talking when oral/perioral jerks occur. It is extremely rare for patients with primary reading epilepsy to have more than 1–5 GTCS or spontaneous seizures, non-related to reading. It is also rare for reading epilepsy to present with other types of ictal manifestations (mainly visual hallucinations) in addition to the jaw myoclonic seizures. Hand myoclonic jerking is common among those with precipitation of seizures by writing.

Precipitating factors: Reading, silently or aloud, is the defining precipitant stimulus. In many patients, clinically identical seizures can also be provoked by the other linguistic activities – justifying the term language-induced epilepsy.[767] One quarter of the patients may have also similar jaw jerks provoked by talking (particularly if this is fast or argumentative), writing, reading music or chewing.

Aetiology: Primary reading epilepsy is probably genetically determined and has been reported in identical twins and among first degree relatives.

Diagnostic procedures: All tests except EEG are normal.

Electroencephalography: The interictal EEG is usually normal. Ictal EEG manifestations may be inconspicuous and difficult to detect because of muscle activity from the jaw muscles and head, but more frequently they consist of a brief burst of sharp waves, which is bilateral with left side preponderance in the temporo-parietal regions (Figure 9.7).

Prognosis: The prognosis of primary reading epilepsy appears to be good because seizures are usually minor and they are related to a precipitant stimulus which can be modified.

Management: Clonazepam (0.5–1 mg nocte) is highly effective. A 40-year-old woman, the sister of one of my patients with reading epilepsy, also had reading epilepsy, never sought medical advice for her condition and never had GTCS but controlled her condition by modifying her way of reading and talking.

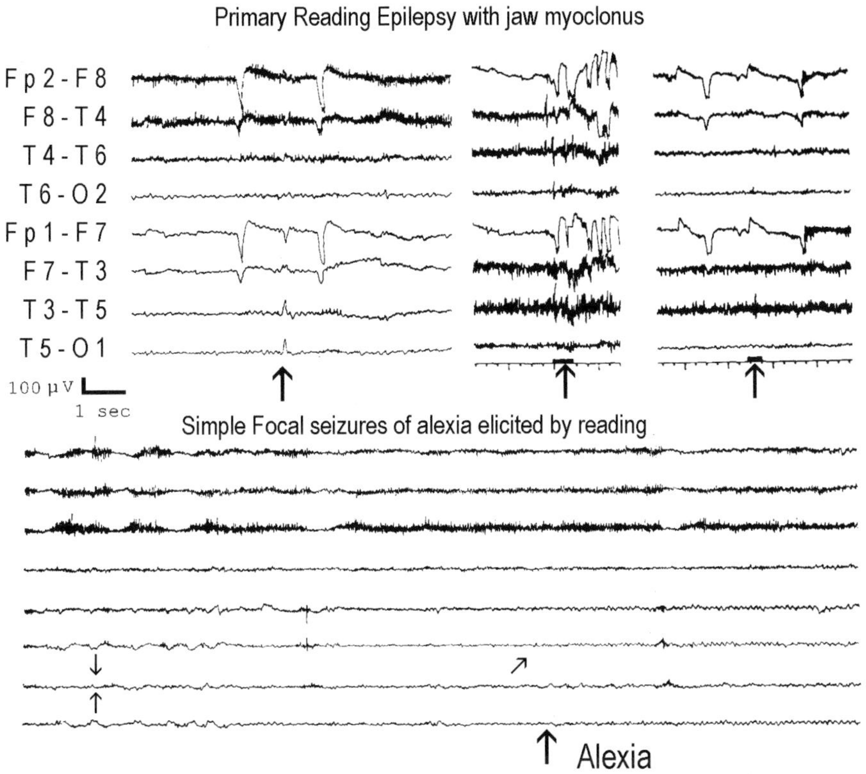

Figure 9.7 Two types of reading-induced seizures; jaw myoclonus or alexia.

Top left: EEG of a woman with jaw jerks (arrow) while reading (case 8 in ref [767]). She was successfully treated with clonazepam 0.5 mg nocte. Her sister also suffered from jaw jerks, mainly when involved in argumentative and fast talk.

Top middle and right: Video-EEG of another woman with jaw jerks (bars and arrows) while reading (case 10 in ref [767]). The EEG shows no detectable abnormality when jerks are mild (middle) and possible changes are obscured by muscle activity (right).

Bottom: Video-EEG of a 24-year-old man with simple focal seizures manifested with alexia (inability to understand written words) and four nocturnal GTCS (case 17 in ref [767]). Interictal EEG during reading showed sharp and slow waves focused in the left temporal regions (midway between middle and posterior temporal electrode). When the patient indicated his inability to understand text (big arrow), the EEG showed low-amplitude fast rhythms (around 10–11 Hz) localised in the left middle temporal regions. This lasted 70 seconds before clinical recovery. MRI and PET scan were normal. The patient was effectively treated with carbamazepine.

Modified from Panayiotopoulos (1996)[435] with the permission of the Editor S. Wallace and the publishers Chapman & Hall.

REFERENCES

1 Hauser WA, Hesdorffer DDC. *Epilepsy: frequency causes and consequences.* New York: Demos, 1990.

2 Hauser WA. Epidemiology of epilepsy in children. *Neurosurg Clin North Am* 1995;**6**:419–29.

3 Jallon P. Epilepsy and epileptic disorders, an epidemiological marker? Contribution of descriptive epidemiology. *Epileptic Disord* 2002;**4**:1–13.

4 Shorvon SD. Epidemiology, classification, natural history, and genetics of epilepsy. *Lancet* 1990;**336**:93–6.

5 Hauser WA, Annegers JF, Kurland LT. Incidence of epilepsy and unprovoked seizures in Rochester, Minnesota: 1935–1984. *Epilepsia* 1993;**34**:453–68.

6 Morrell MJ, Pedley TA. "The scarlet E": epilepsy is still a burden. *Neurology* 2000;**54**:1882–3.

7 Panayiotopoulos CP. Treatment of typical absence seizures and related epileptic syndromes. *Paediatr Drugs* 2001;**3**:379–403.

8 Commission of Classification and Terminology of the International League Against Epilepsy. Proposal for revised clinical and electroencephalographic classification of epileptic seizures. *Epilepsia* 1981;**22**:489–501.

9 Commission on Classification and Terminology of the International League Against Epilepsy. Proposal for revised classification of epilepsies and epileptic syndromes. *Epilepsia* 1989;**30**:389–99.

10 Engel J Jr. A proposed diagnostic scheme for people with epileptic seizures and with epilepsy: Report of the ILAE Task Force on Classification and Terminology. *Epilepsia* 2001;**42**:796–803.

11 Blume WT, Luders HO, Mizrahi E, Tassinari C, van Emde BW, Engel J Jr. Glossary of descriptive terminology for ictal semiology: report of the ILAE task force on classification and terminology. *Epilepsia* 2001;**42**:1212–8.

12 Lempert T. Recognizing syncope: pitfalls and surprises. *J R Soc Med* 1996;**89**:372–5.

13 Kapoor WN. Syncope. *N Engl J Med* 2000;**343**:1856–62.

14 Stephenson JB. *Fits and faints.* London: MacKeith Press, 1990.

15 Dreyfus FE. Classification of epileptic seizures. In Engel J jr, Pedley TA, eds. *Epilepsy. A comprehensive textbook,* pp 517-24. Lippincott-Raven, 1997.

16 Hauser WA, Rich SS, Annegers JF, Anderson VE. Seizure recurrence after a 1st unprovoked seizure: an extended follow-up. *Neurology* 1990;**40**:1163–70.

17 Panayiotopoulos CP. Importance of specifying the type of epilepsy. *Lancet* 1999;**354**:2002–3.

18 Adie WJ. Pyknolepsy: a form of epilepsy occurring in children with a good prognosis. *Brain* 1924;**47**:96–102.

19 Merlis JK. Proposal for an international classification of the epilepsies. *Epilepsia* 1970;**11**:114–19.

20 Roger J, Bureau M, Dravet C, Genton P, Tassinari CA, Wolf P, eds. *Epileptic syndromes in infancy, childhood and adolescence,* 3rd edn. London: John Libbey & Co Ltd, 2002.

21 Commission on Classification and Terminology of the International League Against Epilepsy. Proposal for classification of epilepsy and epileptic syndromes. *Epilepsia* 1985;**26**: 268–78.

22 Wolf P. Historical aspects: the concept of idiopathy. In: Malafose A, Genton P, Hirsch E, Marescaux C, Broglin D, Bernasconi R, eds. *Idiopathic generalised epilepsies: clinical, experimental and genetic aspects,* pp 3–6. London: John Libbey & Company, 1994.

23 Grunewald RA, Panayiotopoulos CP. The diagnosis of epilepsies. *J R Coll Physicians Lond* 1996;**30**:122–7.

24 Benbadis SR, Luders HO. Epileptic syndromes: an underutilized concept [editorial]. *Epilepsia* 1996;**37**:1029–34.

25 Panayiotopoulos CP. *Benign childhood partial seizures and related epileptic syndromes.* London: John Libbey & Company Ltd, 1999.

26 Niedermeyer E, Lopes da Silva F. *Electroencephalography. Basic principles,clinical applications, and related fields,* 4th edn. Baltimore: Williams & Wilkins, 1999.

27 Blume WT. Current trends in electroencephalography. *Curr Opin Neurol* 2001;**14**:193–7.

28 Binnie CD, Prior PF. Electroencephalography. *J Neurol Neurosurg Psychiatr* 1994;**57**:1308–19.

29 Chadwick D. Diagnosis of epilepsy. *Lancet* 1990;**336**:291–5.

30 Panayiotopoulos CP. Significance of the EEG after the first afebrile seizure. *Arch Dis Child* 1998;**78**:575–6.

31 Commission on Neuroimaging of the International League Against Epilepsy. Recommendations for neuroimaging of patients with epilepsy. *Epilepsia* 1997;**38**:1255–6.

32   Commission on Neuroimaging of the International League Against Epilepsy. Guidelines for neuroimaging evaluation of patients with uncontrolled epilepsy considered for surgery. *Epilepsia* 1998;**39**:1375–6.

33   Commission on Diagnostic Strategies: recommendations for functional neuroimaging of persons with epilepsy. *Epilepsia* 2000;**41**:1350–6.

34   Giannakodimos S, Ferrie CD, Panayiotopoulos CP. Qualitative and quantitative abnormalities of breath counting during brief generalized 3 Hz spike and slow wave 'subclinical' discharges. *Clin Electroencephalogr* 1995;**26**:200–3.

35   Cross J. Significance of the EEG after the first afebrile seizure: Commentary. *Arch Dis Child* 1998;**78**:576–7.

36   Panayiotopoulos CP. *Panayiotopoulos syndrome: a common and benign childhood epileptic syndrome.* London: John Libbey & Co., 2002.

37   Panayiotopoulos CP, Agathonikou A, Sharoqi IA, Parker AP. Vigabatrin aggravates absences and absence status. *Neurology* 1997;**49**:1467.

38   Panayiotopoulos CP. Efficacy of lamotrigine (LTG) monotherapy [letter; comment]. *Epilepsia* 2000;**41**:357–9.

39   Hirtz D, Ashwal S, Berg A, Bettis D, Camfield C, Camfield P et al. Practice parameter: evaluating a first nonfebrile seizure in children: report of the quality standards subcommittee of the American Academy of Neurology, The Child Neurology Society, and The American Epilepsy Society. *Neurology* 2000;**55**:616–23.

40   King MA, Newton MR, Jackson GD, Berkovic SF. Epileptology of the first-seizure presentation: a clinical, electroencephalographic, and magnetic imaging study of 300 consecutive patients. *Lancet* 1998;**352**:1007–11.

41   Berg AT, Shinnar S. The risk of seizure recurrence following a first unprovoked seizure: a quantitative review. *Neurology* 1991;**41**:965–72.

42   Hart YM, Sander JW, Johnson AL, Shorvon SD. National General Practice Study of Epilepsy: recurrence after a first seizure. *Lancet* 1990;**336**:1271–4.

43   Shinnar S, Kang H, Berg AT, Goldensohn ES, Hauser WA, Moshe SL. EEG abnormalities in children with a first unprovoked seizure. *Epilepsia* 1994;**35**:471–6.

44   Shinnar S, Berg AT, Moshe SL, O'Dell C, Alemany M, Newstein D et al. The risk of seizure recurrence after a first unprovoked afebrile seizure in childhood: an extended follow-up. *Pediatrics* 1996;**98**:216–25.

45   Hopkins A, Garman A, Clarke C. The first seizure in adult life. Value of clinical features, electroencephalography, and computerised tomographic scanning in prediction of seizure recurrence. *Lancet* 1988;**1**:721–6.

46   Hoekelman RA. A pediatrician's view. The first seizure – a terrifying event [editorial]. *Pediatr Ann* 1991;**20**:9–10.

47   Duncan JS. Imaging and epilepsy. *Brain* 1997;**120** (Pt 2):339–77.

48   Ryvlin P, Bouvard S, Le Bars D, De Lamerie G, Gregoire MC, Kahane P et al. Clinical utility of flumazenil–PET versus [18F]fluorodeoxyglucose-PET and MRI in refractory partial epilepsy. A prospective study in 100 patients. *Brain* 1998;**121** (Pt 11):2067–81.

49   Jackson GD, Connelly A. New NMR measurements in epilepsy. T2 relaxometry and magnetic resonance spectroscopy. *Adv Neurol* 1999;**79**:931–7.

50   Cendes F. Radiological evaluation of hippocampal sclerosis. In: Oxbury JM, Polkey CE, Duchowny M, eds. *Intractable focal epilepsy*, pp 571–94. London: WB Saunders, 2000.

51   Chiron C, Hertz-Pannier L. Cerebral imaging in childhood epilepsy: what's new? *Epileptic Disord* 2001;**3** Spec No. 2:SI25–SI36.

52   Connor SE, Jarosz JM. Magnetic resonance imaging of patients with epilepsy. *Clin Radiol* 2001;**56**:787–801.

53   Duncan JS. Neuroimaging. In: Duncan JS, Sisodiya S, Smalls JE, eds. *Epilepsy 2001. From science to patient*, pp 173–216. Oxford: Meritus Communications, 2001.

54   Kuzniecky RI. Neuroimaging in pediatric epileptology. In: Pellock JM, Dodson WE, Bourgeois BFD, eds. *Pediatric epilepsy*, pp 133–43. New York: Demos, 2001.

55   Ruggieri PM, Najm IM. MR imaging in epilepsy. *Neurol Clin* 2001;**19**:477–89.

56   Wright NB. Imaging in epilepsy: a paediatric perspective. *Br J Radiol* 2001;**74**:575–89.

57   Briellmann RS, Kalnins R, Berkovic S, Jackson GD. Hippocampal pathology in refractory temporal lobe epilepsy; T2-weighted signal change reflects dentate gliosis. *Neurology* 2002;**58**:265–71.

58   Chuang NA, Otsubo H, Chuang SH. Magnetic resonance imaging in pediatric epilepsy. *Top Magn Reson Imaging* 2002;**13**:39–60.

59   Meiners LC. Role of MR imaging in epilepsy. *Eur Radiol* 2002;**12**:499–501.

60   Ferrie CD, Jackson GD, Giannakodimos S, Panayiotopoulos CP. Posterior agyria-pachygyria with polymicrogyria: evidence for an inherited neuronal migration disorder. *Neurology* 1995;**45**:150–3.

61   Volpe JJ. *Neonatal seizures.* Philadelphia: WB Saunders, 1995.

62 Lombroso CT. Neonatal seizures: historic note and present controversies. *Epilepsia* 1996;**37** Suppl 3:5–13.

63 Mizrahi EM. Treatment of neonatal seizures. In: Engel J Jr, Pedley TA, eds. *Epilepsy. A comprehensive textbook*, pp 1295–303. Philadephia: Lippincott-Raven, 1997.

64 Mizrahi EM, Plouin P, Kellaway P. Neonatal seizures. In: Engel J Jr, Pedley TA, eds. *Epilepsy. A comprehensive textbook*, pp 647–63. Philadelphia: Lippincott-Raven, 1997.

65 Rennie JM. Neonatal seizures. *Eur J Pediatr* 1997;**156**:83–7.

66 Hirsch E, Saint-Martin A, Marescaux C. Benign familial neonatal convulsions: a model of idiopathic epilepsy. *Rev Neurol (Paris)* 1999;**155**:463–7.

67 Ronen GM, Penney S, Andrews W. The epidemiology of clinical neonatal seizures in Newfoundland: a population-based study. *J Pediatr* 1999;**134**:71–5.

68 Schmid R, Tandon P, Stafstrom CE, Holmes GL. Effects of neonatal seizures on subsequent seizure-induced brain injury. *Neurology* 1999;**53**:1754–61.

69 Watanabe K, Miura K, Natsume J, Hayakawa F, Furune S, Okumura A. Epilepsies of neonatal onset: seizure type and evolution. *Dev Med Child Neurol* 1999;**41**:318–22.

70 Levene M. The clinical conundrum of neonatal seizures. *Arch Dis Child Fetal Neonatal Ed* 2002;**86**:F75–F77.

71 Mizrahi EM, Kellaway P. *Diagnosis and management of neonatal seizures*. Hagerstown: Lippincott Williams & Wilkins, 1999.

72 Hill A. Neonatal seizures. *Pediatr Rev* 2000;**21**:117–21.

73 Leppert M. Novel K+ channel genes in benign familial neonatal convulsions. *Epilepsia* 2000;**41**:1066–7.

74 Holmes GL, Khazipov R, Ben Ari Y. New concepts in neonatal seizures. *Neuroreport* 2002;**13**:A3–A8.

75 Scher MS. Controversies regarding neonatal seizure recognition. *Epileptic Disord* 2002;**4**:139–58.

76 Volpe JJ. Neonatal seizures: current concepts and revised classification. *Pediatrics* 1989;**84**:422–8.

77 Boylan GB, Panerai RB, Rennie JM, Evans DH, Rabe-Hesketh S, Binnie CD. Cerebral blood flow velocity during neonatal seizures. *Arch Dis Child Fetal Neonatal Ed* 1999;**80**:F105–F110.

78 D'Arceuil HE, de Crespigny AJ, Rother J, Seri S, Moseley ME, Stevenson DK *et al*. Diffusion and perfusion magnetic resonance imaging of the evolution of hypoxic ischemic encephalopathy in the neonatal rabbit. *J Magn Reson Imaging* 1998;**8**:820–8.

79 Leth H, Toft PB, Herning M, Peitersen B, Lou HC. Neonatal seizures associated with cerebral lesions shown by magnetic resonance imaging. *Arch Dis Child Fetal Neonatal Ed* 1997;**77**:F105–F110.

80 Barr PA, Buettiker VE, Antony JH. Efficacy of lamotrigine in refractory neonatal seizures. *Pediatr Neurol* 1999;**20**:161–3.

81 Massingale TW, Buttross S. Survey of treatment practices for neonatal seizures. *J Perinatol* 1993;**13**:107–10.

82 Brod SA, Ment LR, Ehrenkranz RA, Bridgers S. Predictors of success for drug discontinuation following neonatal seizures. *Pediatr Neurol* 1988;**4**:13–17.

83 Ellison PH, Horn JL, Franklin S, Jones MG. The results of checking a scoring system for neonatal seizures. *Neuropediatrics* 1986;**17**:152–7.

84 Plouin P. Benign familial neonatal convulsions and benign idiopathic neonatal convulsions. In: Engel J Jr, Pedley TA, eds. *Epilepsy. A comprehensive textbook*, pp 2247–55. Philadelphia: Lippincott–Raven, 1997.

85 Hirsch E, Velez A, Sellal F, Maton B, Grinspan A, Malafosse A *et al*. Electroclinical signs of benign neonatal familial convulsions. *Ann Neurol* 1993;**34**:835–41.

86 Ballaban KR, Plouin P, Moshe SL. Benign neonatal familial seizures. In: Gilman S, ed. *Medlink Neurology*. San Diego, CA: Arbor Publishing, 2002.

87 Castaldo P, del Giudice EM, Coppola G, Pascotto A, Annunziato L, Taglialatela M. Benign familial neonatal convulsions caused by altered gating of KCNQ2/KCNQ3 potassium channels. *J Neurosci* 2002;**22**:RC199.

88 Biervert C, Steinlein OK. Structural and mutational analysis of KCNQ2, the major gene locus for benign familial neonatal convulsions. *Hum Genet* 1999;**104**:234–40.

89 Berkovic SF, Kennerson ML, Howell RA, Scheffer IE, Hwang PA, Nicholson GA. Phenotypic expression of benign familial neonatal convulsions linked to chromosome 20. *Arch Neurol* 1994;**51**:1125–8.

90 Lee WL, Biervert C, Hallmann K, Tay A, Dean JC, Steinlein OK. A KCNQ2 splice site mutation causing benign neonatal convulsions in a Scottish family. *Neuropediatrics* 2000;**31**:9–12.

91 Singh NA, Charlier C, Stauffer D, DuPont BR, Leach RJ, Melis R *et al*. A novel potassium channel gene, KCNQ2, is mutated in an inherited epilepsy of newborns. *Nat Genet* 1998;**18**:25–9.

92 Dehan M, Quilleron D, Navelet Y *et al*. Les

convulsions du cinquieme jour de vie: un nouveau syndrome? *Arch Fr Pediatr* 1977;**37**:730–42.

93 Plouin P. Benign neonatal convulsions (familial and non-familial). In: Roger J, Bureau M, Dravet C, Dreifuss FE, Perret A, Wolf P, eds. *Epileptic syndromes in infancy, childhood and adolescence*, pp 2–11. London: John Libbey & Co., 1992.

94 Aicardi J. Early myoclonic encephalopathy (neonatal myoclonic encephalopathy). In: Roger J, Bureau M, Dravet C, Dreifuss FE, Perret A, Wolf P, eds. *Epileptic syndromes in infancy, childhood and adolescence*, pp 13–23. London: John Libbey & Co., 1992.

95 Lombroso CT. Early myoclonic encephalopathy, early infantile epileptic encephalopathy, and benign and severe infantile myoclonic epilepsies: a critical review and personal contributions. *J Clin Neurophysiol* 1990;**7**:380–408.

96 Dalla Bernardina B, Dulac O, Fejerman N, Dravet C, Capovilla G, Bondavalli S *et al*. Early myoclonic epileptic encephalopathy (E.M.E.E.). *Eur J Pediatr* 1983;**140**:248–52.

97 Bruel H, Boulloche J, Chabrolle JP, Layet V, Poinsot J. Early myoclonic epileptic encephalopathy and non-ketotic hyperglycemia in the same family. *Arch Pediatr* 1998;**5**:397–9.

98 Fusco L, Pachatz C, Di Capua M, Vigevano F. Video/EEG aspects of early-infantile epileptic encephalopathy with suppression-bursts (Ohtahara syndrome). *Brain Dev* 2001;**23**:708–14.

99 Yamatogi Y, Ohtahara S. Early-infantile epileptic encephalopathy with suppression-bursts, Ohtahara syndrome; its overview referring to our 16 cases. *Brain Dev* 2002;**24**:13–23.

100 Romann D, Golz N, Garbe W. Ohtahara syndrome. *Geburtshilfe Frauenheilkd* 1996;**56**:393–5.

101 Murakami N, Ohtsuka Y, Ohtahara S. Early infantile epileptic syndromes with suppression-bursts: early myoclonic encephalopathy vs. Ohtahara syndrome. *Jpn J Psychiatry Neurol* 1993;**47**:197–200.

102 Komaki H, Sugai K, Maehara T, Shimizu H. Surgical treatment of early-infantile epileptic encephalopathy with suppression-bursts associated with focal cortical dysplasia. *Brain Dev* 2001;**23**:727–31.

103 Di Capua M, Fusco L, Ricci S, Vigevano F. Benign neonatal sleep myoclonus: clinical features and video- polygraphic recordings. *Mov Disord* 1993;**8**:191–4.

104 Daoust-Roy J, Seshia SS. Benign neonatal sleep myoclonus. A differential diagnosis of neonatal seizures. *Am J Dis Child* 1992;**146**:1236–41.

105 Caraballo R, Yepez I, Cersosimo R, Fejerman N. Benign neonatal sleep myoclonus. *Rev Neurol* 1998;**26**:540–4.

106 Sheldon SH. Benign neonatal sleep myoclonus. In: Gilman S, ed. *Medlink*. San Diego, CA: Arbor Publishing, 2002.

107 Lombroso CT, Fejerman N. Benign myoclonus of early infancy. *Ann Neurol* 1977;**1**:138–43.

108 Pachatz C, Fusco L, Vigevano F. Benign myoclonus of early infancy. *Epileptic Disord* 1999;**1**:57–61.

109 Maydell BV, Berenson F, Rothner AD, Wyllie E, Kotagal P. Benign myoclonus of early infancy: an imitator of West's syndrome. *J Child Neurol* 2001;**16**:109–12.

110 Ballaban KR, Moshe SL. Benign nonepileptic infantile spasms. In: Gilman S, ed. *Medlink Neurology*. San Diego, CA: Arbor Publishing, 2002.

111 Kanazawa O. Shuddering attacks – report of four children. *Pediatr Neurol* 2000;**23**:421–4.

112 Andermann F, Keene DL, Andermann E, Quesney LF. Startle disease or hyperekplexia: further delineation of the syndrome. *Brain* 1980;**103**:985–97.

113 Ryan SG, Sherman SL, Terry JC, Sparkes RS, Torres MC, Mackey RW. Startle disease, or hyperekplexia: response to clonazepam and assignment of the gene (STHE) to chromosome 5q by linkage analysis. *Ann Neurol* 1992;**31**:663–8.

114 Tijssen MA, Schoemaker HC, Edelbroek PJ, Roos RA, Cohen AF, van Dijk JG. The effects of clonazepam and vigabatrin in hyperekplexia. *J Neurol Sci* 1997;**149**:63–7.

115 Vergouwe MN, Tijssen MA, Peters AC, Wielaard R, Frants RR. Hyperekplexia phenotype due to compound heterozygosity for GLRA1 gene mutations. *Ann Neurol* 1999;**46**:634–8.

116 Saul B, Kuner T, Sobetzko D, Brune W, Hanefeld F, Meinck HM *et al*. Novel GLRA1 missense mutation (P250T) in dominant hyperekplexia defines an intracellular determinant of glycine receptor channel gating. *J Neurosci* 1999;**19**:869–77.

117 Shiang R, Ryan SG, Zhu YZ, Fielder TJ, Allen RJ, Fryer A *et al*. Mutational analysis of familial and sporadic hyperekplexia. *Ann Neurol* 1995;**38**:85–91.

118 Bernasconi A, Regli F, Schorderet DF, Pescia G. Familial hyperekplexia: startle disease. Clinical, electrophysiological and genetic study of a family. *Rev Neurol (Paris)* 1996;**152**:447–50.

119 de Groen JH, Kamphuisen HA. Periodic nocturnal myoclonus in a patient with hyperexplexia (startle disease). *J Neurol Sci* 1978;**38**:207–13.

120 Nigro MA, Lim HC. Hyperekplexia and sudden neonatal death. *Pediatr Neurol* 1992;**8**:221–5.

121 Nelson KB, Ellenberg JH. Predictors of epilepsy in children who have experienced febrile seizures. *N Engl J Med* 1976;**295**:1029–33.

122 Nelson KB, Ellenberg JH. Prognosis in children with febrile seizures. *Pediatrics* 1978;**61**:720–7.

123 Wallace SJ. *The child with febrile seizures.* London: Butterworth, 1988.

124 Joint Working Group of the Research Unit of the Royal College of Physicians and the British Paediatric Association. Guidelines for the management of convulsions with fever. Joint Working Group of the Research Unit of the Royal College of Physicians and the British Paediatric Association. *BMJ* 1991;**303**:634–6.

125 Fukuyama Y, Seki T, Ohtsuka C, Miura H, Hara M. Practical guidelines for physicians in the management of febrile seizures. *Brain Dev* 1996;**18**:479–84.

126 American Academy of Pediatrics. Practice parameter: the neurodiagnostic evaluation of the child with a first simple febrile seizure. American Academy of Pediatrics. Provisional Committee on Quality Improvement, Subcommittee on Febrile Seizures. *Pediatrics* 1996;**97**:769–72.

127 Berg AT, Shinnar S, Darefsky AS, Holford TR, Shapiro ED, Salomon ME *et al.* Predictors of recurrent febrile seizures. A prospective cohort study. *Arch Pediatr Adolesc Med* 1997;**151**:371–8.

128 Hirtz DG, Camfield CS, Camfield PR. Febrile convulsions. In: Engel J Jr, Pedley TA, eds. *Epilepsy:A comprehensive textbook*, pp 2483–8. Philadelphia: Lippincott-Raven, 1998.

129 American Academy of Pediatrics. Practice parameter: long-term treatment of the child with simple febrile seizures. American Academy of Pediatrics. Committee on Quality Improvement, Subcommittee on Febrile Seizures. *Pediatrics* 1999;**103**:1307–9.

130 Baumann RJ. Technical report: treatment of the child with simple febrile seizures. *Pediatrics* 1999;**103**:e86.

131 Baumann RJ, Duffner PK. Treatment of children with simple febrile seizures: the AAP practice parameter. American Academy of Pediatrics. *Pediatr Neurol* 2000;**23**:11–17.

132 Knudsen FU. Febrile seizures: treatment and prognosis. *Epilepsia* 2000;**41**:2–9.

133 Verity CM. Febrile convulsions – a practical guide. In: Duncan JS, Sisodiya S, Smalls JE, eds. *Epilepsy 2001. From science to patient*, pp 87–100. Oxford: Meritus Communications, 2001.

134 Shinnar S, Pellock JM, Berg AT, O'Dell C, Driscoll SM, Maytal J *et al.* Short-term outcomes of children with febrile status epilepticus. *Epilepsia* 2001;**42**:47–53.

135 Berkovic SF, Scheffer IE. Febrile seizures: genetics and relationship to other epilepsy syndromes. *Curr Opin Neurol* 1998;**11**:129–34.

136 Johnson EW, Dubovsky J, Rich SS, O'Donovan CA, Orr HT, Anderson VE *et al.* Evidence for a novel gene for familial febrile convulsions, FEB2, linked to chromosome 19p in an extended family from the Midwest. *Hum Mol Genet* 1998;**7**:63–7.

137 Kugler SL, Stenroos ES, Mandelbaum DE, Lehner T, McKoy VV, Prossick T *et al.* Hereditary febrile seizures: phenotype and evidence for a chromosome 19p locus. *Am J Med Genet* 1998;**79**:354–61.

138 Nakayama J, Hamano K, Iwasaki N, Nakahara S, Horigome Y, Saitoh H *et al.* Significant evidence for linkage of febrile seizures to chromosome 5q14-q15. *Hum Mol Genet* 2000;**9**:87–91.

139 Peiffer A, Thompson J, Charlier C, Otterud B, Varvil T, Pappas C *et al.* A locus for febrile seizures (FEB3) maps to chromosome 2q23-24. *Ann Neurol* 1999;**46**:671–8.

140 Wallace RH, Berkovic SF, Howell RA, Sutherland GR, Mulley JC. Suggestion of a major gene for familial febrile convulsions mapping to 8q13-21. *J Med Genet* 1996;**33**:308–12.

141 Scheffer IE, Wallace RH, Mulley JC, Berkovic SF. Locus for febrile seizures. *Ann Neurol* 2000;**47**:840–1.

142 Watanabe K, Yamamoto N, Negoro T, Takaesu E, Aso K, Furune S *et al.* Benign complex partial epilepsies in infancy. *Pediatr Neurol* 1987;**3**:208–11.

143 Watanabe K, Yamamoto N, Negoro T, Takahashi I, Aso K, Maehara M. Benign infantile epilepsy with complex partial seizures. *J Clin Neurophysiol* 1990;**7**:409–16.

144 Vigevano F, Fusco L, Di Capua M, Ricci S, Sebastianelli R, Lucchini *et al.* Benign infantile familial convulsions. *Eur J Pediatr* 1992;**151**:608–12.

145 Vigevano F, Cusmai R, Ricci S, Watanabe K. Benign epilepsies of infancy. In: Engel J Jr, Pedley TA, eds. *Epilepsy. A comprehensive textbook*, pp 2267–76. Philadelphia: Lippincott-Raven, 1997.

146 Watanabe K. Benign partial epilepsies in infancy and early childhood: clinical description and genetic background. In: Berkovic SF, Genton P, Hirsch E, Plouin P, eds. *Genetics of focal epilepsies*, pp 73–8. London: John Libbey & Co., 1999.

147 Gennaro E, Malacarne M, Carbone I, Riggio MC, Bianchi A, Bonanni P *et al.* No evidence of a major locus for benign familial infantile convulsions on chromosome 19q12-q13.1. *Epilepsia* 1999;**40**:1799–803.

148 Gautier A, Pouplard F, Bednarek N, Motte J, Berquin P, Billard C *et al*. Benign infantile convulsions. French collaborative study. *Arch Pediatr* 1999;**6**:32–9.

149 Okumura A, Hayakawa F, Kato T, Kuno K, Negoro T, Watanabe K. Early recognition of benign partial epilepsy in infancy. *Epilepsia* 2000;**41**:714–7.

150 Vigevano F. Benign epilepsy of infancy with partial seizures. In: Gilman S, ed. *Medlink Neurology*. San Diego, CA: Arbor Publishing, 2002.

151 Watanabe K, Okumura A. Benign partial epilepsies in infancy. *Brain Dev* 2000;**22**:296–300.

152 Watanabe K, Negoro T, Aso K. Benign partial epilepsy with secondarily generalized seizures in infancy. *Epilepsia* 1993;**34**:635–8.

153 Dravet C, Bureau M. The benign myoclonic epilepsy of infancy. *Rev Electroencephalogr Neurophysiol Clin* 1981;**11**:438–44.

154 Dravet C, Bureau M, Genton P. Benign myoclonic epilepsy of infancy: electroclinical symptomatology and differential diagnosis from the other types of generalized epilepsy of infancy. *Epilepsy Res Suppl* 1992;**6**:131–5.

155 Ricci S, Cusmai R, Fusco L, Vigevano F. Reflex myoclonic epilepsy in infancy: a new age-dependent idiopathic epileptic syndrome related to startle reaction. *Epilepsia* 1995;**36**:342–8.

156 Fejerman N. Benign myoclonic epilepsy in infancy. In: Wallace S, ed. *Epilepsy in children*, pp 235–9. London: Chapman & Hall, 1996.

157 Lin Y, Itomi K, Takada H, Kuboda T, Okumura A, Aso K *et al*. Benign myoclonic epilepsy in infants: video-EEG features and long-term follow-up. *Neuropediatrics* 1998;**29**:268–71.

158 Dravet C, Bureau M. Benign myoclonic epilepsy in infancy. In: Gilman S, ed. *Medlink Neurology*. San Diego, CA: Arbor Publishing, 2002.

159 Watanabe K, Iwase K, Hara K. The evolution of EEG features in infantile spasms: a prospective study. *Dev Med Child Neurol* 1973;**15**:584–96.

160 Negoro T, Matsumoto A, Sugiura M, Iwase K, Watanabe K, Hara K *et al*. Long-term prognosis of 200 cases of infantile spasms. Part II: Electroencephalographic findings at the ages between 5–7. *Folia Psychiatr Neurol Jpn* 1980;**34**:346–7.

161 Hakamada S, Watanabe K, Hara K, Miyazaki S. Brief atonia associated with electroencephalographic paroxysm in an infant with infantile spasms. *Epilepsia* 1981;**22**:285–8.

162 Matsumoto A, Watanabe K, Negoro T, Sugiura M, Iwase K, Hara K *et al*. Infantile spasms: etiological factors, clinical aspects, and long term prognosis in 200 cases. *Eur J Pediatr* 1981;**135**:239–44.

163 Matsumoto A, Watanabe K, Negoro T, Sugiura M, Iwase K, Hara K *et al*. Long-term prognosis after infantile spasms: a statistical study of prognostic factors in 200 cases. *Dev Med Child Neurol* 1981;**23**:51–65.

164 Matsumoto A, Watanabe K, Negoro T, Sugiura M, Iwase K, Hara K *et al*. Prognostic factors of infantile spasms from the etiological viewpoint. *Brain Dev* 1981;**3**:361–4.

165 Plouin P, Jalin C, Dulac O, Chiron C. Ambulatory 24-hour EEG recording in epileptic infantile spasms. *Rev Electroencephalogr Neurophysiol Clin* 1987;**17**:309–18.

166 Donat JF, Wright FS. Clinical imitators of infantile spasms. *J Child Neurol* 1992;**7**:395–9.

167 Jacobi G, Neirich U. Symptomatology and electroencephalography of the 'genuine' type of the West syndrome and its differential diagnosis from the other benign generalized epilepsies of infancy. *Epilepsy Res Suppl* 1992;**6**:145–51.

168 Watanabe K, Negoro T, Okumura. Symptomatology of infantile spasms. *Brain Dev.* 2001;**23**:453–66.

169 Vigevano F, Fusco L, Cusmai R, Claps D, Ricci S, Milani L. The idiopathic form of West syndrome. *Epilepsia* 1993;**34**:743–6.

170 Aicardi J. *Epilepsy in children*. New York: Raven Press, 1994.

171 Baram TZ, Mitchell WG, Brunson K, Haden E. Infantile spasms: hypothesis-driven therapy and pilot human infant experiments using corticotropin-releasing hormone receptor antagonists. *Dev Neurosci* 1999;**21**:281–9.

172 West Syndrome and other Infantile Epileptic Encephalopathies. Proceedings of an International Symposium. Tokyo, Japan, February 9–11, 2001. *Brain Dev* 2001;**23**:441–769.

173 Chugani HT. Pathophysiology of infantile spasms. *Adv Exp Med Biol* 2002;**497**:111–21.

174 Chiron C, Dulac O. Drug therapy for West's syndrome. *Adv Exp Med Biol* 2002;**497**:51–6.

175 Dulac O, Chugani HT, Dalla Bernardina B, eds. *Infantile spasms and West syndrome*. London: WB Saunders, 2002.

176 Hoffman HJ. Surgery for West's syndrome. *Adv Exp Med Biol* 2002;**497**:57–9.

177 Hrachovy RA. West's syndrome (infantile spasms). Clinical description and diagnosis. *Adv Exp Med Biol* 2002;**497**:33–50.

178 Itomi K, Okumura A, Negoro T, Watanabe K, Natsume J, Takada H *et al*. Prognostic value of positron emission tomography in cryptogenic West syndrome. *Dev Med Child Neurol* 2002;**44**:107–11.

179 Shields WD. West's syndrome. *J Child Neurol* 2002;**17** Suppl 1:S76–S79.

179a West WJ. On a peculiar form of infantile convulsions. *Lancet* 1841;**1**:724–5.

180 Tassinari CA, Michelucci R, Shigematsu H, Seino M. Atonic and falling seizures. In: Engel J Jr, Pedley TA, eds. *Epilepsy: A comprehensive extbook*, pp 605–16. Philadelphia: Lippincott–Raven, 1997.

181 Janz D, Inoue Y, Seino M. Myoclonic seizures. In: Engel J Jr, Pedley TA, eds. *Epilepsy: A comprehensive textbook*, pp 591–603. Philadelphia: Lippincott-Raven, 1997.

182 Werhahn KJ, Noachtar S. Epileptic negative myoclonus. In: Luders HO, Noachtar S, eds. *Epileptic seizures. Pathophysiology and clinical semiology*, pp 473–83. New York: Churchill Livingstone, 2000.

183 Tassinari CA, Rubboli G, Parmeggiani L, Valzania F, Plasmati R, Riguzzi P *et al.* Epileptic negative myoclonus. *Adv Neurol* 1995;**67**:181–97.

184 Vigevano F, Fusco L, Yagi K, Seino M. Tonic seizures. In: Engel J Jr, Pedley TA, eds. *Epilepsy: A comprehensive textbook*, pp 617–25. Philadelphia: Lippincott-Raven, 1997.

185 Holmes GL, Vigevano F. Infantile spasms. In: Engel J Jr, Pedley TA, eds. *Epilepsy: A comprehensive textbook*, pp 627–42. Philadelphia: Lippincott-Raven, 1997.

186 Shields MD, Hicks EM, Macgregor DF, Richey S. Infantile spasms associated with theophylline toxicity. *Acta Paediatr* 1995;**84**:215–17.

187 Yasuhara A, Ochi A, Harada Y, Kobayashi Y. Infantile spasms associated with a histamine H1 antagonist. *Neuropediatrics* 1998;**29**:320–1.

188 Dravet C, Giraud N, Bureau M, Roger J, Gobbi G, Dalla Bernardina B. Benign myoclonus of early infancy or benign non-epileptic infantile spasms. *Neuropediatrics* 1986;**17**:33–8.

189 Noone PG, King M, Loftus BG. Benign neonatal sleep myoclonus. *Irish Med J* 1998;**88**:172.

190 Dravet C. Les epilepsies graves de l'enfant. *Vie Med* 1978;**8**:543–8.

191 Dravet C, Bureau M, Guerrini R, Giraud N, Roger J. Severe myoclonic epilepsy in infants. In: Roger J, Bureau M, Dravet C, Dreifuss FE, Perret A, Wolf P, eds. *Epileptic syndromes in infancy, childhood and adolescence*, pp 75–8. London: John Libbey & Co., 1992.

192 Wakai S, Ikehata M, Nihira H, Ito N, Sueoka H, Kawamoto Y *et al.* "Obtundation status (Dravet)" caused by complex partial status epilepticus in a patient with severe myoclonic epilepsy in infancy. *Epilepsia* 1996;**37**:1020–2.

193 Guerrini R, Dravet C. Severe epileptic encephalopathies of infancy, other than the West syndrome. In: Engel J Jr, Pedley TA, eds. *Epilepsy: A comprehensive textbook.*, pp 2285–302. Philadelphia: Lippincott-Raven, 1997.

194 Nieto-Barrera M, Lillo MM, Rodriguez-Collado C, Candau R, Correa A. Severe myoclonic epilepsy in childhood. Epidemiologic analytical study. *Rev Neurol* 2000;**30**:620–4.

195 Oguni H, Hayashi K, Awaya Y, Fukuyama Y, Osawa M. Severe myoclonic epilepsy in infants – a review based on the Tokyo Women's Medical University series of 84 cases. *Brain Dev* 2001;**23**:736–48.

196 Scheffer IE, Wallace R, Mulley JC, Berkovic SF. Clinical and molecular genetics of myoclonic-astatic epilepsy and severe myoclonic epilepsy in infancy (Dravet syndrome). *Brain Dev* 2001;**23**:732–5.

197 Dravet C. Dravet syndrome (Severe myoclonic epilepsy in infancy). In: Gilman S, ed. *Medlink Neurology*. San Diego, CA: Arbor Publishing, 2002.

198 Peled N, Shorer Z, Peled E, Pillar G. Melatonin effect on seizures in children with severe neurologic deficit disorders. *Epilepsia* 2001;**42**:1208–10.

199 Gastaut H, Broughton R. *Epileptic seizures. Clinical and electrographic features, diagnosis and treatment*. Illinois: Charles C Thomas, 1972.

200 Mori Y. Anatomopathology and pathogeny of the hemiconvulsion-hemiplegia-epilepsy syndrome. Part II. *J Neurosurg Sci* 1979;**23**:1–22.

201 Salih MA, Kabiraj M, Al Jarallah AS, El Desouki M, Othman S, Palkar VA. Hemiconvulsion-hemiplegia-epilepsy syndrome. A clinical, electroencephalographic and neuroradiological study. *Child Nerv Syst* 1997;**13**:257–63.

202 Roger J, Dravet C, Bureau M. Unilateral seizures: hemiconvulsions-hemiplegia syndrome (HH) and hemiconvulsions-hemiplegia-epilepsy syndrome (HHE). *Electroencephalogr Clin Neurophysiol Suppl* 1982;211–21.

203 Freeman JL, Coleman LT, Smith LJ, Shield LK. Hemiconvulsion-hemiplegia-epilepsy syndrome: characteristic early magnetic resonance imaging findings. *J Child Neurol* 2002;**17**:10–16.

204 Herbst F, Heckmann M, Reiss I, Hugens-Penzel M, Gortner L, Neubauer B. Hemiconvulsion-Hemiplegia-Epilepsy-Syndrome (HHE). *Klin Padiatr* 2002;**214**:126–7.

205 Arzimanoglou A, Dravet C. Hemiconvulsion-hemiplegia syndrome. In: Gilman S, ed. *Medlink Neurology*. San Diego, CA: Arbor Publishing, 2002.

206 Tanaka Y, Nakanishi Y, Hamano S, Nara T, Aihara T. Brain perfusion in acute infantile hemiplegia studied with single photon emission computed tomography. *No To Hattatsu* 1994;**26**:68–73.

207   Coppola G, Plouin P, Chiron C, Robain O, Dulac O. Migrating partial seizures in infancy: a malignant disorder with developmental arrest. *Epilepsia* 1995;**36**:1017–24.

208   Okuda K, Yasuhara A, Kamei A, Araki A, Kitamura N, Kobayashi Y. Successful control with bromide of two patients with malignant migrating partial seizures in infancy. *Brain Dev* 2000;**22**:56–9.

209   Dalla Bernardina B, Fontana E, Sgro M, Colamaria V, Elia M. Myoclonic epilepsy ('myoclonic status') in non-progressive encephalopathies. In: Roger J, Bureau M, Dravet C, Dreifuss FE, Perret A, Wolf P, eds. *Epileptic syndromes in infancy, childhood and adolescence*, pp 89–96. London: John Libbey & Co., 1992.

210   Dalla Bernardina B, Fontana E, Darra F. Myoclonic status in nonprogressive encephalopathies. In: Gilman S, ed. *Medlink Neurology*. San Diego, CA: Arbor Publishing, 2002.

211   Chiron C, Plouin P, Dulac O, Mayer M, Ponsot G. Myoclonic epilepsy with non-progressive encephalopathy. *Neurophysiol Clin* 1988;**18**:513–24.

212   Gastaut H. The Lennox-Gastaut syndrome: comments on the syndrome's terminology and nosological position amongst the secondary generalized epilepsies of childhood. *Electroencephalogr Clin Neurophysiol Suppl* 1982;71–84.

213   Beaumanoir A. The Lennox-Gastaut syndrome: a personal study. *Electroencephalogr Clin Neurophysiol Suppl* 1982;85–99.

214   Roger J, Remy C, Bureau M, Oller-Daurella L, Beaumanoir A, Favel P *et al.* Lennox-Gastaut syndrome in the adult. *Rev Neurol (Paris)* 1987;**143**:401–5.

215   Niedermeyer E, Degen R, eds. *The Lennox-Gastaut syndrome*. New York: Alan R Liss, 1988.

216   Aicardi J, Levy Gomes A. Clinical and electroencephalographic symptomatology of the 'genuine' Lennox-Gastaut syndrome and its differentiation from other forms of epilepsy of early childhood. *Epilepsy Res Suppl* 1992;**6**:185–93.

217   Beaumanoir A, Dravet C. The Lennox-Gastaut syndrome. In: Roger J, Bureau M, Dravet C, Dreifuss FE, Perret A, Wolf P, eds. *Epileptic syndromes in infancy, childhood and adolescence*, pp 115–32. London: John Libbey & Co., 1992.

218   Oguni H, Hayashi K, Osawa M. Long-term prognosis of Lennox-Gastaut syndrome. *Epilepsia* 1996;**37** Suppl 3:44–7.

219   Genton P, Dravet C. Lennox-Gastaut syndrome and other childhood epileptic encephalopathies. In: Engel J Jr, Pedley TA, eds. *Epilepsy: A comprehensive textbook.*, pp 2355–66. Philadelphia: Lippincott-Raven, 1997.

220   Aicardi J. Lennox-Gastaut syndrome. In: Wallace S, ed. *Epilepsy in children*, pp 249–61. London: Chapman & Hall, 1996.

221   Blume WT. Pathogenesis of Lennox-Gastaut syndrome: considerations and hypotheses. *Epileptic Disord* 2001;**3**:183–96.

222   Niedermeyer E. Lennox-Gastaut syndrome. Clinical description and diagnosis. *Adv Exp Med Biol* 2002;**497**:61–75.

223   Farrell K. Drug therapy in Lennox-Gastaut syndrome. *Adv Exp Med Biol* 2002;**497**:77–86.

224   Doose H. Myoclonic-astatic epilepsy [Review]. *Epilepsy Res Suppl* 1992;**6**:163–8.

225   Aicardi J. Myoclonic epilepsies difficult to classify either as Lennox-Gastaut syndrome or myoclonic-astatic epilepsy. In: Wallace S, ed. *Epilepsy in children*, pp 271–3. London: Chapman & Hall, 1996.

226   Doose H. Myoclonic-astatic epilepsy. *Epilepsy Res Suppl* 1992;**6**:163–8.

227   Doose H. Myoclonic astatic epilepsy of early childhood. In: Roger J, Dravet C, Bureau M, Dreifuss FE, Wolf P, eds. *Epileptic syndromes in infancy, childhood and adolescence*, pp 103–14. London: John Libbey & Co., 1985.

228   Doose H, Baier WK. Epilepsy with primarily generalized myoclonic-astatic seizures: a genetically determined disease. *Eur J Pediatr* 1987;**146**:550–4.

229   Goldsmith IL, Zupanc ML, Buchhalter JR. Long-term seizure outcome in 74 patients with Lennox-Gastaut syndrome: effects of incorporating MRI head imaging in defining the cryptogenic subgroup. *Epilepsia* 2000;**41**:395–9.

230   Trevathan E, Murphy CC, Yeargin-Allsopp M. Prevalence and descriptive epidemiology of Lennox-Gastaut syndrome among Atlanta children. *Epilepsia* 1997;**38**:1283–8.

231   Rantala H, Putkonen T. Occurrence, outcome, and prognostic factors of infantile spasms and Lennox-Gastaut syndrome. *Epilepsia* 1999;**40**:286–9.

232   Heiskala H. Community-based study of Lennox-Gastaut syndrome. *Epilepsia* 1997;**38**:526–31.

233   Ikeno T, Shigematsu H, Miyakoshi M, Ohba A, Yagi K, Seino M. An analytic study of epileptic falls. *Epilepsia* 1985;**26**:612–21.

234   Parker AP, Ferrie CD, Keevil S, Newbold M, Cox T, Maisey M *et al.* Neuroimaging and spectroscopy in children with epileptic encephalopathies. *Arch Dis Child* 1998;**79**:39–43.

235   Ferrie CD, Marsden PK, Maisey MN, Robinson RO. Cortical and subcortical glucose metabolism in childhood epileptic encephalopathies. *J Neurol Neurosurg Psychiatry* 1997;**63**:181–7.

236 Ferrie CD, Marsden PK, Maisey MN, Robinson RO. Visual and semiquantitative analysis of cortical FDG-PET scans in childhood epileptic encephalopathies. *J Nucl Med* 1997;**38**:1891–4.

237 Chugani HT, Mazziotta JC, Engel J Jr, Phelps ME. The Lennox-Gastaut syndrome: metabolic subtypes determined by 2-deoxy-2[18F]fluoro-D-glucose positron emission tomography. *Ann Neurol* 1987;**21**:4–13.

238 Fitzgerald LF, Stone JL, Hughes JR, Melyn MA, Lansky LL. The Lennox-Gastaut syndrome: electroencephalographic characteristics, clinical correlates, and follow-up studies. *Clin Electroencephalogr* 1992;**23**:180–9.

239 Velasco AL, Boleaga B, Santos N, Velasco F, Velasco M. Electroencephalographic and magnetic resonance correlations in children with intractable seizures of Lennox-Gastaut syndrome and epilepsia partialis continua. *Epilepsia* 1993;**34**:262–70.

240 Hughes JR, Patil VK. Long-term electro-clinical changes in the Lennox-Gastaut syndrome before, during, and after the slow spike-wave pattern. *Clin Electroencephalogr* 2002;**33**:1–7.

241 Kotagal P. Multifocal independent Spike syndrome: relationship to hypsarrhythmia and the slow spike-wave (Lennox-Gastaut) syndrome. *Clin Electroencephalogr* 1995;**26**:23–9.

242 Ogawa K, Kanemoto K, Ishii Y, Koyama M, Shirasaka Y, Kawasaki J et al. Long-term follow-up study of Lennox-Gastaut syndrome in patients with severe motor and intellectual disabilities: with special reference to the problem of dysphagia. *Seizure* 2001;**10**:197–202.

243 Yagi K. Evolution of Lennox-Gastaut syndrome: a long-term longitudinal study. *Epilepsia* 1996;**37** Suppl 3:48–51.

244 Ohtahara S, Ohtsuka Y, Kobayashi K. Lennox-Gastaut syndrome: a new vista. *Psychiatry Clin Neurosci* 1995;**49**:S179–S183.

245 Ohtsuka Y, Amano R, Mizukawa M, Ohtahara S. Long-term prognosis of the Lennox-Gastaut syndrome. *Jpn J Psychiatry Neurol* 1990;**44**:257–64.

246 Yagi K, Seino M. Lennox-Gastaut syndrome – clinical seizure outcome and social prognosis. *Jpn J Psychiatry Neurol* 1990;**44**:374–5.

247 Schmidt D, Bourgeois B. A risk-benefit assessment of therapies for Lennox-Gastaut syndrome. *Drug Saf* 2000;**22**:467–77.

248 Crumrine PK. Lennox-Gastaut syndrome. *J Child Neurol* 2002;**17** Suppl 1:S70–S75.

249 Glauser TA, Levisohn PM, Ritter F, Sachdeo RC. Topiramate in Lennox-Gastaut syndrome: open-label treatment of patients completing a randomized controlled trial. Topiramate YL Study Group. *Epilepsia* 2000;**41** Suppl 1:S86–S90.

250 Siegel H, Kelley K, Stertz B, Reeves-Tyer P, Flamini R, Malow B et al. The efficacy of felbamate as add-on therapy to valproic acid in the Lennox-Gastaut syndrome. *Epilepsy Res* 1999;**34**:91–7.

251 Dulac O, N'Guyen T. The Lennox-Gastaut syndrome. *Epilepsia* 1993;**34** Suppl 7:S7–S17.

252 Parker AP, Polkey CE, Binnie CD, Madigan C, Ferrie CD, Robinson RO. Vagal nerve stimulation in epileptic encephalopathies. *Pediatrics* 1999;**103**:778–82.

253 Engel J Jr, ed. *Surgical treatment of the epilepsies.* New York: Raven, 1993.

254 Gates JR. Surgery in Lennox-Gastaut syndrome. Corpus callosum division for children. *Adv Exp Med Biol* 2002;**497**:87–98.

255 Beaumanoir A. The Landau-Kleffner syndrome. In: Roger J, Bureau M, Dravet C, Dreifuss FE, Perret A, Wolf P, eds. *Epileptic syndromes in infancy, childhood and adolescence*, pp 231–43. London: John Libbey & Co., 1992.

256 Smith MC. Landau-Kleffner syndrome and continuous spikes and waves during slow sleep. In: Engel J Jr, Pedley TA, eds. *Epilepsy: A comprehensive textbook*, Philadelphia: Lippincott-Raven, 1997.

257 Dugas M, Franc S, Gerard CL, Lecendreux M. Evolution of acquired epileptic aphasia with or without continuous spikes and waves during slow sleep. In: Beaumanoir A, Bureau M, Deonna T, Mira L, Tassinari CA, eds. *Continuous spikes and waves during slow sleep. Electrical status epilepticus during slow sleep. Acquired epileptic aphasia and related conditions*, pp 47–55. John Libbey & Co., 1995.

258 Deonna T, Roulet E. Acquired epileptic aphasia (AEA): definition of the syndrome and current problems. In: Beaumanoir A, Bureau M, Deonna T, Mira L, Tassinari CA, eds. *Continuous spikes and waves during slow sleep. Electrical status epilepticus during slow sleep. Acquired epileptic aphasia and related conditions*, pp 37–45. John Libbey & Co., 1995.

259 Morrell F, Whisler WW, Smith MC, Hoeppner TJ, de Toledo-Morrell L, Pierre-Louis SJ et al. Landau-Kleffner syndrome. Treatment with subpial intracortical transection. *Brain* 1995;**118**:1529–46.

260 Beaumanoir A, Bureau M, Mira L. Identification of the syndrome. In: Beaumanoir A, Bureau M, Deonna T, Mira L, Tassinari CA, eds. *Continuous spikes and waves during slow sleep. Electrical status epilepticus during slow sleep. Acquired epileptic aphasia and related conditions*, pp 243–9. John Libbey & Co., 1995.

261 da Silva EA, Chugani DC, Muzik O, Chugani HT. Landau-Kleffner syndrome: metabolic

abnormalities in temporal lobe are a common feature. *J Child Neurol* 1997;**12**:489–95.

262 Genton P, Guerrini R. What differentiates Landau-Kleffner syndrome from the syndrome of continuous spikes and waves during slow sleep? [letter; comment]. *Arch Neurol* 1993;**50**:1008–9.

263 Sawhney IM, Robertson IJ, Polkey CE, Binnie CD, Elwes RD. Multiple subpial transection: a review of 21 cases. *J Neurol Neurosurg Psychiatr* 1995;**58**:344–9.

264 Bureau M. 'Continuous spikes and waves during slow sleep'(CSWS): definition of the syndrome. In: Beaumanoir A, Bureau M, Deonna T, Mira L, Tassinari CA, eds. *Continuous spikes and waves during slow sleep. Electrical status epilepticus during slow sleep. Acquired epileptic aphasia and related conditions*, pp 17–26. London: John Libbey & Co., 1995.

265 Tassinari CA. The problems of 'continuous spikes and waves during slow sleep' or 'electrical status epilepticus during slow sleep' today. In: Beaumanoir A, Bureau M, Deonna T, Mira L, Tassinari CA, eds. *Continuous spikes and waves during slow sleep. Electrical status epilepticus during slow sleep. Acquired epileptic aphasia and related conditions*, pp 251–5. London: John Libbey & Co., 1995.

266 Beaumanoir A, Bureau M, Deonna T, Mira L, Tassinari CA. *Continuous spike and waves during slow sleep. Electrical status epilepticus during slow sleep*. London: John Libbey & Co., 1995.

267 Tassinari CA, Volpi L, Michellluchi R. Electrical status epilepticus during slow sleep. In: Gilman S, ed. *Medlink Neurology*. San Diego, CA: Arbor Publishing, 2002.

268 Tassinari CA, Bureau M, Dravet C, Dalla Bernardina B, Roger J. Epilepsy with continuous spikes amd waves during slow sleep – otherwise described as ESES (epilepsy with electrical status epilepticus during slow sleep). In: Roger J, Bureau M, Dravet C, Dreifuss FE, Perret A, Wolf P, eds. *Epileptic syndromes in infancy, childhood and adolescence*, pp 245–56. London: John Libbey & Co., 1992.

269 Koutroumanidis M. Panayiotopoulos syndrome: a common benign but underdiagnosed and unexplored early childhood seizure syndrome [Editorial]. *BMJ* 2002;**324**:1228–9.

270 Ferrie CD, Grunewald RA. Panayiotopoulos syndrome: a common and benign childhood epilepsy [Commentary]. *Lancet* 2001;**357**:821–3.

271 Lada C, Skiadas K, Theodorou V, Covanis A. A study of 43 patients with Panayiotopoulos syndrome: a common and benign childhood seizure suceptibility. *Epilepsia* (in press) 2002.

272 Lerman P. Benign childhood epilepsy with centrotemporal spikes. In: Engel J Jr, Pedley TA, eds. *Epilepsy: A comprehensive textbook*, pp

2307–14. Philadelphia: Lippincott-Raven, 1997.

273 Beaussart M, Loiseau P. The discovery of "benign rolandic epilepsy". In: Berkovic SF, Genton P, Hirsch E, Plouin P, eds. *Genetics of focal epilepsies*, pp 3–6. London: John Libbey & Co., 1998.

274 Loiseau P, Duche B. Benign rolandic epilepsy [Review]. *Adv Neurol* 1992;**57**:411–17.

275 Bouma PA, Bovenkerk AC, Westendorp RG, Brouwer OF. The course of benign partial epilepsy of childhood with centrotemporal spikes: a meta-analysis. *Neurology* 1997;**48**:430–7.

276 Stephani U, ed. Spectrum of rolandic epilepsy: agreements, disagreements and open questions. *Epileptic Disord* 2000;**2** (Suppl 1).

277 Neubauer BA, Fiedler B, Himmelein B, Kampfer F, Lassker U, Schwabe G et al. Centrotemporal spikes in families with rolandic epilepsy: linkage to chromosome 15q14. *Neurology* 1998;**51**:1608–12.

278 Legarda S, Jayakar P, Duchowny M, Alvarez L, Resnick T. Benign rolandic epilepsy: high central and low central subgroups. *Epilepsia* 1994;**35**:1125–9.

279 Baglietto MG, Battaglia FM, Nobili L, Tortorelli S, De Negri E, Calevo MG et al. Neuropsychological disorders related to interictal epileptic discharges during sleep in benign epilepsy of childhood with centrotemporal or Rolandic spikes. *Dev Med Child Neurol* 2001;**43**:407–12.

280 Yung AW, Park YD, Cohen MJ, Garrison TN. Cognitive and behavioral problems in children with centrotemporal spikes. *Pediatr Neurol* 2000;**23**:391–5.

281 Fejerman N, Caraballo R, Tenembaum SN. Atypical evolutions of benign partial epilepsy of infancy with centro-temporal spikes. *Rev Neurol* 2000;**31**:389–96.

282 Fejerman N, Caraballo R, Tenembaum SN. Atypical evolutions of benign localization-related epilepsies in children: are they predictable? *Epilepsia* 2000;**41**:380–90.

283 Panayiotopoulos CP. Inhibitory effect of central vision on occipital lobe seizures. *Neurology* 1981;**31**:1330–3.

284 Panayiotopoulos CP. Vomiting as an ictal manifestation of epileptic seizures and syndromes. *J Neurol Neurosurg Psychiatr* 1988;**51**:1448–51.

285 Ferrie CD, Beaumanoir A, Guerrini R, Kivity S, Vigevano F, Takaishi Y et al. Early-onset benign occipital seizure susceptibility syndrome. *Epilepsia* 1997;**38**:285–93.

286 Oguni H, Hayashi K, Imai K, Hirano Y, Mutoh A, Osawa M. Study on the early-onset variant

of benign childhood epilepsy with occipital paroxysms otherwise described as early-onset benign occipital seizure susceptibility syndrome. *Epilepsia* 1999;**40**:1020–30.

287 Kivity S, Ephraim T, Weitz R, Tamir A. Childhood epilepsy with occipital paroxysms: clinical variants in 134 patients. *Epilepsia* 2000;**41**:1522–3.

288 Caraballo R, Cersosimo R, Medina C, Fejerman N. Panayiotopoulos-type benign childhood occipital epilepsy: a prospective study. *Neurology* 2000;**55**:1096–100.

289 Berg AT, Panayiotopoulos CP. Diversity in epilepsy and a newly recognized benign childhood syndrome [Editorial]. *Neurology* 2000;**55**:1073–4.

290 Vigevano F, Lispi ML, Ricci S. Early onset benign occipital susceptibility syndrome: video-EEG documentation of an illustrative case. *Clin Neurophysiol* 2000;**111** Suppl 2:S81–S86.

291 Martinovic Z. Panayiotopoulos syndrome. *Lancet* 2001;**358**:69.

292 Oguni H. Panayiotopoulos syndrome. *Lancet* 2001;**358**:69.

293 Panayiotopoulos CP. Benign childhood occipital seizures (Panayiotopoulos syndrome). In: Gilman S, ed. *Medlink Neurology*. San Diego, CA: Arbor Publishing, 2002.

294 Lada C, Covanis A, Skiadas K, Loli N, Theodorou V. Panayiotopoulos syndrome: benign childhood seizures with ictal vomiting, occipital and extra-occipital spikes or normal EEG. *Epileptic Disord* 2002;**4**:58.

295 Luders HO, Noachtar S, Burgess RC. Semiologic classification of epileptic seizures. In: Luders HO, Noachtar S, eds. *Epileptic seizures. Pathophysiology and clinical semiology*, pp 263–85. New York: Churchill Livingstone, 2000.

296 Burgess RC. Autonomic signs associated with seizures. In: Luders HO, Noachtar S, eds. *Epileptic seizures. Pathophysiology and clinical semiology*, pp 631–41. New York: Churchill Livingstone, 2000.

297 Panayiotopoulos CP. Panayiotopoulos syndrome. *Lancet* 2001;**358**:68–9.

298 Wieser HG. Aura Continua. In: Engel J Jr, Fejerman N, Williamson PD, eds. *Epilepsy International Leaque against Epilepsy Task Force on Classification*. San Diego, CA: Arbor Publishing, 2001.

299 Beaumanoir A. Semiology of occipital seizures in infants and children. In: Andermann F, Beaumanoir A, Mira L, Roger J, Tassinari CA, eds. *Occipital seizures and epilepsies in children*, pp 71–86. London: John Libbey and Co., 1993.

300 Ferrie CD, Panayiotopoulos CP. Idiopathic generalised epilepsy with generalised tonic clonic seizures on awakening. In: Wallace SJ, Farrell K, eds. *Epilepsy in children*, 2nd edn. London: Edward Arnold, 2002.

301 Caraballo RH, Astorino F, Cersosimo R, Soprano AM, Fejerman N. Atypical evolution in childhood epilepsy with occipital paroxysms (Panayiotopoulos type). *Epileptic Disord* 2001;**3**:157–62.

302 Gastaut H. A new type of epilepsy: benign partial epilepsy of childhood with occipital spike-waves. *Clin Electroencephalogr* 1982;**13**:13–22.

303 Gastaut H, Zifkin BG. Benign epilepsy of childhood with occipital spike and wave complexes. In: Andermann F, Lugaresi E, eds. *Migraine and epilepsy*, pp 47–81. Boston: Butterworths, 1987.

304 Gastaut H, Roger J, Bureau M. Benign epilepsy of childhood with occipital paroxysms. Up-date. In: Roger J, Bureau M, Dravet C, Dreifuss FE, Perret A, Wolf P, eds. *Epileptic syndromes in infancy, childhood and adolescence*, pp 201–17. London: John Libbey & Co., 1992.

305 Panayiotopoulos CP. Idiopathic childhood occipital epilepsies. In: Roger J, Bureau M, Dravet C, Genton P, Tassinari CA, Wolf P, eds. *Epileptic syndromes in infancy, childhood and adolescence*, 3rd edn. pp 203–28. London: John Libbey & Co., 2002.

306 Panayiotopoulos CP. Elementary visual hallucinations, blindness, and headache in idiopathic occipital epilepsy: differentiation from migraine. *J Neurol Neurosurg Psychiatry* 1999;**66**:536–40.

307 Gobbi G, Bertani G, Italian Working Group on Coeliac Disease and Epilepsy. Coeliac disease and epilepsy. In: Gobbi G, Andermann F, Naccarato S, Banchini G, eds. *Epilepsy and other neurological disorders in coeliac disease*, pp 65–79. London: John Libbey & Co., 1997.

308 Guerrini R, Bonanni P, Parmeggiani A. Idiopathic photosensitive occipital lobe epilepsy. In: Gilman S, ed. *Medlink Neurology*. San Diego, CA: Arbor Publishing, 2002.

309 Guerrini R, Bonanni P, Parmeggiani L, Thomas P, Mattia D, Harvey AS *et al.* Induction of partial seizures by visual stimulation. Clinical and electroencephalographic features and evoked potential studies. *Adv Neurol* 1998;**75**:159–78.

310 Dalla Bernardina B, Colamaria V, Chiamenti C, Capovilla G, Trevisan E, Tassinari CA. Benign partial epilepsy with affective symptoms ('benign psychomotor epilepsy'). In: Roger J, Bureau M, Dravet C, Dreifuss FE, Perret A, Wolf P, eds. *Epileptic syndromes in infancy, childhood and adolescence*, pp 219–23. London: John Libbey & Co., 1992.

311 Tassinari CA, De Marco P. Benign partial epilepsy with extreme somato-sensory evoked

potentials. In: Roger J, Bureau M, Dravet C, Dreifuss FE, Wolf P, Perret A, eds. *Epileptic syndromes in infancy, childhood and adolescence*, pp 225–9. London: John Libbey & Co., 1992.

312 Fonseca LC, Tedrus GM. Somatosensory evoked spikes and epileptic seizures: a study of 385 cases. *Clin Electroencephalogr* 2000;**31**:71–5.

313 Beaumanoir A, Nahory A. Benign partial epilepsies: 11 cases of frontal partial epilepsy with favorable prognosis. *Revue d'Electroencephalographie et de Neurophysiologie Clinique* 1983;**13**:207–11.

314 Martin-Santidrian MA, Garaizar C, Prats-Vinas JM. Frontal lobe epilepsy in infancy: is there a benign partial frontal lobe epilepsy?. *Rev Neurol* 1998;**26**:919–23.

315 Bagdorf R, Lee SI. Midline spikes: is it another benign EEG pattern of childhood? *Epilepsia* 1993;**34**:271–4.

316 Mitchell WG. Status epilepticus and acute repetitive seizures in children, adolescents, and young adults: etiology, outcome, and treatment. *Epilepsia* 1996;**37** Suppl 1:S74–S80.

317 Koren G. Intranasal midazolam for febrile seizures. A step forward in treating a common and distressing condition. *BMJ* 2000;**321**:64–5.

318 Lahat E, Goldman M, Barr J, Bistritzer T, Berkovitch M. Comparison of intranasal midazolam with intravenous diazepam for treating febrile seizures in children: prospective randomised study. *BMJ* 2000;**321**:83–6.

319 Scott RC, Besag FM, Neville BG. Intranasal midazolam for treating febrile seizures in children. Buccal midazolam should be preferred to nasal midazolam. *BMJ* 2001;**322**:107.

320 Balslev T. Parental reactions to a child's first febrile convulsion. A follow-up investigation. *Acta Paediatr Scand* 1991;**80**:466–9.

321 Panayiotopoulos CP. Benign childhood partial epilepsies: benign childhood seizure susceptibility syndromes [editorial]. *J Neurol Neurosurg Psychiatry* 1993;**56**:2–5.

322 Loiseau P, Orgogozo JM. An unrecognized syndrome of benign focal epileptic seizures in teenagers? *Lancet* 1978;**2**:1070–1.

323 Loiseau P, Louiset P. Benign partial seizures of adolescence. In: Roger J, Bureau M, Dravet C, Dreifuss FE, Perret A, Wolf P, eds. *Epileptic syndromes in infancy, childhood and adolescence*, pp 343–5. London: John Libbey & Co., 1992.

324 Panayiotopoulos CP. Benign partial seizures of adolescence. In: Wallace S, ed. *Epilepsy in children*, pp 377–8. London: Chapman & Hall, 1996.

325 Caraballo R, Galicchio S, Granana N, Cersosimo R, Fejerman N. Benign partial convulsions in adolescence. *Rev Neurol* 1999;**28**:669–71.

326 King MA, Newton MR, Berkovic SF. Benign partial seizures of adolescence. *Epilepsia* 1999;**40**:1244–7.

327 Capovilla G, Gambardella A, Romeo A, Beccaria F, Montagnini A, Labate A *et al*. Benign partial epilepsies of adolescence: a report of 37 new cases. *Epilepsia* 2001;**42**:1549–52.

328 Loiseau P, Jallon P. Isolated partial seizures of adolescence. In: Roger J, Bureau M, Dravet C, Genton P, Tassinari CA, Wolf P, eds. *Epileptic syndromes in infancy, childhood and adolescence*, 3rd edn. pp 327–30. London: John Libbey & Co., 2002.

329 Mauri JA, Iniguez C, Jerico I, Morales F. Benign partial seizures of adolescence. *Epilepsia* 1996;**37** Suppl 4:102.

330 Jallon P, Loiseau J, Loiseau P, de Zelicourt M, Motte J, Vallee L *et al*. The risk of recurrence after a first unprovoked seizure in adolescence. *Epilepsia* 1999;**40** Suppl 7:87–8.

331 Malafosse A, Genton P, Hirsch E, Marescaux C, Broglin D, Bernasconi R, eds. *Idiopathic generalised epilepsies*. London: John Libbey & Co., 1994.

332 Duncan JS, Panayiotopoulos CP, eds. *Typical absences and related epileptic syndromes*. London: Churchill Communications Europe, 1995.

333 Delgado-Escueta AV, Medina MT, Serratosa JM, Castroviejo IP, Gee MN, Weissbecker K *et al*. Mapping and positional cloning of common idiopathic generalized epilepsies: juvenile myoclonus epilepsy and childhood absence epilepsy. *Adv Neurol* 1999;**79**:351–74.

334 Durner M, Keddache MA, Tomasini L, Shinnar S, Resor SR, Cohen J *et al*. Genome scan of idiopathic generalized epilepsy: evidence for major susceptibility gene and modifying genes influencing the seizure type. *Ann Neurol* 2001;**49**:328–35.

335 Panayiotopoulos CP. Absence epilepsies. In: Engel J Jr, Pedley TA, eds. *Epilepsy: A comprehensive textbook*, pp 2327–46. Philadelphia: Lippincott-Raven, 1997.

336 Panayiotopoulos CP. Typical absence seizures. In: Gilman S, ed. *Medlink Neurology*. San Diego, CA: Arbor Publishing, 2002.

337 Snead OC III, Depaulis A, Vergnes M, Marescaux C. Absence epilepsy: advances in experimental animal models. *Adv Neurol* 1999;**79**:253–78.

338 Loiseau P, Panayiotopoulos CP, Hirsch E. Childhood absence epilepsy and related syndromes. In: Roger J, Bureau M, Dravet C, Genton P, Tassinari CA, Wolf P, eds. *Epileptic syndromes in infancy, childhood and adolescence*, 3rd edn. pp 285–304. London: John Libbey & Co., 2002.

339 Panayiotopoulos CP, Koutroumanidis M, Giannakodimos S, Agathonikou A. Idiopathic generalised epilepsy in adults manifested by phantom absences, generalised tonic-clonic seizures, and frequent absence status. *J Neurol Neurosurg Psychiatr* 1997;**63**:622–7.

340 Janz D, Durner M. Juvenile myoclonic epilepsy. In: Engel J Jr, Pedley TA, eds. *Epilepsy: A comprehensive textbook*, pp 2389–400. Philadelphia: Lippincott-Raven, 1997.

341 Panayiotopoulos CP, Obeid T, Tahan AR. Juvenile myoclonic epilepsy: a 5-year prospective study. *Epilepsia* 1994;**35**:285–96.

342 Diagnosing juvenile myoclonic epilepsy [editorial]. *Lancet* 1992;**340**:759–60.

343 Wolf P. Epilepsy with grand mal on awakening. In: Roger J, Bureau M, Dravet C, Dreifuss FE, Perret A, Wolf P, eds. *Epileptic syndromes in infancy, childhood and adolescence*, pp 329–41. London: John Libbey & Co., 1992.

344 Shorvon SD. Status epilepticus: its clinical features and treatment in children and adults. Cambridge: Cambridge University Press, 1994.

345 Shorvon S. Absence status epilepticus. In: Duncan JS, Panayiotopoulos CP, eds. *Typical absences and related epileptic syndromes*, pp 263–74. London: Churchill Communications Europe, 1995.

346 Agathonikou A, Panayiotopoulos CP, Giannakodimos S, Koutroumanidis M. Typical absence status in adults: diagnostic and syndromic considerations. *Epilepsia* 1998;**39**:1265–76.

347 Panayiotopoulos CP. Absence status epilepticus. In: Gilman S, ed. *Medlink Neurology*. San Diego, CA: Arbor Publishing, 2002.

348 Thomas P, Andermann F. Late-onset absence status epilepticus is most often situation-related. In: Malafosse A, Genton P, Hirsch E, Marescaux C, Broglin D, Bernasconi R, eds. *Idiopathic generalized epilepsies*, pp 95–109. London: John Libbey & Co., 1994.

349 Thomas P. Absence status epilepsy. *Rev Neurol (Paris)* 1999;**155**:1023–38.

350 Engel J Jr. Classifications of the International League Against Epilepsy: time for reappraisal [comment]. *Epilepsia* 1998;**39**:1014–17.

351 Engel J Jr. Classification of Epileptic Disorders. *Epilepsia* 2001;**42**:316.

352 Andermann F, Berkovic SF. Idiopathic generalized epilepsy with generalised and other seizures in adolescence. *Epilepsia* 2001;**42**:317–20.

353 Doose H. Das akinetische petit mal. *Arch Psychiatr Nervenkr* 1965;**205**:638–54.

354 Doose H, Gerken H, Leonhardt T, Volz E, Volz C. Centrencephalic myoclonic-astatic petit mal. Clinical and genetic investigation. *Neuropaediatrie* 1970;**2**:59–78.

355 Aicardi J. Myoclonic-astatic epilepsy. In: Wallace S, ed. *Epilepsy in children*, pp 263–70. London: Chapman & Hall, 1996.

356 Oguni H, Fukuyama Y, Tanaka T, Hayashi K, Funatsuka M, Sakauchi M *et al.* Myoclonic-astatic epilepsy of early childhood – clinical and EEG analysis of myoclonic-astatic seizures, and discussions on the nosology of the syndrome. *Brain Dev* 2001;**23**:757–64.

357 Dulac O, Dreifuss F. Myoclonic-astatic epilepsy of childhood. In: Gilman S, ed. *Medlink Neurology*. San Diego, CA: Arbor Publishing, 2002.

358 Kaminska A, Ickowicz A, Plouin P, Bru MF, Dellatolas G, Dulac O. Delineation of cryptogenic Lennox-Gastaut syndrome and myoclonic astatic epilepsy using multiple correspondence analysis. *Epilepsy Res* 1999;**36**:15–29.

359 Aicardi J, Chevrie JJ. Atypical benign partial epilepsy of childhood. *Dev Med Child Neurol* 1982;**24**:281–92.

360 Fejerman N. Atypical evolution of benign partial epilepsy in children. *Rev Neurol* 1996;**24**:1415–20.

361 Loiseau P, Panayiotopoulos CP. Childhood absence epilepsy. In: Gilman S, ed. *Medlink Neurology*. San Diego, CA: Arbor Publishing, 2002.

362 Crunelli V, Leresche N. Childhood absence epilepsy: genes, channels, neurons and networks. *Nat Rev Neurosci* 2002;**3**:371–82.

363 Lennox WG, Lennox MA. *Epilepsy and related disorders*. Boston: Little, Brown & Co., 1960.

364 Tassinari CA, Rubboli G, Michellluchi R. Epilepsy with myoclonic absences. In: Gilman S, ed. *Medlink Neurology*. San Diego, CA: Arbor Publishing, 2002.

365 Verrotti A, Greco R, Chiarelli F, Domizio S, Sabatino G, Morgese G. Epilepsy with myoclonic absences with early onset: a follow-up study. *J Child Neurol* 1999;**14**:746–9.

366 Tassinari CA, Bureau M, Thomas P. Epilepsy with myoclonic absences. In: Roger J, Bureau M, Dravet C, Dreifuss FE, Perret A, Wolf P, eds. *Epileptic syndromes in infancy, childhood and adolescence*, pp 151–60. London: John Libbey & Co., 1992.

367 Tassinari CA, Michelucci R, Rubboli G, Passarelli D, Riguzzi P, Parmeggiani L *et al.* Myoclonic absence epilepsy. In: Duncan JS, Panayiotopoulos CP, eds. *Typical absences and related epileptic syndromes*, pp 187–95. London: Churchill Communications Europe, 1995.

368 Panayiotopoulos CP, Obeid T, Waheed G. Differentiation of typical absence seizures in epileptic syndromes. A video EEG study of 224 seizures in 20 patients. *Brain* 1989;**112**:1039–56.

369 Elia M, Guerrini R, Musumeci SA, Bonanni P, Gambardella A, Aguglia U. Myoclonic absence-like seizures and chromosome abnormality syndromes. *Epilepsia* 1998;**39**:660–3.

370 Ferrie CD, Giannakodimos S, Robinson RO, Panayiotopoulos CP. Symptomatic typical absence seizures. In: Duncan JS, Panayiotopoulos CP, eds. *Typical absences and related epileptic syndromes*, pp 241–52. London: Churchill Communications Europe, 1995.

371 Wolf P. Juvenile absence epilepsy. In: Roger J, Bureau M, Dravet C, Dreifuss FE, Perret A, Wolf P, eds. *Epileptic syndromes in infancy, childhood and adolescence*, pp 307–12. London: John Libbey & Co., 1992.

372 Obeid T. Clinical and genetic aspects of juvenile absence epilepsy. *J Neurol* 1994;**241**:487–91.

373 Panayiotopoulos CP, Giannakodimos S, Chroni E. Typical absences in adults. In: Duncan JS, Panayiotopoulos CP, eds. *Typical absences and related epileptic syndromes*, pp 289–99. London: Churchill Communications Europe, 1995.

374 Osservatorio Regionale per L'Epilessia (OREp) L. ILAE classification of epilepsies: its applicability and practical value of different diagnostic categories. Osservatorio Regionale per L'Epilessia (OREp), Lombardy. *Epilepsia* 1996;**37**:1051–9.

375 Doose H, Volzke E, Scheffner D. Verlaufsformen kindlicher epilepsien mit spike wave-absencen. *Arch Psychiatr Nervenkr* 1965;**207**:394–415.

376 Oller L. Prospective study of the differences between the syndromes of infantile absence epilepsy and syndromes of juvenile absence epilepsy. *Rev Neurol* 1996;**24**:930–6.

377 Berkovic SF, Howell RA, Hay DA, Hopper JL. Epilepsies in twins. In: Wolf P, ed. *Epileptic seizures and syndromes*, pp 157–64. London: John Libbey & Co., 1994.

378 Bianchi A, and the Italian LAE Collaborative Group. Study of concordance of symptoms in families with absence epilepsies. In: Duncan JS, Panayiotopoulos CP, eds. *Typical absences and related epileptic syndromes*, pp 328–37. London: Churchill Communications Europe, 1995.

379 Durner M, Zhou G, Fu D, Abreu P, Shinnar S, Resor SR et al. Evidence for linkage of adolescent-onset idiopathic generalized epilepsies to chromosome 8-and genetic heterogeneity. *Am J Hum Genet* 1999;**64**:1411–19.

380 Sander T, Hildmann T, Kretz R, Furst R, Sailer U, Bauer G et al. Allelic association of juvenile absence epilepsy with a GluR5 kainate receptor gene (GRIK1) polymorphism. *Am J Med Genet* 1997;**74**:416–21.

381 Meencke HJ, Janz D. The significance of microdysgenesia in primary generalized epilepsy: an answer to the considerations of Lyon and Gastaut. *Epilepsia* 1985;**26**:368–71.

382 Woermann FG, Sisodiya SM, Free SL, Duncan JS. Quantitative MRI in patients with idiopathic generalized epilepsy. Evidence of widespread cerebral structural changes. *Brain* 1998;**121**:1661–7.

383 Panayiotopoulos CP, Chroni E, Daskalopoulos C, Baker A, Rowlinson S, Walsh P. Typical absence seizures in adults: clinical, EEG, video-EEG findings and diagnostic/syndromic considerations. *J Neurol Neurosurg Psychiatr* 1992;**55**:1002–8.

384 Grunewald RA, Panayiotopoulos CP. Juvenile myoclonic epilepsy. A review. *Arch Neurol* 1993;**50**:594–8.

385 Genton P, Gelisse P. Juvenile myoclonic epilepsy. *Arch Neurol* 2001;**58**:1487–90.

386 Schmitz B, Sander T, eds. *Juvenile myoclonic epilepsy: the Janz syndrome*. Petersfield. Wrightson Biomedical, 1999.

387 Janz D, Christian W. Impulsiv-Petit mal. Zeitschrift f Nervenheilkunde.1957;176:346–386. [Translated into English by Genton P]. In: Malafosse A, Genton P, Hirsch E, Marescaux C, Broglin D, Bernasconi R, eds. *Idiopathic generalised epilepsies*, pp 229–51. London: John Libbey & Co., 1957.

388 Delgado-Escueta AV, Enrile-Bacsal F. Juvenile myoclonic epilepsy of Janz. *Neurology* 1984;**34**:285–94.

389 Panayiotopoulos CP. Juvenile myoclonic epilepsy: an underdiagnosed syndrome. In: Wolf P, ed. *Epileptic seizures and syndromes*, pp 221–30. London: John Libbey & Co., 1994.

390 Oguni H, Mukahira K, Oguni M, Uehara T, Su YH, Izumi T et al. Video-polygraphic analysis of myoclonic seizures in juvenile myoclonic epilepsy. *Epilepsia* 1994;**35**:307–16.

391 Panayiotopoulos CP, Obeid T, Waheed G. Absences in juvenile myoclonic epilepsy: a clinical and video- electroencephalographic study. *Ann Neurol* 1989;**25**:391–7.

392 Canevini MP, Mai R, Di Marco C, Bertin C, Minotti L, Pontrelli V et al. Juvenile myoclonic epilepsy of Janz: clinical observations in 60 patients. *Seizure* 1992;**1**:291–8.

393 Salas Puig J, Tunon A, Vidal JA, Mateos V, Guisasola LM, Lahoz CH. Janz's juvenile myoclonic epilepsy: a little-known frequent syndrome. A study of 85 patients. *Med Clin (Barc)* 1994;**103**:684–9.

394 Panayiotopoulos CP, Obeid T. Juvenile myoclonic epilepsy: an autosomal recessive disease. *Ann Neurol* 1989;**25**:440–3.

395 Janz D. Juvenile myoclonic epilepsy. Epilepsy with impulsive petit mal. *Cleve Clin J Med* 1989;**56** Suppl Pt 1:S23–S33; discussion S40–S42.

396 Serratosa JM, Delgado-Escueta AV, Medina MT, Zhang Q, Iranmanesh R, Sparkes RS. Clinical and genetic analysis of a large pedigree with juvenile myoclonic epilepsy. *Ann Neurol* 1996;**39**:187–95.

397 Tsuboi T, Christian W. On the genetics of the primary generalised epilepsy with sporadic myoclonus of impulsive petit mal type. *Humangenetik* 1973;**19**:155–82.

398 Delgado-Escueta AV, Greenberg D, Weissbecker K, Liu A, Treiman L, Sparkes R *et al.* Gene mapping in the idiopathic generalized epilepsies: juvenile myoclonic epilepsy, childhood absence epilepsy, epilepsy with grand mal seizures, and early childhood myoclonic epilepsy. *Epilepsia* 1990;**31** Suppl 3:S19–29:S19–S29.

399 Elmslie FV, Rees M, Williamson MP, Kerr M, Kjeldsen MJ, Pang KA *et al.* Genetic mapping of a major susceptibility locus for juvenile myoclonic epilepsy on chromosome 15q. *Hum Mol Genet* 1997;**6**:1329–34.

400 Taske NL, Williamson MP, Makoff A, Bate L, Curtis D, Kerr M *et al.* Evaluation of the positional candidate gene CHRNA7 at the juvenile myoclonic epilepsy locus (EJM2) on chromosome 15q13-14. *Epilepsy Res* 2002;**49**:157–72.

401 Suzuki T, Ganesh S, Agarwala KL, Morita R, Sugimoto Y, Inazawa J *et al.* A novel gene in the chromosomal region for juvenile myoclonic epilepsy on 6p12 encodes a brain-specific lysosomal membrane protein. *Biochem Biophys Res Commun* 2001;**288**:626–36.

402 Greenberg DA, Durner M, Shinnar S, Resor S, Rosenbaum D, Klotz I *et al.* Association of HLA class II alleles in patients with juvenile myoclonic epilepsy compared with patients with other forms of adolescent-onset generalized epilepsy. *Neurology* 1996;**47**:750–5.

403 Obeid T, el Rab MO, Daif AK, Panayiotopoulos CP, Halim K, Bahakim H *et al.* Is HLA-DRW13 (W6) associated with juvenile myoclonic epilepsy in Arab patients? *Epilepsia* 1994;**35**:319–21.

404 Le Hellard S, Neidhart E, Thomas P, Feingold J, Malafosse A, Tafti M. Lack of association between juvenile myoclonic epilepsy and HLA-DR13. *Epilepsia* 1999;**40**:117–19.

405 Woermann FG, Free SL, Koepp MJ, Sisodiya SM, Duncan JS. Abnormal cerebral structure in juvenile myoclonic epilepsy demonstrated with voxel-based analysis of MRI. *Brain* 1999;**122**:2101–8.

406 Panayiotopoulos CP, Tahan R, Obeid T. Juvenile myoclonic epilepsy: factors of error involved in the diagnosis and treatment. *Epilepsia* 1991;**32**:672–6.

407 Grunewald RA, Chroni E, Panayiotopoulos CP. Delayed diagnosis of juvenile myoclonic epilepsy. *J Neurol Neurosurg Psychiatry* 1992;**55**:497–9.

408 Wirrell EC, Camfield CS, Camfield PR, Gordon KE, Dooley JM. Long-term prognosis of typical childhood absence epilepsy: remission or progression to juvenile myoclonic epilepsy. *Neurology* 1996;**47**:912–18.

409 Penry JK, Dean JC, Riela AR. Juvenile myoclonic epilepsy: long-term response to therapy. *Epilepsia* 1989;30 Suppl 4:S19–S23; discussion S24–S27.

410 Gelisse P, Genton P, Thomas P, Rey M, Samuelian JC, Dravet C. Clinical factors of drug resistance in juvenile myoclonic epilepsy. *J Neurol Neurosurg Psychiatry* 2001;**70**:240–3.

411 Obeid T, Panayiotopoulos CP. Clonazepam in juvenile myoclonic epilepsy. *Epilepsia* 1989;**30**:603–6.

412 Buchanan N. The use of lamotrigine in juvenile myoclonic epilepsy. *Seizure* 1996;**5**:149–51.

413 Isojarvi JI, Rattya J, Myllyla VV, Knip M, Koivunen R, Pakarinen AJ *et al.* Valproate, lamotrigine, and insulin-mediated risks in women with epilepsy. *Ann Neurol* 1998;**43**:446–51.

414 Genton P, Bauer J, Duncan S, Taylor AE, Balen AH, Eberle A *et al.* On the association between valproate and polycystic ovary syndrome. *Epilepsia* 2001;**42**:295–304.

415 Roger J, Bureau M, Oller Ferrer-Vidal L, Oller-Daurella L, Saltarelli A, Genton P. Clinical and electroencephalographic characteristics of idiopathic generalised epilepsies. In: Malafosse A, Genton P, Hirsch E, Marescaux C, Broglin D, Bernasconi R, eds. *Idiopathic generalised epilepsies*, pp 7–18. London: John Libbey & Co., 1994.

416 Oller-Daurella LF-V, Oller L. *5000 epilepticos. Clinica y evolucion.* Barcelona: Ciba-Geigy, 1994.

417 Janz D. Epilepsy with grand mal on awakening and sleep-waking cycle. *Clin Neurophysiol* 2000;**111** Suppl 2:S103–S110.

418 Janz D. Pitfalls in the diagnosis of grand mal on awakening. In: Wolf P, ed. *Epileptic seizures and syndromes*, pp 213–20. London: John Libbey & Co., 1994.

419 Janz D. Die epilepsien: Spezielle pathologie and therapie. Stuttgart: Georg Thieme, 1969.

420 Greenberg DA, Durner M, Resor S, Rosenbaum D, Shinnar S. The genetics of

idiopathic generalized epilepsies of adolescent onset: differences between juvenile myoclonic epilepsy and epilepsy with random grand mal and with awakening grand mal. *Neurology* 1995;**45**:942–6.

421 Scheffer IE, Berkovic SF. Generalized epilepsy with febrile seizures plus. A genetic disorder with heterogeneous clinical phenotypes. *Brain* 1997;**120**:479–90.

422 Baulac S, Gourfinkel-An I, Picard F, Rosenberg-Bourgin M, Prudhomme JF, Baulac M *et al.* A second locus for familial generalized epilepsy with febrile seizures plus maps to chromosome 2q21-q33. *Am J Hum Genet* 1999;**65**:1078–85.

423 Singh R, Scheffer IE, Crossland K, Berkovic SF. Generalized epilepsy with febrile seizures plus: a common childhood-onset genetic epilepsy syndrome. *Ann Neurol* 1999;**45**:75–81.

424 Lopes-Cendes I, Scheffer IE, Berkovic SF, Rousseau M, Andermann E, Rouleau GA. A new locus for generalized epilepsy with febrile seizures plus maps to chromosome 2. *Am J HumGenet* 2000;**66**:698–701.

425 Escayg A, Heils A, MacDonald BT, Haug K, Sander T, Meisler MH. A novel SCN1A mutation associated with generalized epilepsy with febrile seizures plus – and prevalence of variants in patients with epilepsy. *Am J Hum Genet* 2001;**68**:866–73.

426 Wallace RH, Scheffer IE, Barnett S, Richards M, Dibbens L, Desai RR *et al.* Neuronal sodium-channel alpha1-subunit mutations in generalized epilepsy with febrile seizures plus. *Am J Hum Genet* 2001;**68**:859–65.

427 Baier WK, Doose H. Petit mal-absences of childhood onset: familial prevalences of migraine and seizures. *Neuropediatrics* 1985;**16**:80–3.

428 Doose H. Absence epilepsy of early childhood – genetic aspects. *Eur J Pediatr* 1994;**153**:372–7.

429 Doose H. Absence epilepsy of early childhood. In: Wolf P, ed. *Epileptic seizures and syndromes*, pp 133–5. London: John Libbey & Co., 1994.

430 Panayiotopoulos CP, Ferrie CD, Giannakodimos S, Robinson RO. Perioral myoclonia with absences: a new syndrome. In: Wolf P, ed. *Epileptic seizures and syndromes*, pp 143–53. London: John Libbey & Co., 1994.

431 Panayiotopoulos CP. Typical absences are syndrome related. In: Duncan JS, Panayiotopoulos CP, eds. *Typical absences and related epileptic syndromes*, pp 304–10. London: Churchill Communications Europe, 1995.

432 Genton P. Epilepsy with 3Hz spike-and-waves without clinically evident absences. In: Duncan JS, Panayiotopoulos CP, eds. *Typical absences and related epileptic syndromes*, pp 231–8. London: Churchill Communications Europe, 1995.

433 Panayiotopoulos CP. Epilepsy with generalised tonic-clonic seizures on awakening. In: Wallace S, ed. *Epilepsy in children*, pp 349–53. London: Chapman & Hall, 1996.

434 Harding GFA, Jeavons PM. *Photosensitive epilepsy*. London: MacKeith Press, 1994.

435 Panayiotopoulos CP. Epilepsies characterized by seizures with specific modes of precipitation (reflex epilepsies). In: Wallace S, ed. *Epilepsy in children*, pp 355–75. London: Chapman & Hall, 1996.

436 Isojarvi JI, Tauboll E, Tapanainen JS, Pakarinen AJ, Laatikainen TJ, Knip M *et al.* On the association between valproate and polycystic ovary syndrome: a response and an alternative view. *Epilepsia* 2001;**42**:305–10.

437 Kasteleijn-Nolst Trenite DG, Marescaux C, Stodieck S, Edelbroek PM, Oosting J. Photosensitive epilepsy: a model to study the effects of antiepileptic drugs. Evaluation of the piracetam analogue, levetiracetam. *Epilepsy Res* 1996;**25**:225–30.

438 Montouris G, Biton V, Rosenfeld W, and the Topiramate YTC/YTCE study group. Nonfocal generalized tonic-clonic seizures: response during long-term topiramate treatment. *Epilepsia* 2000;**41** Suppl 1:S77–S81.

439 Leppik IE. Zonisamide. *Epilepsia* 1999;**40** Suppl 5:S23–S29.

440 Chadwick D, Leiderman DB, Sauermann W, Alexander J, Garofalo E. Gabapentin in generalized seizures. *Epilepsy Res* 1996;**25**:191–7.

441 Chaisewikul R, Privitera MD, Hutton JL, Marson AG. Levetiracetam add-on for drug-resistant localization related (partial) epilepsy (Cochrane Review). *Cochrane Database Syst Rev* 2001;**1**:CD001901.

441a Greenhill L, Betts T, Smith K. Effect of levetiracetam on resistant juvenile myoclonic epilepsy. *Epilepsia* 2002;**42** Suppl 7:179.

442 Genton P, Gelisse P. Antimyoclonic effect of levetiracetam. *Epileptic Disord* 2000;**2**:209–12.

443 Klitgaard H, Matagne A, Gobert J, Wulfert E. Evidence for a unique profile of levetiracetam in rodent models of seizures and epilepsy. *Eur J Pharmacol* 1998;**353**:191–206.

444 Scott RC, Neville BG. Pharmacological management of convulsive status epilepticus in children. *Dev Med Child Neurol* 1999;**41**:207–10.

445 Shorvon S. *Handbook of epilepsy treatment*. Oxford: Blackwell Science, 2000.

446 Smith BJ. Treatment of status epilepticus. *Neurol Clin* 2001;**19**:347–69.

447 Lowenstein DH, Alldredge BK, Allen F, Neuhaus J, Corry M, Gottwald M *et al.* The prehospital treatment of status epilepticus

(PHTSE) study: design and methodology. *Control Clin Trials* 2001;**22**:290–309.

448 Shorvon S. The management of status epilepticus. *J Neurol Neurosurg Psychiatry* 2001;**70** Suppl 2:II22–II27.

449 Alldredge BK, Gelb AM, Isaacs SM, Corry MD, Allen F, Ulrich S *et al*. A comparison of lorazepam, diazepam, and placebo for the treatment of out-of-hospital status epilepticus. *N Engl J Med* 2001;**345**:631–7.

450 Hirsch LJ, Claassen J. The current state of treatment of status epilepticus. *Curr Neurol Neurosci Rep* 2002;**2**:345–56.

451 De Negri M, Baglietto MG. Treatment of status epilepticus in children. *Paediatr Drugs* 2001;**3**:411–20.

452 Walker MC. Diagnosis and treatment of nonconvulsive status epilepticus. *CNS Drugs* 2001;**15**:931–9.

453 Scott RC, Besag FM, Neville BG. Buccal midazolam and rectal diazepam for treatment of prolonged seizures in childhood and adolescence: a randomised trial. *Lancet* 1999;**353**:623–6.

454 Berkovic SF, Genton P, Hirsch E, Picard F. *Genetics of focal epilepsies*, pp 85–93. London: John Libbey & Co., 1999.

455 Berkovic SF, Ottman R. Molecular genetics of the idiopathic epilepsies: the next steps. *Epileptic Disord* 2000;**2**:179–81.

456 Scheffer IE, Berkovic SF. Genetics of the epilepsies. *Curr Opin Pediatr* 2000;**12**:536–42.

457 Ottman R. Progress in the genetics of the partial epilepsies. *Epilepsia* 2001;**42** Suppl 5:24–30.

458 Celesia GG. Disorders of membrane channels or channelopathies. *Clin Neurophysiol* 2001;**112**:2–18.

459 Scheffer IE. Autosomal dominant nocturnal frontal lobe epilepsy. In: Berkovic SF, Genton P, Hirsch E, Picard F, eds. *Genetics of focal epilepsies*, pp 81–4. London: John Libbey & Co., 1999.

460 Bertrand D. Neuronal nicotinic acetylcholine receptors: their properties and alterations in autosomal dominant nocturnal frontal lobe epilepsy. *Rev Neurol (Paris)* 1999;**155**:457–62.

461 Hirose S, Iwata H, Akiyoshi H, Kobayashi K, Ito M, Wada K *et al*. A novel mutation of CHRNA4 responsible for autosomal dominant nocturnal frontal lobe epilepsy. *Neurology* 1999;**53**:1749–53.

462 Provini F, Plazzi G, Tinuper P, Vandi S, Lugaresi E, Montagna P. Nocturnal frontal lobe epilepsy. A clinical and polygraphic overview of 100 consecutive cases. *Brain* 1999;**122** (Pt 6):1017–31.

463 Nakken KO, Magnusson A, Steinlein OK. Autosomal dominant nocturnal frontal lobe epilepsy: an electroclinical study of a Norwegian family with ten affected members. *Epilepsia* 1999;**40**:88–92.

464 Picard F, Chauvel P. Autosomal dominant nocturnal frontal lobe epilepsy: the syndrome. *Rev Neurol (Paris)* 1999;**155**:445–9.

465 Ito M, Kobayashi K, Fujii T, Okuno T, Hirose S, Iwata H *et al*. Electroclinical picture of autosomal dominant nocturnal frontal lobe epilepsy in a Japanese family. *Epilepsia* 2000;**41**:52–8.

466 Steinlein OK, Stoodt J, Mulley J, Berkovic S, Scheffer IE, Brodtkorb E. Independent occurrence of the CHRNA4 Ser248Phe mutation in a Norwegian family with nocturnal frontal lobe epilepsy. *Epilepsia* 2000;**41**:529–35.

467 Duga S, Asselta R, Bonati MT, Malcovati M, Dalpra L, Oldani A *et al*. Mutational analysis of nicotinic acetylcholine receptor beta2 subunit gene (CHRNB2) in a representative cohort of Italian probands affected by autosomal dominant nocturnal frontal lobe epilepsy. *Epilepsia* 2002;**43**:362–4.

468 Motamedi GK, Lesser RP. Autosomal dominant nocturnal frontal lobe epilepsy. *Adv Neurol* 2002;**89**:463–73.

469 Scheffer IE, Bhatia KP, Lopes-Cendes I, Fish DR, Marsden CD, Andermann F *et al*. Autosomal dominant frontal epilepsy misdiagnosed as sleep disorder. *Lancet* 1994;**343**:515–17.

470 Phillips HA, Favre I, Kirkpatrick M, Zuberi SM, Goudie D, Heron SE *et al*. CHRNB2 is the second acetylcholine receptor subunit associated with autosomal dominant nocturnal frontal lobe epilepsy. *Am J Hum Genet* 2001;**68**:225–31.

471 Lugaresi E, Cirignotta F, Montagna P. Nocturnal paroxysmal dystonia. *Epilepsy Res Suppl* 1991;**2**:137–40.

472 Vigevano F, Fusco L. Hypnic tonic postural seizures in healthy children provide evidence for a partial epileptic syndrome of frontal lobe origin. *Epilepsia* 1993;**34**:110–19.

473 Berkovic SF, Howell RA, Hopper JL. Familial temporal lobe epilepsy: a new syndrome with adolescent/adult onset and a benign course. In: Wolf P, ed. *Epileptic seizures and syndromes*, pp 257–63. London: John Libbey & Co., 1994.

474 Berkovic SF, McIntosh A, Howell RA, Mitchell A, Sheffield LJ, Hopper JL *et al*. Familial temporal lobe epilepsy: a common disorder identified in twins. *Ann Neurol* 1996;**40**:227–35.

475 Tassinari CA, Michelucci R. Familial frontal and temporal lobe epilepsies. In: Engel J Jr, Pedley TA, eds. *Epilepsy: A comprehensive textbook*, pp 2427–31. Philadelphia: Lippincott-Raven, 1997.

476 Cendes F, Lopes-Cendes I, Andermann E, Andermann F. Familial temporal lobe epilepsy:

a clinically heterogeneous syndrome. *Neurology* 1998;**50**:554–7.

477 Berkovic SF. Familial temporal lobe epilepsy. In: Berkovic SF, Genton P, Hirsch E, Picard F, eds. *Genetics of focal epilepsies*, pp 85–93. London: John Libbey & Co., 1999.

478 Gordon N. Familial temporal-lobe epilepsy. *Dev Med Child Neurol* 1999;**41**:501–2.

479 Gambardella A, Messina D, Le Piane E, Oliveri RL, Annesi G, Zappia M et al. Familial temporal lobe epilepsy autosomal dominant inheritance in a large pedigree from southern Italy. *Epilepsy Res* 2000;**38**:127–32.

480 Brodtkorb E, Gu W, Nakken KO, Fischer C, Steinlein OK. Familial temporal lobe epilepsy with aphasic seizures and linkage to chromosome 10q22-q24. *Epilepsia* 2002;**43**:228–35.

481 Winawer MR, Ottman R, Hauser WA, Pedley TA. Autosomal dominant partial epilepsy with auditory features: defining the phenotype. *Neurology* 2000;**54**:2173–6.

482 Ottman R, Risch N, Hauser WA, Pedley TA, Lee JH, Barker-Cummings C et al. Localization of a gene for partial epilepsy to chromosome 10q. *Nat Genet* 1995;**10**:56–60.

483 Depondt C, van Paesschen W, Matthijs G, Legius E, Martens K, Demaerel P et al. Familial temporal lobe epilepsy with febrile seizures. *Neurology* 2002;**58**:1429–33.

484 Berkovic SF, Steinlein OK. Genetics of partial epilepsies. *Adv Neurol* 1999;**79**:375–81.

485 Scheffer IE, Phillips HA, O'Brien CE, Saling MM, Wrennall JA, Wallace RH et al. Familial partial epilepsy with variable foci: a new partial epilepsy syndrome with suggestion of linkage to chromosome 2. *Ann Neurol* 1998;**44**:890–9.

486 Scheffer IE. Familial partial epilepsy with variable foci. In: Berkovic SF, Genton P, Hirsch E, Picard F, eds. *Genetics of focal epilepsies*, pp 103–8. London: John Libbey & Co., 1999.

487 Xiong L, Labuda M, Li DS, Hudson TJ, Desbiens R, Patry G et al. Mapping of a gene determining familial partial epilepsy with variable foci to chromosome 22q11-q12. *Am J Hum Genet* 1999;**65**:1698–710.

488 Picard F, Baulac S, Kahane P, Hirsch E, Sebastianelli R, Thomas P et al. Dominant partial epilepsies. A clinical, electrophysiological and genetic study of 19 European families. *Brain* 2000;**123** (Pt 6):1247–62.

489 Scheffer IE, Jones L, Pozzebon M, Howell RA, Saling MM, Berkovic SF. Autosomal dominant rolandic epilepsy and speech dyspraxia: a new syndrome with anticipation. *Ann Neurol* 1995;**38**:633–42.

490 Scheffer IE. Autosomal dominant rolandic epilepsy with speech dyspraxia. *Epileptic Disord* 2000;**2** Suppl 1:S19–S22.

491 Kinton L, Johnson MR, Smith SJM, Farrell F, Stevens J, Rance JB et al. Partial epilepsy with pericentral spikes: a new familial epilepsy syndrome with evidence for linkage to chromosome 4p15. *Ann Neurol* 2002;**51**:740–9.

492 Ottman R, Barker-Cummings C, Lee JH, Ranta S. Genetics of autosomal dominant partial epilepsy with auditory features. In: Berkovic SF, Genton P, Hirsch E, Picard F, eds. *Genetics of focal epilepsies*, pp 95–102. London: John Libbey & Co., 1999.

493 Ikeda A, Kunieda T, Miyamoto S, Fukuyama H, Shibasaki H. Autosomal dominant temporal lobe epilepsy in a Japanese family. *J Neurol Sci* 2000;**176**:162–5.

494 Michelucci R, Passarelli D, Pitzalis S, Dal Corso G, Tassinari CA, Nobile C. Autosomal dominant partial epilepsy with auditory features: description of a new family. *Epilepsia* 2000;**41**:967–70.

495 Kalachikov S, Evgrafov O, Ross B, Winawer M, Barker-Cummings C, Boneschi FM et al. Mutations in LGI1 cause autosomal-dominant partial epilepsy with auditory features. *Nat Genet* 2002;**30**:335–41.

496 Winawer MR, Boneschi FM, Barker-Cummings C, Lee JH, Liu J, Mekios C et al. Four new families with autosomal dominant partial epilepsy with auditory features: clinical description and linkage to chromosome 10q24. *Epilepsia* 2002;**43**:60–7.

497 Morante-Redolat JM, Gorostidi-Pagola A, Piquer-Sirerol S, Saenz A, Poza JJ, Galan J et al. Mutations in the LGI1/Epitempin gene on 10q24 cause autosomal dominant lateral temporal epilepsy. *Hum Mol Genet* 2002;**11**:1119–28.

498 Guerrini R, Bonanni P, Nardocci N, Parmeggiani L, Piccirilli M, De Fusco M et al. Autosomal recessive rolandic epilepsy with paroxysmal exercise-induced dystonia and writer's cramp: delineation of the syndrome and gene mapping to chromosome 16p12-11.2. *Ann Neurol* 1999;**45**:344–52.

499 Hauser WA. Incidence and prevalence of epilepsy. In: Engel J Jr, Pedley TA, eds. *Epilepsy: A comprehensive textbook*, pp 47–57. Philadelphia: Lippincott-Raven, 1997.

500 Crawford PM. Epidemiology of intractable focal epilepsy. In: Oxbury JM, Polkey CE, Duchowny M, eds. *Intractable focal epilepsy*, pp 25–40. London: WB Saunders, 2000.

501 Wiebe S. Epidemiology of temporal lobe epilepsy. *Can J Neurol Sci* 2000;**27** Suppl 1:S6–S10.

502 Engel J Jr, Williamson PD, Wieser HG. Mesial temporal lobe epilepsy. In: Engel J Jr, Pedley TA, eds. *Epilepsy: A comprehensive textbook*, pp 2417–26. Philadelphia: Lippincott-Raven, 1997.

503 Gil-Nagel A, Risinger MW. Ictal semiology in hippocampal versus extrahippocampal temporal lobe epilepsy. *Brain* 1997;**120** (Pt 1):183–92.

504 Elger CE. Semeiology of temporal lobe seizures. In: Oxbury JM, Polkey CE, Duchowny M, eds. *Intractable focal epilepsy*, pp 63–8. London: WB Saunders, 2000.

505 Wieser HG, Hajek M, Gooss A, Aguzzi A. Mesial temporal lobe epilepsy syndrome with hippocampal and amygdala sclerosis. In: Oxbury JM, Polkey CE, Duchowny M, eds. *Intractable focal epilepsy*, pp 131–58. London: WB Saunders, 2000.

506 Williamson PD. Mesial temporal lobe epilepsy. In: Gilman S, ed. *Medlink*. San Diego, CA: Arbor Publishing, 2002.

507 Babb TL. Synaptic reorganizations in human and rat hippocampal epilepsy. *Adv Neurol* 1999;**79**:763–79.

508 Jackson JH. On the anatomical, physiological and pathological investigation of the epilepsies. *West Riding Lunatic Asylum Medical Reports* 1873;**3**:315–39 (In: Taylor J, ed. *Selected writings of John Hughlings Jackson*, pp 90–111. London: Hodder and Stoughton, 1958.)

509 Gloor P, Olivier A, Quesney LF, Andermann F, Horowitz S. The role of the limbic system in experiential phenomena of temporal lobe epilepsy. *Ann Neurol* 1982;**12**:129–44.

510 Gastaut H. *Dictionary of epilepsies. Part I: Definitions*. Geneva: World Health Organization, 1973.

511 Fisher PD, Sperber EF, Moshe SL. Hippocampal sclerosis revisited. *Brain Dev* 1998;**20**:563–73.

512 Lewis DV. Febrile convulsions and mesial temporal sclerosis. *Curr Opin Neurol* 1999;**12**:197–201.

513 Jefferys JG. Hippocampal sclerosis and temporal lobe epilepsy: cause or consequence? [editorial; comment]. *Brain* 1999;**122** (Pt 6):1007–8.

514 Lado FA, Laureta EC, Moshe SL. Seizure-induced hippocampal damage in the mature and immature brain. *Epileptic Disord* 2002;**4**:83–97.

515 Fernandez G, Effenberger O, Vinz B, Steinlein O, Elger CE, Dohring W et al. Hippocampal malformation as a cause of familial febrile convulsions and subsequent hippocampal sclerosis. *Neurology* 1998;**50**:909–17.

516 VanLandingham KE, Heinz ER, Cavazos JE, Lewis DV. Magnetic resonance imaging evidence of hippocampal injury after prolonged focal febrile convulsions. *Ann Neurol* 1998;**43**:413–26.

517 Mohamed A, Luders HO. Magnetic resonance imaging in temporal lobe epilepsy: usefulness for the etiological diagnosis of temporal lobe epilepsy. *Neurol Med Chir (Tokyo)* 2000;**40**:1–15.

518 Moser DJ, Bauer RM, Gilmore RL, Dede DE, Fennell EB, Algina JJ et al. Electroencephalographic, volumetric, and neuropsychological indicators of seizure focus lateralization in temporal lobe epilepsy. *Arch Neurol* 2000;**57**:707–12.

519 Koutroumanidis M, Hennessy MJ, Seed PT, Elwes RD, Jarosz J, Morris RG et al. Significance of interictal bilateral temporal hypometabolism in temporal lobe epilepsy. *Neurology* 2000;**54**:1811–21.

520 Lamusuo S, Pitkanen A, Jutila L, Ylinen A, Partanen K, Kalviainen R et al. [11 C]Flumazenil binding in the medial temporal lobe in patients with temporal lobe epilepsy: correlation with hippocampal MR volumetry, T2 relaxometry, and neuropathology. *Neurology* 2000;**54**:2252–60.

521 Koepp MJ, Hammers A, Labbe C, Woermann FG, Brooks DJ, Duncan JS. 11C-flumazenil PET in patients with refractory temporal lobe epilepsy and normal MRI. *Neurology* 2000;**54**:332–9.

522 Li LM, Cendes F, Antel SB, Andermann F, Serles W, Dubeau F et al. Prognostic value of proton magnetic resonance spectroscopic imaging for surgical outcome in patients with intractable temporal lobe epilepsy and bilateral hippocampal atrophy. *Ann Neurol* 2000;**47**:195–200.

523 Hogan RE, Bucholz RD, Choudhuri I, Mark KE, Butler CS, Joshi S. Shape analysis of hippocampal surface structure in patients with unilateral mesial temporal sclerosis. *J Digit Imaging* 2000;**13**:39–42.

524 Li LM, Caramanos Z, Cendes F, Andermann F, Antel SB, Dubeau F et al. Lateralization of temporal lobe epilepsy (TLE) and discrimination of TLE from extra-TLE using pattern analysis of magnetic resonance spectroscopic and volumetric data. *Epilepsia* 2000;**41**:832–42.

525 Williamson PD, French JA, Thadani VM, Kim JH, Novelly RA, Spencer SS et al. Characteristics of medial temporal lobe epilepsy: II. Interictal and ictal scalp electroencephalography, neuropsychological testing, neuroimaging, surgical results, and pathology. *Ann Neurol* 1993;**34**:781–7.

526 Koutroumanidis M, Binnie CD, Elwes RD, Polkey CE, Seed P, Alarcon G et al. Interictal regional slow activity in temporal lobe epilepsy correlates with lateral temporal hypometabolism as imaged with 18FDG PET: neurophysiological and metabolic implications. *J Neurol Neurosurg Psychiatry* 1998;**65**:170–6.

527 Meyer MA, Zimmerman AW, Miller CA. Temporal lobe epilepsy presenting as panic attacks: detection of interictal hypometabolism with positron emission tomography. *J Neuroimaging* 2000;**10**:120–2.

528 Lin YY, Su MS, Yiu CH, Shih YH, Yen DJ, Kwan SY et al. Relationship between mesial temporal seizure focus and elevated serum prolactin in temporal lobe epilepsy. *Neurology* 1997;**49**:528–32.

529 Engel J Jr. Introduction to temporal lobe epilepsy. *Epilepsy Res* 1996;**26**:141–50.

530 Engel J Jr. Clinical evidence for the progressive nature of epilepsy. *Epilepsy Res Suppl* 1996;**12**:9–20.

531 Blume WT, Hwang PA. Pediatric candidates for temporal lobe epilepsy surgery. *Can J Neurol Sci* 2000;**27** Suppl 1:S14–S19.

532 Polkey CE. Temporal lobe resections. In: Oxbury JM, Polkey CE, Duchowny M, eds. *Intractable focal epilepsy*, pp 667–95. London: WB Saunders, 2000.

533 Engel J Jr. The timing of surgical intervention for mesial temporal lobe epilepsy: a plan for a randomized clinical trial. *Arch Neurol* 1999;**56**:1338–41.

534 Mathern GW, Babb TL, Pretorius JK, Melendez M, Levesque MF. The pathophysiologic relationships between lesion pathology, intracranial ictal EEG onsets, and hippocampal neuron losses in temporal lobe epilepsy. *Epilepsy Res* 1995;**21**:133–47.

535 Harvey AS, Berkovic SF, Wrennall JA, Hopkins IJ. Temporal lobe epilepsy in childhood: clinical, EEG, and neuroimaging findings and syndrome classification in a cohort with new-onset seizures. *Neurology* 1997;**49**:960–8.

536 Foldvary N, Lee N, Thwaites G, Mascha E, Hammel J, Kim H et al. Clinical and electrographic manifestations of lesional neocortical temporal lobe epilepsy. *Neurology* 1997;**49**:757–63.

537 Salanova V, Morris HH, Van Ness P, Kotagal P, Wyllie E, Luders H. Frontal lobe seizures: electroclinical syndromes. *Epilepsia* 1995;**36**:16–24.

538 Chauvel P, Delgado-Escueta AV, Halgren E, Bancaud J, eds. Frontal lobe seizures and epilepsies. *Adv Neurol* 1992;1–750.

539 Bancaud J, Talairach J. Clinical semiology of frontal lobe seizures. *Adv Neurol* 1992;**57**:3–58.

540 Jasper H, Riggio S, Goldman-Rakie P. *Epilepsy and the functional anatomy of the frontal lobe.* New York: Raven Press, 1995.

541 Chauvel P, Kliemann F, Vignal JP, Chodkiewicz JP, Talairach J, Bancaud J. The clinical signs and symptoms of frontal lobe seizures. Phenomenology and classification. *Adv Neurol* 1995;**66**:115–25.

542 Williamson PD. Frontal lobe epilepsy. Some clinical characteristics. *Adv Neurol* 1995;**66**:127–50.

543 Kotagal P, Arunkumar GS. Lateral frontal lobe seizures. *Epilepsia* 1998;**39** Suppl 4:S62–S68.

544 Niedermeyer E. Frontal lobe epilepsy: the next frontier. *Clin Electroencephalogr* 1998;**29**:163–9.

545 Bartolomei F, Chauvel P. Seizure symptoms and cerebral localization: frontal lobe and rolandic seizures. In: Oxbury JM, Polkey CE, Duchowny M, eds. *Intractable focal epilepsy*, pp 55–62. London: WB Saunders, 2000.

546 Blume WT, Ociepa D, Kander V. Frontal lobe seizure propagation: scalp and subdural EEG studies. *Epilepsia* 2001;**42**:491–503.

547 Goldman-Rakie P. Anatomical and functional circuits in prefrontal cortex of non-human primates. Relevance to epilepsy. *Adv Neurol* 1995;**66**:51–65.

548 Rasmussen T. Characteristics of a pure culture of frontal lobe epilepsy. *Epilepsia* 1983;**24**:482–93.

549 Manford M, Hart YM, Sander JW, Shorvon SD. National General Practice Study of Epilepsy (NGPSE): partial seizure patterns in a general population. *Neurology* 1992;**42**:1911–17.

550 Laich E, Kuzniecky R, Mountz J, Liu HG, Gilliam F, Bebin M et al. Supplementary sensorimotor area epilepsy. Seizure localization, cortical propagation and subcortical activation pathways using ictal SPECT. *Brain* 1997;**120**:855–64.

551 Baumgartner C, Flint R, Tuxhorn I, Van Ness PC, Kosalko J, Olbrich A et al. Supplementary motor area seizures: propagation pathways as studied with invasive recordings. *Neurology* 1996;**46**:508–14.

552 King DW, Smith JR. Supplementary sensorimotor area epilepsy in adults. *Adv Neurol* 1996;**70**:285–91.

553 Spencer DD, Schumacher J. Surgical management of patients with intractable supplementary motor area seizures. The Yale experience. *Adv Neurol* 1996;**70**:445–50.

554 Connolly MB, Langill L, Wong PK, Farrell K. Seizures involving the supplementary sensorimotor area in children: a video–EEG analysis. *Epilepsia* 1995;**36**:1025–32.

555 So NK. Supplementary motor area epilepsy: the clinical syndrome. In: Wolf P, ed. *Epileptic seizures and syndromes*, pp 299–317. London: John Libbey & Co., 1994.

556 Holthausen H, Hoppe M. Hypermotor seizures. In: Luders HO, Noachtar S, eds. *Epileptic seizures. Pathophysiology and clinical semiology*, pp 439–48. New York: Churchill Livingstone, 2000.

557 Penfield W. The supplementary motor area in the cerebral cortex of man. *Arch Psychiatr* 1950;**185**:670–4.

558 Marchesi GF, Macchi G, Cianchetti C, Chinzari P. Supplementary motor areas in the cat: electrophysiological studies of the suprasylvian

and ectosylvian regions. *Boll Soc Ital Biol Sper* 1972;**48**:70–4.

559 Van Ness PC, Bleasel A, Tuxhorn I. Supplementary motor seizures: localization of the epileptogenic zone. In: Wolf P, ed. *Epileptic seizures and syndromes*, pp 319–30. London: John Libbey & Co., 1994.

560 Bancaud J. Kojewnikow's syndrome (epilepsia partialis continua) in children. In: Roger J, Bureau M, Dravet C, Dreifuss FE, Perret A, Wolf P, eds. *Epileptic syndromes in infancy, childhood and adolescence*, pp 363–74. London: John Libbey & Co., 1992.

561 Foerster O, Penfield W. The structural basis of traumatic epilepsy and results of radical operation. *Assoc Res Nev Ment Dis* 1929;**7**:569–91.

562 Bancaud J. Physiopathogenesis of generalised epilepsies of organic nature (stereo-electroencephalographic study). In: Gastaut H, Jasper H, Bancaud J, Waltregny A, eds. *The physiopathogenesis of the epilepsies*, pp 158–85. Springfield: Charles C Thomas, 1969.

563 Chauvel P, Bancaud J. The spectrum of frontal lobe seizures: with a note of frontal lobe syndromatology. In: Wolf P, ed. *Epileptic seizures and syndromes*, pp 331–4. London: John Libbey & Co., 1994.

564 Gastaut H, Jasper H, Bancaud J, Waltregny A. *The physiopathogenesis of the epilepsies*. Springfield, IL: Charles C Thomas,1969.

565 Penfield W, Jasper HH. *Epilepsy and the functional anatomy of the human brain*. Boston: Little, Brown & Co., 1954.

566 Penfield W, Perot P. The brain's record of auditory and visual experience. *Brain* 1963;**86**:595–696.

567 Janszky J, Jokeit H, Schulz R, Hoppe M, Ebner A. EEG predicts surgical outcome in lesional frontal lobe epilepsy. *Neurology* 2000;**54**:1470–6.

568 Bautista RE, Spencer DD, Spencer SS. EEG findings in frontal lobe epilepsies. *Neurology* 1998;**50**:1765–71.

569 Williamson A, Spencer SS, Spencer DD. Depth electrode studies and intracellular dentate granule cell recordings in temporal lobe epilepsy. *Ann Neurol* 1995;**38**:778–87.

570 Fahn S. The early history of paroxysmal dyskinesias. *Adv Neurol* 2002;**89**:377–85.

571 Jankovic J, Demirkiran M. Classification of paroxysmal dyskinesias and ataxias. *Adv Neurol* 2002;**89**:387–400.

572 Guerrini R. Idiopathic epilepsy and paroxysmal dyskinesia. *Epilepsia* 2001;**42** Suppl 3:36–41.

573 LeWitt PA. Psychogenic movement disorders. In: Gilman S, ed. *Neurobase*. San Diego, CA: Arbor Publishing, 2000.

574 Matsuo H, Kamakura K, Matsushita S, Ohmori T, Okano M, Tadano Y *et al*. Mutational analysis of the anion exchanger 3 gene in familial paroxysmal dystonic choreoathetosis linked to chromosome 2q. *Am J Med Genet* 1999;**88**:733–7.

575 Houser MK, Soland VL, Bhatia KP, Quinn NP, Marsden CD. Paroxysmal kinesigenic choreoathetosis: a report of 26 patients. *J Neurol* 1999;**246**:120–6.

576 Sadamatsu M, Masui A, Sakai T, Kunugi H, Nanko S, Kato N. Familial paroxysmal kinesigenic choreoathetosis: an electrophysiologic and genotypic analysis. *Epilepsia* 1999;**40**:942–9.

577 Tomita H, Nagamitsu S, Wakui K, Fukushima Y, Yamada K, Sadamatsu M *et al*. Paroxysmal kinesigenic choreoathetosis locus maps to chromosome 16p11.2-q12.1. *Am J Hum Genet* 1999;**65**:1688–97.

578 Escayg A, De Waard M, Lee DD, Bichet D, Wolf P, Mayer T *et al*. Coding and noncoding variation of the human calcium-channel beta4-subunit gene CACNB4 in patients with idiopathic generalized epilepsy and episodic ataxia. *Am J Hum Genet* 2000;**66**:1531–9.

579 Boland LM, Price DL, Jackson KA. Episodic ataxia/myokymia mutations functionally expressed in the Shaker potassium channel. *Neuroscience* 1999;**91**:1557–64.

580 Denier C, Ducros A, Vahedi K, Joutel A, Thierry P, Ritz A *et al*. High prevalence of CACNA1A truncations and broader clinical spectrum in episodic ataxia type 2. *Neurology* 1999;**52**:1816–21.

581 Zuberi SM, Eunson LH, Spauschus A, De Silva R, Tolmie J, Wood NW *et al*. A novel mutation in the human voltage-gated potassium channel gene (Kv1.1) associates with episodic ataxia type 1 and sometimes with partial epilepsy. *Brain* 1999;**122** (Pt 5):817–25.

582 Lance JW. Familial paroxysmal dystonic choreoathetosis and its differentiation from related syndromes. *Ann Neurol* 1977;**2**:285–93.

583 Hayashi R, Hanyu N, Yahikozawa H, Yanagisawa N. Ictal muscle discharge pattern and SPECT in paroxysmal kinesigenic choreoathetosis. *Electromyogr Clin Neurophysiol* 1997;**37**:89–94.

584 Wein T, Andermann F, Silver K, Dubeau F, Andermann E, Rourke-Frew F *et al*. Exquisite sensitivity of paroxysmal kinesigenic choreoathetosis to carbamazepine. *Neurology* 1996;**47**:1104–6.

585 Hamada Y, Hattori H, Okuno T. [Eleven cases of paroxysmal kinesigenic choreoathetosis; correlation with benign infantile convulsions.] *No To Hattatsu* 1998;**30**:483–8.

586 Andermann F, Hart Y. Rasmussen's syndrome. In: Gilman S, ed. *Medlink*. San Diego, CA: Arbor Publishing, 2002.

587 Panayiotopoulos CP. Kozhevnikov-Rasmussen syndrome and the new proposal on classification. *Epilepsia* 2002;**43**:928–9.

588 Obeso JA, Rothwell JC, Marsden CD. The spectrum of cortical myoclonus. From focal reflex jerks to spontaneous motor epilepsy. *Brain* 1985;**108** (Pt 1):193–24.

589 Wieser HG. Epilepsia partialis continua. In: Gilman S, ed. *Medlink*. San Diego, CA: Arbor Publishing, 2002.

590 Molyneux PD, Barker RA, Thom M, van Paesschen W, Harkness WF, Duncan JS. Successful treatment of intractable epilepsia partialis continua with multiple subpial transections [letter]. *J Neurol Neurosurg Psychiatry* 1998;**65**:137–8.

591 Biraben A, Chauvel P. Epilepsia Partialis Continua. In: Engel J Jr, Pedley TA, eds. *Epilepsy: A comprehensive textbook*, pp 2447–53. Philadelphia: Lippincott-Raven, 1997.

592 Shigeto H, Tobimatsu S, Morioka T, Yamamoto T, Kobayashi T, Kato M. Jerk-locked back averaging and dipole source localization of magnetoencephalographic transients in a patient with epilepsia partialis continua. *Electroencephalogr Clin Neurophysiol* 1997;**103**:440–4.

593 Cockerell OC, Rothwell J, Thompson PD, Marsden CD, Shorvon SD. Clinical and physiological features of epilepsia partialis continua. Cases ascertained in the UK. *Brain* 1996;**119** (Pt 2):393–407.

594 Schomer DL. Focal status epilepticus and epilepsia partialis continua in adults and children. *Epilepsia* 1993;**34** Suppl 1:S29–S36.

595 Bancauc JRJBM. Kojewnikow's syndrome (epilepsia partialis continua) in children: Update. In: Roger J, Bureau M, Dravet C, Dreifuss FE, Perret A, Wolf P, eds. *Epileptic syndromes in infancy, childhood and adolescence*, pp 374–9. London: John Libbey & Co., 1992.

596 Dereux J. *Le syndrome de Kojewnikow (epilepsie partialis continue)*. Paris: Thesis, 1955.

597 Kozhevnikov AY. A peculiar type of cortical epilepsy (epilepsia corticalis sive partialis continua). *Miditsinskoe Obozreni* 1894;**42/14**:33–62.

598 Rasmussen T, Olszweski J, Lloyd-Smith DL. Focal seizures due to chronic localized encephalitis. *Neurology* 1958;**8**:435–55.

599 Andermann F, ed. *Chronic encephalitis and epilepsy: Rasmussen's syndrome*. Boston: Butterworth-Heinemann, 1991.

600 Aarli JA. Rasmussen's encephalitis: a challenge to neuroimmunology [editorial]. *Curr Opin Neurol* 2000;**13**:297–9.

601 Kaiboriboon K, Cortese C, Hogan RE. Magnetic resonance and positron emission tomography changes during the clinical progression of Rasmussen encephalitis. *J Neuroimaging* 2000;**10**:122–5.

602 Bhatjiwale MG, Polkey C, Cox TC, Dean A, Deasy N. Rasmussen's encephalitis: neuroimaging findings in 21 patients with a closer look at the basal ganglia. *Pediatr Neurosurg* 1998;**29**:142–8.

603 Williamson PD, Boon PA, Thadani VM, Darcey TM, Spencer DD, Spencer SS *et al.* Parietal lobe epilepsy: diagnostic considerations and results of surgery. *Ann Neurol* 1992;**31**:193–201.

604 Cascino GD, Hulihan JF, Sharbrough FW, Kelly PJ. Parietal lobe lesional epilepsy: electroclinical correlation and operative outcome. *Epilepsia* 1993;**34**:522–7.

605 Sveinbjornsdottir S, Duncan JS. Parietal and occipital lobe epilepsy: a review. *Epilepsia* 1993;**34**:493–521.

606 Ho SS, Berkovic SF, Newton MR, Austin MC, McKay WJ, Bladin PF. Parietal lobe epilepsy: clinical features and seizure localization by ictal SPECT. *Neurology* 1994;**44**:2277–84.

607 Salanova V, Andermann F, Rasmussen T, Olivier A, Quesney LF. Parietal lobe epilepsy. Clinical manifestations and outcome in 82 patients treated surgically between 1929 and 1988. *Brain* 1995;**118** (Pt 3):607–27.

608 Salanova V, Andermann F, Rasmussen T, Olivier A, Quesney LF. Tumoral parietal lobe epilepsy. Clinical manifestations and outcome in 34 patients treated between 1934 and 1988. *Brain* 1995;**118** (Pt 5):1289–304.

609 Abou-Khalil B, Fakhoury T, Jennings M, Moots P, Warner J, Kessler RM. Inhibitory motor seizures: correlation with centroparietal structural and functional abnormalities. *Acta Neurol Scand* 1995;**91**:103–8.

610 Olivier A, Boling W Jr. Surgery of parietal and occipital lobe epilepsy. *Adv Neurol* 2000;**84**:533–75.

611 Siegel AM, Williamson PD. Parietal lobe epilepsy. *Adv Neurol* 2000;**84**:189–99.

612 Tuxhorn I, Kerdar MS. Somatosensory auras. In: Luders HO, Noachtar S, eds. *Epileptic seizures. Pathophysiology and clinical semiology*, pp 286–97. New York: Churchill Livingstone, 2000.

613 Calleja J, Carpizo R, Berciano J. Orgasmic epilepsy. *Epilepsia* 1988;**29**:635–9.

614 Lesser RP, Lueders H, Conomy JP, Furlan AJ, Dinner DS. Sensory seizure mimicking a psychogenic seizure. *Neurology* 1983;**33**:800–2.

615 Poeck K. [Differential diagnosis of "migraine accompagnee" and sensory Jacksonian seizures]. *Dtsch Med Wochenschr* 1972;**97**:637–41.

616 Andermann F, Beaumanoir A, Mira E, Roger J, Tassinari CA. *Occipital seizures and epilepsies in children*, pp 1–246. London: John Libbey & Co., 1993.

617 Salanova V, Andermann F, Rasmussen TB. Occipital lobe epilesy. In: Wyllie E, ed. *The treatment of epilepsy*, pp 533–40. Philadelphia: Lee & Febiger, 1993.

618 Williamson PD. Seizures with origin in the occipital or parietal lobes. In: Wolf P, ed. *Epileptic seizures and syndromes*, pp 383–90. London: John Libbey & Co., 1994.

619 Kuzniecky R, Gilliam F, Morawetz R, Faught E, Palmer C, Black L. Occipital lobe developmental malformations and epilepsy: clinical spectrum, treatment, and outcome. *Epilepsia* 1997;**38**:175–81.

620 Kuzniecky R. Symptomatic occipital lobe epilepsy. *Epilepsia* 1998;**39** Suppl 4:S24–S31.

621 Panayiotopoulos CP. Visual phenomena and headache in occipital epilepsy: a review, a systematic study and differentiation from migraine. *Epileptic Disord* 1999;**1**:205–16.

622 Manford M, Hart YM, Sander JW, Shorvon SD. The National General Practice Study of Epilepsy. The syndromic classification of the International League Against Epilepsy applied to epilepsy in a general population. *Arch Neurol* 1992;**49**:801–8.

623 Walker MC, Smith SJ, Sisodiya SM, Shorvon SD. Case of simple partial status epilepticus in occipital lobe epilepsy misdiagnosed as migraine: clinical, electrophysiological, and magnetic resonance imaging characteristics. *Epilepsia* 1995;**36**:1233–6.

624 Plazzi G, Tinuper P, Cerullo A, Provini F, Lugaresi E. Occipital lobe epilepsy: a chronic condition related to transient occipital lobe involvement in eclampsia. *Epilepsia* 1994;**35**:644–7.

625 Berkovic SF. Progressive myoclonic epilepsies. In: Engel J Jr, Pedley TA, eds. *Epilepsy: A comprehensive textbook*, pp 2455–68. Philadelphia: Lippincott-Raven, 1997.

626 Roger J, Genton P, Bureau M, Dravet C. Progressive myoclonus epilepsies in childhood and adolescence. In: Roger J, Bureau M, Dravet C, Dreifuss FE, Perret A, Wolf P, eds. *Epileptic syndromes in childhood and adolescence*, pp 381–400. London: John Libbey & Co., 1992.

627 Minassian BA. Lafora's disease: towards a clinical, pathologic, and molecular synthesis. *Pediatr Neurol* 2001;**25**:21–9.

628 Hirano M, DiMauro S. Primary mitochondrial diseases. In: Engel J Jr, Pedley TA, eds. *Epilepsy. A comprehensive textbook*, pp 2563–70. Philadelphia: Lippincott-Raven, 1997.

629 Kim SK, Lee DS, Lee SK, Kim YK, Kang KW, Chung CK et al. Diagnostic performance of [18F]FDG-PET and ictal [99mTc]-HMPAO SPECT in occipital lobe epilepsy. *Epilepsia* 2001;**42**:1531–40.

630 Salanova V, Andermann F, Olivier A, Rasmussen T, Quesney LF. Occipital lobe epilepsy: electroclinical manifestations, electrocorticography, cortical stimulation and outcome in 42 patients treated between 1930 and 1991. Surgery of occipital lobe epilepsy. *Brain* 1992;**115**:1655–80.

631 Williamson PD, Thadani VM, Darcey TM, Spencer DD, Spencer SS, Mattson RH et al. Occipital lobe epilepsy: clinical characteristics, seizure spread patterns, and results of surgery. *Ann Neurol* 1992;**31**:3–13.

632 Rasmussen T. Surgery for central, parietal and occipital epilepsy. *Can J Neurol Sci* 1991;**18**:611–16.

633 Tassinari CA, Riguzzi P, Rizzi R, Passarelli D, Volpi L. Gelastic seizures. In: Tuxhorn I, Holthausen H, Boenigk H, eds. *Paediatric epilepsy syndromes and their surgical treatment*, pp 429–46. London: John Libbey & Co., 1997.

634 Munari C, Quarato P, Kahane P, Tassi L, Minotti L, Hoffman D et al. Gelastic and dacrystic seizures. In: Luders HO, Noachtar S, eds. *Epileptic seizures. Pathophysiology and clinical semiology*, pp 458–71. New York: Churchill Livingstone, 2000.

635 Striano S, Striano P, Cirillo S, Nocerino C, Bilo L, Meo R et al. Small hypothalamic hamartomas and gelastic seizures. *Epileptic Disord* 2002;**4**:129–33.

636 Feeks EF, Murphy GL, Porter HO. Laughter in the cockpit: gelastic seizures – a case report. *Aviat Space Environ Med* 1997;**68**:66–8.

637 Thom M, Gomez-Anson B, Revesz T, Harkness W, O'Brien CJ, Kett-White R et al. Spontaneous intralesional haemorrhage in dysembryoplastic neuroepithelial tumours: a series of five cases. *J Neurol Neurosurg Psychiatry* 1999;**67**:97–101.

638 Cerullo A, Tinuper P, Provini F, Contin M, Rosati A, Marini C et al. Autonomic and hormonal ictal changes in gelastic seizures from hypothalamic hamartomas. *Electroencephalogr Clin Neurophysiol* 1998;**107**:317–22.

639 Berkovic SF, Andermann F, Melanson D, Ethier RE, Feindel W, Gloor P. Hypothalamic hamartomas and ictal laughter: evolution of a characteristic epileptic syndrome and diagnostic value of magnetic resonance imaging. *Ann Neurol* 1988;**23**:429–39.

640 Rosenfeld JV, Harvey AS, Wrennall J, Zacharin M, Berkovic SF. Transcallosal resection of hypothalamic hamartomas, with control of seizures, in children with gelastic epilepsy. *Neurosurgery* 2001;**48**:108–18.

641 Berkovic SF, Kuzniecky RI, Andermann F. Human epileptogenesis and hypothalamic

hamartomas: new lessons from an experiment of nature [editorial]. *Epilepsia* 1997;**38**:1–3.

642 Munari C, Kahane P, Francione S, Hoffmann D, Tassi L, Cusmai R *et al.* Role of the hypothalamic hamartoma in the genesis of gelastic fits (a video-stereo-EEG study). *Electroencephalogr Clin Neurophysiol* 1995;**95**:154–60.

643 Zaatreh M, Tennison M, Greenwood RS. Successful treatment of hypothalamic seizures and precocious puberty with GnRH analogue. *Neurology* 2000;**55**:1908–10.

644 Panayiotopoulos CP. Gelastic epilepsy. *Materia Medica Greca* 1979;**7**:570–5.

645 Dreyer R, Wehmeyer W. Laughing in complex partial seizure epilepsy. A video tape analysis of 32 patients with laughing as symptom of an attack. *Fortschr Neurol Psychiatr Grenzgeb* 1978;**46**:61–75.

646 Sartori E, Biraben A, Taussig D, Bernard AM, Scarabin JM. Gelastic seizures: video-EEG and scintigraphic analysis of a case with a frontal focus; review of the literature and pathophysiological hypotheses. *Epileptic Disord* 1999;**1**:221–8.

647 Arroyo S, Lesser RP, Gordon B, Uematsu S, Hart J, Schwerdt P *et al.* Mirth, laughter and gelastic seizures. *Brain* 1993;**116** (Pt 4):757–80.

648 Deonna T, Ziegler AL. Hypothalamic hamartoma, precocious puberty and gelastic seizures: a special model of "epileptic" developmental disorder. *Epileptic Disord* 2000;**2**:33–7.

649 Kuzniecky R, Guthrie B, Mountz J, Bebin M, Faught E, Gilliam F *et al.* Intrinsic epileptogenesis of hypothalamic hamartomas in gelastic epilepsy. *Ann Neurol* 1997;**42**:60–7.

650 Fukuda M, Kameyama S, Wachi M, Tanaka R. Stereotaxy for hypothalamic hamartoma with intractable gelastic seizures: technical case report. *Neurosurgery* 1999;**44**:1347–50.

651 Kramer G. The limitations of antiepileptic drug monotherapy. *Epilepsia* 1997;**38** Suppl 5:S9–S13.

652 Cockerell OC, Johnson AL, Sander JW, Shorvon SD. Prognosis of epilepsy: a review and further analysis of the first nine years of the British National General Practice Study of Epilepsy, a prospective population-based study. *Epilepsia* 1997;**38**:31–46.

653 Wyllie E, ed. *The treatment of epilepsy. Principles and practice.* Philadelphia: Lee & Febiger, 1993.

654 Shorvon S, Dreifuss FE, Fish D, Thomas DE. *The treatment of epilepsy.* Oxford: Blackwell Science, 1996.

655 Oxbury JM, Polkey CE, Duchowny M, eds. *Intractable focal epilepsy.* London: WB Saunders, 2000.

656 Pellock JM, Dodson WE, Bourgeois BFDE. *Pediatric epilepsy.* New York: Demos, 2001.

657 Leach JP, Marson T, Chadwick D. New antiepileptic drugs: revolution or marketing spin? *Practical Neurology* 2001;**1**:70–81.

658 Marson AG, Chadwick DW. New drug treatments for epilepsy. *J Neurol Neurosurg Psychiatry* 2001;**70**:143–7.

659 Marson AG, Hutton JL, Leach JP, Castillo S, Schmidt D, White S *et al.* Levetiracetam, oxcarbazepine, remacemide and zonisamide for drug resistant localization-related epilepsy: a systematic review. *Epilepsy Res* 2001;**46**:259–70.

660 Baulac M. [New antiepileptic drugs: new therapeutic options.] *Rev Neurol (Paris)* 2002;**158**:46–54.

661 Bialer M, Walker MC, Sander JW. Pros and cons for the development of new antiepileptic drugs. *CNS Drugs* 2002;**16**:285–9.

662 Bialer M. New antiepileptic drugs currently in clinical trials: is there a strategy in their development? *Ther Drug Monit* 2002;**24**:85–90.

663 Brunbech L, Sabers A. Effect of antiepileptic drugs on cognitive function in individuals with epilepsy: a comparative review of newer versus older agents. *Drugs* 2002;**62**:593–604.

664 Duncan JS. The promise of new antiepileptic drugs. *Br J Clin Pharmacol* 2002;**53**:123–31.

665 Hachad H, Ragueneau-Majlessi I, Levy RH. New antiepileptic drugs: review on drug interactions. *Ther Drug Monit* 2002;**24**:91–103.

666 Leppik IE. Three new drugs for epilepsy: levetiracetam, oxcarbazepine, and zonisamide. *J Child Neurol* 2002;**17** Suppl 1:S53–S57.

667 Perucca E. Marketed new antiepileptic drugs: are they better than old-generation agents? *Ther Drug Monit* 2002;**24**:74–80.

668 Schwabe SK. Challenges in the clinical development of new antiepileptic drugs. *Ther Drug Monit* 2002;**24**:81–4.

669 Temple RJ, Himmel MH. Safety of newly approved drugs: implications for prescribing. *JAMA* 2002;**287**:2273–5.

670 Weinstein SL, Conry J. New antiepileptic drugs: comparative studies of efficacy and cognition. *Curr Neurol Neurosci Rep* 2002;**2**:134–41.

671 Bialer M, Johannessen SI, Kupferberg HJ, Levy RH, Loiseau P, Perucca E. Progress report on new antiepileptic drugs: a summary of the Fifth Eilat Conference (EILAT V). *Epilepsy Res* 2001;**43**:11–58.

672 Smith D, Chadwick D. The management of epilepsy. *J Neurol Neurosurg Psychiatry* 2001;**70** Suppl 2:II15–II21.

673 Walker MC, Sander JW. The impact of new antiepileptic drugs on the prognosis of epilepsy:

seizure freedom should be the ultimate goal. *Neurology* 1996;**46**:912–14.

674 Walker MC, Sander JW. Difficulties in extrapolating from clinical trial data to clinical practice: the case of antiepileptic drugs. *Neurology* 1997;**49**:333–7.

675 Marson AG, Kadir ZA, Chadwick DW. New antiepileptic drugs: a systematic review of their efficacy and tolerability. *BMJ* 1996;**313**:1169–74.

676 Glauser TA. Oxcarbazepine in the treatment of epilepsy. *Pharmacotherapy* 2001;**21**:904–19.

677 Steiner TJ, Dellaportas CI, Findley LJ, Gross M, Gibberd FB, Perkin GD *et al.* Lamotrigine monotherapy in newly diagnosed untreated epilepsy: a double-blind comparison with phenytoin. *Epilepsia* 1999;**40**:601–7.

678 Mullens EL. Lamotrigine monotherapy in epilepsy. *Clin Drug Invest* 1998;**16**:125–33.

679 Marson AG, Williamson PR, Clough H, Hutton JL, Chadwick DW. Carbamazepine versus valproate monotherapy for epilepsy: a meta-analysis. *Epilepsia* 2002;**43**:505–13.

680 Bawden HN, Camfield CS, Camfield PR, Cunningham C, Darwish H, Dooley JM *et al.* The cognitive and behavioural effects of clobazam and standard monotherapy are comparable. Canadian Study Group for Childhood Epilepsy. *Epilepsy Res* 1999;**33**:133–43.

681 Barcs G, Halasz P. Effectiveness and tolerance of clobazam in temporal lobe epilepsy. *Acta Neurol Scand* 1996;**93**:88–93.

682 Morris GL. Gabapentin. *Epilepsia* 1999;**40** Suppl 5:S63–S70.

683 Hardus P, Verduin WM, Postma G, Stilma JS, Berendschot TT, van Veelen CW. Long term changes in the visual fields of patients with temporal lobe epilepsy using vigabatrin. *Br J Ophthalmol* 2000;**84**:788–90.

684 Barron TF, Hunt SL, Hoban TF, Price ML. Lamotrigine monotherapy in children. *Pediatr Neurol* 2000;**23**:160–3.

685 Culy CR, Goa KL. Lamotrigine. A review of its use in childhood epilepsy. *Paediatr Drugs* 2000;**2**:299–330.

686 Messenheimer J, Mullens EL, Giorgi L, Young F. Safety review of adult clinical trial experience with lamotrigine. *Drug Saf* 1998;**18**:281–96.

687 Brodie MJ. Lamotrigine – an update. *Can J Neurol Sci* 1996;**23**:S6–S9.

688 Messenheimer JA. Lamotrigine. *Epilepsia* 1995;**36** Suppl 2:S87–S94.

689 Faught E. Lamotrigine for startle-induced seizures. *Seizure* 1999;**8**:361–3.

690 Frank LM, Enlow T, Holmes GL, Manasco P, Concannon S, Chen C *et al.* Lamictal

(lamotrigine) monotherapy for typical absence seizures in children. *Epilepsia* 1999;**40**:973–9.

691 Faught E, Morris G, Jacobson M, French J, Harden C, Montouris G *et al.* Adding lamotrigine to valproate: incidence of rash and other adverse effects. Postmarketing Antiepileptic Drug Survey (PADS) Group. *Epilepsia* 1999;**40**:1135–40.

692 Guberman AH, Besag FM, Brodie MJ, Dooley JM, Duchowny MS, Pellock JM *et al.* Lamotrigine-associated rash: risk/benefit considerations in adults and children. *Epilepsia* 1999;**40**:985–91.

693 Panayiotopoulos CP, Ferrie CD, Knott C, Robinson RO. Interaction of lamotrigine with sodium valproate [letter]. *Lancet* 1993;**341**:445.

694 Ferrie CD, Panayiotopoulos CP. Therapeutic interaction of lamotrigine and sodium valproate in intractable myoclonic epilepsy. *Seizure* 1994;**3**:157–9.

695 Mikati MA, Holmes GL. Lamotrigine in absence and primary generalized epilepsies. *J Child Neurol* 1997;**12** Suppl 1:S29–S37.

696 Brodie MJ, Yuen AW. Lamotrigine substitution study: evidence for synergism with sodium valproate? 105 Study Group. *Epilepsy Res* 1997;**26**:423–32.

697 Fitton A, Goa KL. Lamotrigine. An update of its pharmacology and therapeutic use in epilepsy. *Drugs* 1995;**50**:691–713.

698 Leppik IE, ed. Pharmacological treatment of epilepsy: current trade-offs and the role of levetiracetam. *Epilepsia* 2001;**42** Suppl 4:1–45.

699 Levetiracetam – a new drug for epilepsy. *Drug Ther Bull* 2002;**40**:30–2.

700 Boon P, Chauvel P, Pohlmann-Eden B, Otoul C, Wroe S. Dose-response effect of levetiracetam 1000 and 2000 mg/day in partial epilepsy. *Epilepsy Res* 2002;**48**:77–89.

701 Glauser TA, Pellock JM, Bebin EM, Fountain NB, Ritter FJ, Jensen CM *et al.* Efficacy and safety of levetiracetam in children with partial seizures: an open-label trial. *Epilepsia* 2002;**43**:518–24.

702 Welty TE, Gidal BE, Ficker DM, Privitera MD. Levetiracetam: a different approach to the pharmacotherapy of epilepsy. *Ann Pharmacother* 2002;**36**:296–304.

703 Klitgaard H. Levetiracetam: the preclinical profile of a new class of antiepileptic drugs? *Epilepsia* 2001;**42** Suppl 4:13–8.

704 Krakow K, Walker M, Otoul C, Sander JW. Long-term continuation of levetiracetam in patients with refractory epilepsy. *Neurology* 2001;**56**:1772–4.

705 Nash EM, Sangha KS. Levetiracetam. *Am J Health Syst Pharm* 2001;**58**:1195–9.

706 Privitera M. Efficacy of levetiracetam: a review of three pivotal clinical trials. *Epilepsia* 2001;**42** Suppl 4:31–5.

707 Gower AJ, Hirsch E, Boehrer A, Noyer M, Marescaux C. Effects of levetiracetam, a novel antiepileptic drug, on convulsant activity in two genetic rat models of epilepsy. *Epilepsy Res* 1995;**22**:207–13.

708 Schauer R, Singer M, Saltuari L, Kofler M. Suppression of cortical myoclonus by levetiracetam. *Mov Disord* 2002;**17**:411–15.

709 Cramer JA, Arrigo C, Van Hammee G, Gauer LJ, Cereghino JJ. Effect of levetiracetam on epilepsy-related quality of life. N132 Study Group. *Epilepsia* 2000;**41**:868–74.

710 French J, Edrich P, Cramer JA. A systematic review of the safety profile of levetiracetam: a new antiepileptic drug. *Epilepsy Res* 2001;**47**:77–90.

711 French J. Use of levetiracetam in special populations. *Epilepsia* 2001;**42** Suppl 4:40–3.

712 Ormrod D, McClellan K. Topiramate: a review of its use in childhood epilepsy. *Paediatr Drugs* 2001;**3**:293–319.

713 Glauser TA. Topiramate in the catastrophic epilepsies of childhood. *J Child Neurol* 2000;**15** Suppl 1:S14–S21.

714 Reife R, Pledger G, Wu SC. Topiramate as add-on therapy: pooled analysis of randomized controlled trials in adults. *Epilepsia* 2000;**41** Suppl 1:S66–S71.

715 Shank RP, Gardocki JF, Streeter AJ, Maryanoff BE. An overview of the preclinical aspects of topiramate: pharmacology, pharmacokinetics, and mechanism of action. *Epilepsia* 2000;**41** Suppl 1:S3–S9.

716 Perucca E. A pharmacological and clinical review on topiramate, a new antiepileptic drug. *Pharmacol Res* 1997;**35**:241–56.

717 Rosenfeld WE. Topiramate: a review of preclinical, pharmacokinetic, and clinical data. *Clin Ther* 1997;**19**:1294–308.

718 Coppola G, Capovilla G, Montagnini A, Romeo A, Spano M, Tortorella G et al. Topiramate as add-on drug in severe myoclonic epilepsy in infancy: an Italian multicenter open trial. *Epilepsy Res* 2002;**49**:45–8.

719 Singh BK, White-Scott S. Role of topiramate in adults with intractable epilepsy, mental retardation, and developmental disabilities. *Seizure* 2002;**11**:47–50.

720 Wang Y, Zhou D, Wang B, Kirchner A, Hopp P, Kerling F et al. Clinical effects of topiramate against secondarily generalized tonic-clonic seizures. *Epilepsy Res* 2002;**49**:121–30.

721 Dooley JM, Camfield PR, Smith E, Langevin P, Ronen G. Topiramate in intractable childhood onset epilepsy – a cautionary note. *Can J Neurol Sci* 1999;**26**:271–3.

722 Baeta E, Santana I, Castro G, Gon AS, Gon AT, Carmo I et al. [Cognitive effects of therapy with topiramate in patients with refractory partial epilepsy.] *Rev Neurol* 2002;**34**:737–41.

723 Banta JT, Hoffman K, Budenz DL, Ceballos E, Greenfield DS. Presumed topiramate-induced bilateral acute angle-closure glaucoma. *Am J Ophthalmol* 2001;**132**:112–14.

724 Aldenkamp AP, Baker G, Mulder OG, Chadwick D, Cooper P, Doelman J et al. A multicenter, randomized clinical study to evaluate the effect on cognitive function of topiramate compared with valproate as add-on therapy to carbamazepine in patients with partial-onset seizures. *Epilepsia* 2000;**41**:1167–78.

725 Montenegro MA, Cendes F, Noronha AL, Mory SB, Carvalho MI, Marques LH et al. Efficacy of clobazam as add-on therapy in patients with refractory partial epilepsy. *Epilepsia* 2001;**42**:539–42.

726 Sheth RD, Ronen GM, Goulden KJ, Penney S, Bodensteiner JB. Clobazam for intractable pediatric epilepsy. *J Child Neurol* 1995;**10**:205–8.

727 Singh A, Guberman AH, Boisvert D. Clobazam in long-term epilepsy treatment: sustained responders versus those developing tolerance. *Epilepsia* 1995;**36**:798–803.

728 Remy C. Clobazam in the treatment of epilepsy: a review of the literature. *Epilepsia* 1994;**35** Suppl 5:S88–S91.

729 Schmidt D. Clobazam for treatment of intractable epilepsy: a critical assessment. *Epilepsia* 1994;**35** Suppl 5:S92–S95.

730 Buchanan N. Clobazam in the treatment of epilepsy: prospective follow-up to 8 years. *J R Soc Med* 1993;**86**:378–80.

731 Munn R, Farrell K. Open study of clobazam in refractory epilepsy. *Pediatr Neurol* 1993;**9**:465–9.

732 Canadian Clobazam Cooperative Group. Clobazam in treatment of refractory epilepsy: the Canadian experience. A retrospective study. *Epilepsia* 1991;**32**:407–16.

733 Canadian Study Group for Childhood Epilepsy. Clobazam has equivalent efficacy to carbamazepine and phenytoin as monotherapy for childhood epilepsy. *Epilepsia* 1998;**39**:952–9.

734 Feely M, Gibson J. Intermittent clobazam for catamenial epilepsy: tolerance avoided. *J Neurol Neurosurg Psychiatry* 1984;**47**:1279–82.

735 Cochrane AL. *Effectiveness and efficiency: random reflections on health services.* Cambridge: Cambridge University Press, 1989.

736 Marson AG. Meta-analysis of antiepileptic drug trials. In: Duncan JS, Sisodiya S, Smalls JE, eds. *Epilepsy 2001. From science to patient*, pp 317–28. Oxford: Meritus Communications, 2001.

737   Faught E, Pellock JMe. Matching the medicine to the patient. *Epilepsia* 2001;**42** Suppl 8:1–38.

738   Kaminska A. [New antiepileptic drugs in childhood epilepsies: indications and limits.] *Epileptic Disord* 2001;**3** Spec No. 2:SI37–SI46.

739   Kopec K. New anticonvulsants for use in pediatric patients (part I). *J Pediatr Health Care* 2001;**15**:81–6.

740   Bourgeois BF. New antiepileptic drugs in children: which ones for which seizures? *Clin Neuropharmacol* 2000;**23**:119–32.

741   Camfield PR, Camfield CS. Treatment of children with "ordinary" epilepsy. *Epileptic Disord* 2000;**2**:45–51.

742   Willmore LJ. Choice and use of newer anticonvulsant drugs in older patients. *Drugs Aging* 2000;**17**:441–52.

743   Crawford P, Appleton R, Betts T, Duncan J, Guthrie E, Morrow J. Best practice guidelines for the management of women with epilepsy. The Women with Epilepsy Guidelines Development Group. *Seizure* 1999;**8**:201–17.

744   Morrell MJ. Epilepsy in women: the science of why it is special. *Neurology* 1999;**53**:S42–S48.

745   Rose VL. New guidelines offer recommendations for women with epilepsy. *Am Fam Physician* 1999;**59**:1681–2.

746   Beaumanoir A, Gastaut H, Roger J, eds. *Reflex seizures and reflex epilepsies*. Geneva: Medecine and Hygiene, 1989.

747   Zifkin B, Andermann F, Rowan AJ, Beaumanoir A, eds. *Reflex epilepsies and reflex seizures*. New York: Lippincott-Raven, 1998.

748   Ferrie CD, De Marco P, Grunewald RA, Giannakodimos S, Panayiotopoulos CP. Video game induced seizures. *J Neurol Neurosurg Psychiatry* 1994;**57**:925–31.

749   Ferrie CD, Robinson RO, Giannakodimos S, Panayiotopoulos CP. Video-game epilepsy [letter; comment]. *Lancet* 1994;**344**:1710–1.

750   Forster FM, Cleeland CS. Somatosensory evoked epilepsy. *Trans Am Neurol Assoc* 1969;**94**:268–9.

751   DeMarco P. Parietal epilepsy with evoked and spontaneous spikes: report on siblings with possible genetic transmission. *Clin Electroencephalogr* 1986;**17**:159–61.

752   Deonna T. Reflex seizures with somatosensory precipitation. Clinical and electroencephalographic patterns and differential diagnosis, with emphasis on reflex myoclonic epilepsy of infancy. *Adv Neurol* 1998;**75**:193–206.

753   Koutroumanidis M, Pearce R, Sadoh DR, Panayiotopoulos CP. Tooth brushing-induced seizures: a case report. *Epilepsia* 2001;**42**:686–8.

754   Ioos C, Fohlen M, Villeneuve N, Badinand-Hubert N, Jalin C, Cheliout-Heraut F *et al.*

755   Satishchandra P, Ullal GR, Shankar SK. Hot water epilepsy. *Adv Neurol* 1998;**75**:283–93.

756   Dreifuss FE. Classification of reflex epilepsies and reflex seizures. *Adv Neurol* 1998;**75**:5–13.

757   Duncan JS, Panayiotopoulos CP. The differentiation of 'eye-closure' from 'eye-closed' EEG abnormalities and their relation to photo- and fixation-off sensitivity. In: Duncan JS, Panayiotopoulos CP, eds. *Eyelid myoclonia with absences*, pp 77–87. London: John Libbey & Co., 1996.

758   Beaumanoir A, Mira L, van Lierde A. Epilepsy or paroxysmal kinesigenic choreoathetosis? *Brain Dev* 1996;**18**:139–41.

759   Senanayake N. 'Eating epilepsy' – a reappraisal. *Epilepsy Res* 1990;**5**:74–9.

760   Remillard GM, Zifkin BG, Andermann F. Seizures induced by eating. *Adv Neurol* 1998;**75**:227–40.

761   Tassinari CA, Rubboli G, Rizzi R, Gardella E, Michelucci R. Self-induction of visually-induced seizures. *Adv Neurol* 1998;**75**:179–92.

762   Panayiotopoulos CP, Giannakodimos S, Agathonikou A, Koutroumanidis M. Eyelid myoclonia is not a manoeuvre for self-induced seizures in eyelid myoclonia with absences. In: Duncan JS, Panayiotopoulos CP, eds. *Eyelid myoclonia with absences*, pp 93–106. London: John Libbey & Co., 1996.

763   Binnie CD, Wilkins AJ. Visually induced seizures not caused by flicker (intermittent light stimulation). *Adv Neurol* 1998;**75**:123–38.

764   Panayiotopoulos CP. Self-induced pattern-sensitive epilepsy. *Arch Neurol* 1979;**36**:48–50.

765   Panayiotopoulos CP. Fixation-off, scotosensitive, and other visual-related epilepsies. *Adv Neurol* 1998;**75**:139–57.

766   Koepp MJ, Hansen ML, Pressler RM, Brooks DJ, Brandl U, Guldin B *et al.* Comparison of EEG, MRI and PET in reading epilepsy: a case report. *Epilepsy Res* 1998;**29**:251–7.

767   Koutroumanidis M, Koepp MJ, Richardson MP, Camfield C, Agathonikou A, Ried S *et al.* The variants of reading epilepsy. A clinical and video-EEG study of 17 patients with reading-induced seizures. *Brain* 1998;**121**:1409–27.

768   Ramani V. Reading epilepsy. *Adv Neurol* 1998;**75**:241–62.

769   Radhakrishnan K, Silbert PL, Klass DW. Reading epilepsy. An appraisal of 20 patients diagnosed at the Mayo Clinic, Rochester, Minnesota, between 1949 and 1989, and delineation of the epileptic syndrome. *Brain* 1995;**118** (Pt 1):75–89.

Hot water epilepsy: a benign and unrecognized form. *J Child Neurol* 2000;**15**:125–8.

770 Wolf P. Reading epilepsy. In: Roger J, Bureau M, Dravet C, Dreifuss FE, Perret A, Wolf P, eds. *Epileptic syndromes in infancy, childhood and adolescence*, pp 281–98. London: John Libbey & Co., 1992.

771 Cirignotta F, Zucconi M, Mondini S, Lugaresi E. Writing epilepsy. *Clin Electroencephalogr* 1986;**17**:21–3.

772 Wieser HG. Seizure induction in reflex seizures and reflex epilepsy. *Adv Neurol* 1998;**75**:69–85.

773 Zifkin BG, Zatorre RJ. Musicogenic epilepsy. *Adv Neurol* 1998;**75**:273–81.

774 Wieser HG, Hungerbuhler H, Siegel AM, Buck A. Musicogenic epilepsy: review of the literature and case report with ictal single photon emission computed tomography. *Epilepsia* 1997;**38**:200–7.

775 Andermann F, Zifkin BG, Andermann E. Epilepsy induced by thinking and spatial tasks. *Adv Neurol* 1998;**75**:263–72.

776 Koutroumanidis M, Agathonikou A, Panayiotopoulos CP. Self induced noogenic seizures in a photosensitive patient [letter]. *J Neurol Neurosurg Psychiatry* 1998;**64**:139–40.

777 Mutani R, Ganga A, Agnetti V. Reflex epilepsy evoked by decision making: report of a case. *Schweiz Arch Neurol Neurochir Psychiatr* 1980;**127**:61–7.

778 Forster FM, Richards JF, Panitch HS, Huisman RE, Paulsen RE. Reflex epilepsy evoked by decision making. *Arch Neurol* 1975;**32**:54–6.

779 Wiebers DO, Westmoreland BF, Klass DW. EEG activation and mathematical calculation. *Neurology* 1979;**29**:1499–503.

780 Gras P, Grosmaire N, Giroud M, Soichot P, Dumas R. Investigation via electroencephalogram with sphenoidal electrodes of a case of reading epilepsy: role of the temporal lobe in the emotional evocation of seizures. *Neurophysiol Clin* 1992;**22**:313–20.

781 Rocand JC, Graveleau D, Etienne M, Le Balle JC, Laplane R. Emotionally precipitated epilepsy. Its relations to hysteroepilepsy and reflex epilepsy. Apropos of a case. *Ann Pediatr (Paris)* 1965;**12**:434–9.

782 Zifkin B, Andermann F. Startle epilepsy. In: Gilman S, ed. *Medlink Neurology*. San Diego, CA: Arbor Publishing, 2002.

783 Vignal JP, Biraben A, Chauvel PY, Reutens DC. Reflex partial seizures of sensorimotor cortex (including cortical reflex myoclonus and startle epilepsy). *Adv Neurol* 1998;**75**:207–26.

784 Wilkins A. *Visual stress*. Oxford: Oxford University Press, 1995.

785 Doose H, Waltz S. Photosensitivity – genetics and clinical significance. *Neuropediatrics* 1993;**24**:249–55.

786 Waltz S, Stephani U. Inheritance of photosensitivity. *Neuropediatrics* 2000;**31**:82–5.

787 Quirk JA, Fish DR, Smith SJ, Sander JW, Shorvon SD, Allen PJ. First seizures associated with playing electronic screen games: a community-based study in Great Britain. *Ann Neurol* 1995;**37**:733–7.

788 Quirk JA, Fish DR, Smith SJ, Sander JW, Shorvon SD, Allen PJ. Incidence of photosensitive epilepsy: a prospective national study. *Electroencephalogr Clin Neurophysiol* 1995;**95**:260–7.

789 Grecory RP, Oates T, Merry RTC. EEG epileptiform abnormalities in candidates for aircrew training. *Electroencephalogr Clin Neurophysiol* 1993;**86**:75–7.

790 Gastaut H, Regis H, Bostem F, Beaussart M. Etude electroencephalographique de 35 sujets ayant presente des crises au cours d' un spectacle televise. *Rev Neurol (Paris)* 1960;**102**:533–4.

791 Kasteleijn-Nolst Trenite DG. Photosensitivity in epilepsy: electrophysiological and clinical correlates. *Acta Neurol Scand Suppl* 1989;**125**:3–149.

792 Kasteleijn-Nolst Trenite DG. Reflex seizures induced by intermittent light stimulation. *Adv Neurol* 1998;**75**:99–121.

793 Kasteleijn-Nolst Trenite DG, Binnie CD, Meinardi H. Photosensitive patients: symptoms and signs during intermittent photic stimulation and their relation to seizures in daily life. *J Neurol Neurosurg Psychiatry* 1987;**50**:1546–9.

794 Benbadis SR, Gerson WA, Harvey JH, Luders HO. Photosensitive temporal lobe epilepsy. *Neurology* 1996;**46**:1540–2.

795 Kasteleijn-Nolst Trenite DG, Binnie CD, Harding GF, Wilkins A, Covanis T, Eeg-Olofsson O et al. Medical technology assessment photic stimulation – standardization of screening methods. *Neurophysiol Clin* 1999;**29**:318–24.

796 Kasteleijn-Nolst Trenite DG, Binnie CD, Harding GF, Wilkins A. Photic stimulation: standardization of screening methods. *Epilepsia* 1999;**40** Suppl 4:75–9.

797 Jeavons PM, Harding GF, Panayiotopoulos CP, Drasdo N. The effect of geometric patterns combined with intermittent photic stimulation in photosensitive epilepsy. *Electroencephalogr Clin Neurophysiol* 1972;**33**:221–4.

798 Agathonikou A, Panayiotopoulos CP, Koutroumanidis M, Rowlinson A. Idiopathic regional occipital epilepsy imitating migraine. *J Epilepsy* 1997;**10**:287–90.

799 Panayiotopoulos CP, Jeavons PM, Harding GF. Occipital spikes and their relation to visual responses in epilepsy, with particular reference to photosensitive epilepsy. *Electroencephalogr Clin Neurophysiol* 1972;**32**:179–90.

800 Panayiotopoulos CP. Effectiveness of photic stimulation on various eye-states in photosensitive epilepsy. *J Neurol Sci* 1974;**23**:165–73.

801 Giannakodimos S, Panayiotopoulos CP. Eyelid myoclonia with absences in adults: a clinical and video- EEG study. *Epilepsia* 1996;**37**:36–44.

802 Panayiotopoulos CP. Fixation-off-sensitive epilepsy in eyelid myoclonia with absence seizures. *Ann Neurol* 1987;**22**:87–9.

803 Graf WD, Chatrian GE, Glass ST, Knauss TA. Video game-related seizures: a report on 10 patients and a review of the literature. *Pediatrics* 1994;**93**:551–6.

804 Kasteleijn-Nolst Trenite DG, da Silva AM, Ricci S, Binnie CD, Rubboli G, Tassinari CA *et al*. Video-game epilepsy: a European study. *Epilepsia* 1999;**40** Suppl 4:70–4.

805 Kasteleijn-Nolst Trenite DG, Silva AM, Ricci S, Rubboli G, Tassinari CA, Lopes J *et al*. Video games are exciting: a European study of video game-induced seizures and epilepsy. [Published with videosequences]. *Epileptic Disord* 2002;**4**:121–8.

806 Binnie CD. Differential diagnosis of eyelid myoclonia with absences and self-induction by eye closure. In: Duncan JS, Panayiotopoulos CP, eds. *Eyelid myoclonia with absences*, pp 89–92. London: John Libbey & Co., 1996.

807 Ames FR, Saffer D. The sunflower syndrome. A new look at "self-induced" photosensitive epilepsy. *J Neurol Sci* 1983;**59**:1–11.

808 Wilkins AJ, Baker A, Amin D, Smith S, Bradford J, Zaiwalla Z *et al*. Treatment of photosensitive epilepsy using coloured glasses. *Seizure* 1999;**8**:444–9.

809 Gastaut H, Regis H, Bostem F. Attacks provoked by television, and their mechanisms. *Epilepsia* 1962;**3**:438–45.

810 Gastaut H, Tassinari CA. Triggering mechanisms in epilepsy. The electroclinical point of view. *Epilepsia* 1966;**7**:85–138.

811 Panayiotopoulos CP. *A study of photosensitive epilepsy with particular reference to occipital spikes induced by intermittent photic stimulation*. Birmingham: Aston University, 1972:1–289.

812 Binnie CD. Simple reflex epilepsies. In: Engel J Jr, Pedley TA, eds. *Epilepsy: A comprehensive textbook*, pp 2489–505. Philadelphia: Lippincott-Raven, 1997.

813 Wolf P, Goosses R. Relation of photosensitivity to epileptic syndromes. *J Neurol Neurosurg Psychiatry* 1986;**49**:1386–91.

814 Gowers WR. *Epilepsies and other chronic convulsive diseases. Their causes, symptoms and treatment*. London: JA Churchill, 1881.

815 Gastaut H, Roger J, Gastaut Y. Les formes experimentales de l' epilepsie humaine: 1. L'

816 Bickford RG, Daly DD, Keith HM. Convulsive effects of light stimulation in children. *Am J Dis Child* 1953;**86**:170–83.

817 Panayiotopoulos CP, Jeavons PM, Harding GF. Relation of occipital spikes evoked by intermittent photic stimulation to visual evoked responses in photosensitive epilepsy. *Nature* 1970;**228**:566–7.

818 Tassinari CA, Rubboli G, Plasmati R, Salvi F, Ambrosetto G, Bianchedi G *et al*. Television-induced epilepsy with occipital seizures. In: Beaumanoir A, Gastaut H, Naquet R, eds. *Reflex seizures and reflex epilepsies*, pp 241–3. Geneva: Editions Medecine & Hygiene, 1989.

819 Aso K, Watanabe K, Negoro T, Furune A, Takahashi I, Yamamoto N *et al*. Photosensitive partial seizure: The origin of abnormal discharges. *J Epilepsy* 1988;**1**:87–93.

820 Guerrini R, Dravet C, Genton P, Bureau M, Bonanni P, Ferrari AR *et al*. Idiopathic photosensitive occipital lobe epilepsy. *Epilepsia* 1995;**36**:883–91.

821 Takada H, Aso K, Watanabe K, Okumura A, Negoro T, Ishikawa T. Epileptic seizures induced by animated cartoon, "Pocket Monster". *Epilepsia* 1999;**40**:997–1002.

822 Sharief M, Howard RO, Panayiotopoulos CP, Koutroumanidis M, Rowlinson S, Sanders S. Occipital photosensitivity with onset of seizures in adulthood: an unrecognised condition of good prognosis. *J Neurol Neurosurg Psychiatry* 2000;**68**:257 (abstracts).

823 Terasaki T, Yamatogi Y, Ohtahara S. Electroclinical delineation of occipital lobe epilepsy in childhood. In: Andermann F, Lugaresi E, eds. *Migraine and epilepsy*, pp 125–37. Boston: Butterworths, 1987.

824 Ricci S, Vigevano F. Occipital seizures provoked by intermittent light stimulation: ictal and interictal findings. *J Clin Neurophysiol* 1993;**10**:197–209.

825 Michelucci R, Tassinari CA. Television-induced occipital seizures. In: Andermann F, Beaumanoir A, Mira L, Roger J, Tassinari CA, eds. *Occipital seizures and epilepsies in children*, pp 141–4. London: John Libbey & Co., 1993.

826 Guerrini R, Bonanni P, Parmeggiani L, Belmonte A. Adolescent onset of idiopathic photosensitive occipital epilepsy after remission of benign Rolandic epilepsy. *Epilepsia* 1997;**38**:777–81.

827 Hishikawa Y, Yamamoto J, Furuya E, Yamada Y, Miyazaki K. Photosensitive epilepsy: relationships between the visual evoked responses and the epileptiform discharges

induced by intermittent photic stimulation. *Electroencephalogr Clin Neurophysiol* 1967;**23**:320–34.

828 Maheshwari MC. The clinical significance of occipital spikes as a sole response to intermittent photic stimulation. *Electroencephalogr Clin Neurophysiol* 1975;**39**:93–5.

829 Holmes G. Sabill memorial oration on focal epilepsy. *Lancet* 1927;**i**:957–62.

830 Guerrini R, Ferrari AR, Battaglia A, Salvadori P, Bonanni P. Occipitotemporal seizures with ictus emeticus induced by intermittent photic stimulation. *Neurology* 1994;**44**:253–9.

831 Wilson J. Migraine and epilepsy. *Dev Med Child Neurol* 1992;**34**:645–7.

832 Donnet A, Bartolomei F. Migraine with visual aura and photosensitive epileptic seizures. *Epilepsia* 1997;**38**:1032–4.

833 Duncan JS, Panayiotopoulos CP, eds. *Eyelid myoclonia with absences*. London: John Libbey & Co., 1996.

834 Panayiotopoulos CP. Eyelid myoclonia with or without absences. In: Gilman S, ed. *Medlink Neurology*. San Diego, CA: Arbor Publishing, 2002.

835 Ferrie CD, Agathonikou A, Parker A, Robinson RO, Panayiotopoulos CP. The spectrum of childhood epilepsies with eyelid myoclonia. In: Duncan JS, Panayiotopoulos CP, eds. *Eyelid myoclonia with absences*, pp 39–48. London: John Libbey & Co., 1996.

836 Parker A, Gardiner RM, Panayiotopoulos CP, Agathonikou A, Ferrie CD. Observations on families with eyelid myoclonia with absences. In: Duncan JS, Panayiotopoulos CP, eds. *Eyelid myoclonia with absences*, pp 107–15. London: John Libbey & Co., 1996.

837 Wilkins A. Towards an understanding of reflex epilepsy and absence. In: Duncan JS, Panayiotopoulos CP, eds. *Typical absences and related epileptic syndromes*, pp 196–205. London: Churchill Communications Europe, 1995.

838 Chatrian GE, Lettich E, Miller LH, Green JR, Kupfer C. Pattern-sensitive epilepsy. 2. Clinical changes, tests of responsiveness and motor output, alterations of evoked potenials and therapeutic measures. *Epilepsia* 1970;**11**:151–62.

839 Chatrian GE, Lettich E, Miller LH, Green JR. Pattern-sensitive epilepsy. I. An electrographic study of its mechanisms. *Epilepsia* 1970;**11**:125–49.

840 Wilkins AJ, Darby CE, Binnie CD. Neurophysiological aspects of pattern-sensitive epilepsy. *Brain* 1979;**102**:1–25.

841 Wilkins AJ, Andermann F, Ives J. Stripes, complex cells and seizures. An attempt to determine the locus and nature of the trigger mechanism in pattern-sensitive epilepsy. *Brain* 1975;**98**:365–80.

842 Krakow K, Baxendale SA, Maguire EA, Krishnamoorthy ES, Lemieux L, Scott CA *et al.* Fixation-off sensitivity as a model of continuous epileptiform discharges: electroencephalographic, neuropsychological and functional MRI findings. *Epilepsy Res* 2000;**42**:1–6.

843 Agathonikou A, Koutroumanidis M, Panayiotopoulos CP. Fixation-off (Scoto) sensitivity combined with photosensitivity. *Epilepsia* 1998;**39**:552–5.

844 Bancaud J, Talairach J, Lamarche M, Bonis A, Trottier S. Neurophysiopathological hypothesis on startle epilepsy in man. *Rev Neurol* 1975;**131**:559–71.

845 Wilkins DE, Hallett M, Wess MM. Audiogenic startle reflex of man and its relationship to startle syndromes. A review. *Brain* 1986;**109** (Pt 3):561–73.

846 Manford MR, Fish DR, Shorvon SD. Startle provoked epileptic seizures: features in 19 patients. *J Neurol Neurosurg Psychiatry* 1996;**61**:151–6.

847 Cokar O, Gelisse P, Livet MO, Bureau M, Habib M, Genton P. Startle response: epileptic or non-epileptic? The case for "flash" SMA reflex seizures. *Epileptic Disord* 2001;**3**:7–12.

848 Cengiz B, Odabasi Z, Ozdag F, Eroglu E, Gokcil Z, Vural O. Essential startle disease may not be a uniform entity. *Clin Electroencephalogr* 2001;**32**:92–5.

849 Guerrini R, Genton P, Bureau M, Dravet C, Roger J. Reflex seizures are frequent in patients with Down syndrome and epilepsy. *Epilepsia* 1990;**31**:406–17.

850 Matsuoka H, Takahashi T, Sasaki M, Matsumoto K, Yoshida S, Numachi Y *et al.* Neuropsychological EEG activation in patients with epilepsy. *Brain* 2000;**123** (Pt 2):318–30.

851 Goossens LA, Andermann F, Andermann E, Remillard GM. Reflex seizures induced by calculation, card or board games, and spatial tasks: a review of 25 patients and delineation of the epileptic syndrome. *Neurology* 1990;**40**:1171–6.

INDEX